T0327499

RADIATION BIOLOGY OF MEDICAL IMAGING

RADIATION BIOLOGY OF MEDICAL IMAGING

CHARLES A. KELSEY PhD
Department of Radiology
University of New Mexico

PHILIP H. HEINTZ PhD
Department of Radiology
University of New Mexico

DANIEL J. SANDOVAL MS
Department of Radiology
University of New Mexico

GREGORY D. CHAMBERS MS
Department of Radiology
University of New Mexico

NATALIE L. ADOLPHI PhD
Department of Radiology
University of New Mexico

KIMBERLY S. PAFFETT MS
Department of Radiology
University of New Mexico

WILEY Blackwell

Published by John Wiley & Sons, Inc., Hoboken, New Jersey.
Published simultaneously in Canada.

Library of Congress Cataloging-in-Publication Data:
  Kelsey, Charles A., author.
  Radiation Biology of Medical Imaging / Charles A. Kelsey, Philip H. Heintz, Daniel J. Sandoval, Gregory D. Chambers, Natalie L. Adolphi, Kimberly S. Paffett
      p. ; cm
  Includes bibliographical references.
  ISBN 978-0-470-55177-6 (cloth)
  I. Heintz, Philip, author.   II. Sandoval, Daniel, author.   III. Chambers, Gregory D. (Gregory Daniel), author.   IV. Adolphi, Natalie, author.   V. Paffett, Kimberly, author.   VI. Title
  [DNLM: 1. Radiobiology. 2. Diagnostic Imaging. 3. Tissues–radiation effects. WN 600]
  QP82.2.R3
  612'.01448–dc23
                                                2013012759

Printed in the United States of America

10 9 8 7 6 5 4 3 2 1

CONTENTS

ACKNOWLEDGMENTS

The authors want to acknowledge and thank the many individuals who contributed their thoughts and views regarding the impact of radiation biology in the practice of medicine. While the authors are fully responsible for the content of this book, we thank these individuals for their generous time and effort in reducing the number and egregiousness of the errors and in suggesting better ways in which to explain things.

In particular, we would like to thank Bret Heintz, PhD, and Phillip Berry, PhD, for their careful review of several chapters, and Ruth Anne Bump, Tanner Adams, and Sage Byrne for their efforts in tirelessly working their way through the seemingly endless revision of the illustrations. And also, we thank the numerous students who struggled through the earlier versions of the course. Their challenging questions and perceptive views have immeasurably improved this text.

The authors would like to thank our spouses and families for their seemingly ever-lasting support in this project, specifically, Judy Kelsey, Lillian Heintz, Kristen Sandoval, Jennifer Chambers, Andrew McDowell, and Michael Paffett.

INTRODUCTION

This book evolved from courses taught over the past several years to medical professionals, technologists, scientists, and engineers at the University of New Mexico. The medical professionals in our classes were primarily radiology and cardiology residents and fellows. Our students included X-ray, nuclear medicine, radiation oncology, and ultrasound technology students. The residents, fellows, and students were studying for board certification or registry examinations to establish their competence to practice their professions. We needed a book for these "users" of radiation with questions of the type they would face in their examinations. The authors consist of a team of scientists and engineers with over 75 years combined experience working with and teaching about radiation. We have included a chapter on radiation therapy because it is also deeply involved in imaging. The biological effects of magnetic resonance and ultrasound are included, although they employ nonionizing radiation because their biological effects may be cause for concern at higher power levels.

Within a year of Roentgen's discovery of X-rays in 1895, their biological effects were evident because radiation burns and ulcers were observed in early users. Clarence Daly, one of Edison's assistants, died from radiation-induced cancer less than 10 years after their discovery. In the years between X-ray's discovery and Watson and Crick's unraveling of the DNA structure in 1953, radiobiology studies concentrated on radiation in the treatment of cancer and on the effects of radiation on those exposed to radiation during World War II. Since 1953, radiobiology studies have focused on radiation damage to the DNA molecule. For a number of years before 9/11, there was a lull in the study of radiation effects. Since 9/11, there has been an increased effort to understand the effect of low levels of ionizing radiation. With recent developments in the study of DNA, now is an exciting time for the field of radiation biology.

Medical radiation, which is responsible for about half the U.S. population exposure, comes primarily from three sources: radiation therapy, interventional/

diagnostic, and nuclear medicine. Radiation therapy, often called radiation oncology, uses high doses to cure cancer. Interventional/diagnostic uses lower doses to guide the insertion of devices into the body or determine what ails the patient. Nuclear medicine follows radioactive materials injected into the body to determine body functions. The effects of medical radiation depend on the dose and the parts of the body irradiated, but do not depend on how or why the radiation was delivered.

The first quarter of the book is designed to establish an essential background knowledge base in biology and physics. For many readers, this will be a straightforward review. The book next covers DNA structure and function, DNA damage and repair, genetic effects, and the characteristics of cancer. The third quarter of the book covers the effects of radiation on various body organs and on the whole body, including a brief discussion of radiation-induced bystander effects. The final quarter concentrates on radiation effects from medical and natural sources of radiation and the regulations designed to protect workers and the general public. Particular attention is directed to the effects of low-dose, long-term exposures and the limitations of the linear no-threshold (LNT) hypothesis. A brief discussion of hormesis is included in this section.

Each chapter contains a clear statement of the chapter goals, a main body with illustrations covering the material, and a summary of the important points covered in the chapter. The chapter is closed with a series of multiple choice questions in the style and difficulty of many national examinations. We hope we have fulfilled our goal of producing a book useful for individuals studying for professional competence examinations and who employ radiation in their professions. With the advent of Maintenance of Certification (MOC) for certified professions, this book may be used to obtain Continuing Medical Education (CME) credits to satisfy some education requirements.

CHAPTER 1

ANATOMY AND PHYSIOLOGY

KEYWORDS

Cell components, homeostasis, tissue growth, tissue repair, organs, organ systems

TOPICS

- Four main components of a cell
- Four tissue groups
- The difference between tissue growth and tissue repair
- Organs and organ systems
- The role of homeostasis

INTRODUCTION

The human body is a complex arrangement of chemicals and chemical reactions. Atoms are combined into specific arrangements creating the chemicals that are used in precise reactions. In addition to orderly reactions, the chemicals combine to form the complex substances that make living cells. Chemicals are nonliving components that allow cells, the basic units of all life, to perform all aspects of life. These characteristics include organization, growth, and reproduction. As can be seen in

Radiation Biology of Medical Imaging, First Edition. Charles A. Kelsey, Philip H. Heintz, Daniel J. Sandoval, Gregory D. Chambers, Natalie L. Adolphi, and Kimberly S. Paffett. © 2014 John Wiley & Sons, Inc. Published 2014 by John Wiley & Sons, Inc.

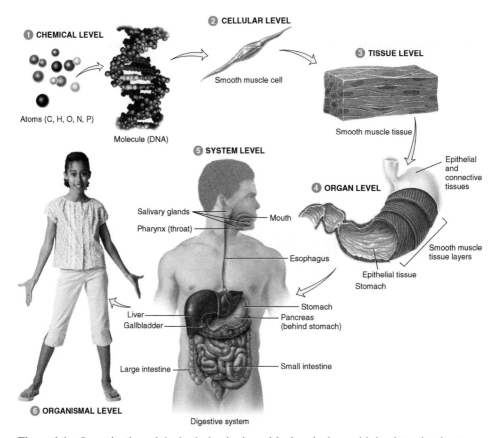

Figure 1.1 Organization of the body, beginning with chemicals combining into simple atoms and progressing through cells, tissues, organs, and, finally, the whole body. From Tortora and Nielsen (2012), figure 1.1, p. 5.

Fig. 1.1, the organization and structure of the body begins with chemicals and progresses through greater levels of organization, beginning simply with cells and ending with the entire human body.

The cell is the simplest structure of the human body. As the levels of organization expand, so does the complexity of the system. Groups of cells with the same, or similar, functions gather to form tissues. For instance, the primary function of pancreatic cells is to produce insulin whereas cells of the kidney aid in the filtration of blood. When a group of similar tissues function together, they become known as an organ. Most organs have several roles and belong to multiple organ systems. An organ system consists of multiple organs that function together and benefit the body as a whole. For example, the respiratory system, which consists primarily of the lungs, allows carbon dioxide to be exchanged for oxygen in the blood. The blood then delivers oxygen to cells throughout the body.

In this chapter, the levels of organization in the human body will be discussed: beginning with the cell, moving through tissue and organ function, and ending with homeostasis.

MAMMALIAN CELL COMPONENTS

Cells are the smallest viable component of all living organisms. Organisms can be either unicellular, containing only one cell, or multicellular, containing many cells. The human body is multicellular and made up of approximately 100 trillion, 10^{14}, cells. These cells are split into over 200 different types within the body. Each cell type is responsible for a specific function, but, despite differences in structure and function, there are four basic components contained in every cell. These features are the cell membrane, cytoplasm, cellular organelles, and genetic material.

The cell membrane, or plasma membrane, is responsible for the separation of the internal environment of the cell from the external environment. The membrane is primarily constructed of phospholipids, which form a bilayer that makes most of the membrane. Phospholipids allow for movement of lipid-soluble substances into and out of the cell by simple diffusion through the membrane itself. In addition to phospholipids, cholesterol is interspersed throughout the membrane. Cholesterol strengthens the structure of the membrane by decreasing its fluidity. Another vital component of the cell membrane is protein. Protein molecules, like cholesterol, are embedded in the membrane. These proteins have several different functions within the membrane. The functions include forming protein channels and acting as transporters and as receptor sites. Protein channels permit passage of molecules, such as water or other ions, into the cell unabated. Transport proteins, or carrier enzymes, also assist with the movement of molecules into or out of the cell. Receptor proteins are primarily located on the outer side of the membrane. The receptors are used to transmit signals into the cell from external signals. These signals include the absorption of hormones or signaling chemicals. Although the plasma membrane is the outer boundary of the cell, it is not a static, wall-like structure. Shown in Fig. 1.2 is the basic structure of a plasma membrane.

In addition to the cell membrane, each cell is filled with cytoplasm. Cytoplasm is an aqueous substance that resides between the outer cell membrane and the nucleus. The cytoplasm is made of water, salts, and organic molecules and accounts for 70% of the cell volume. Many of the chemical reactions that occur within the cell, such as glycolysis, occur within the cytoplasm. Other cell processes, such as cell division, are also contained within the cytoplasm.

Although organelles are contained within the cytoplasm, they are separated into their own class of cellular components. Organelles are specialized subunits within the cell. Each organelle performs a specific function within the cell. For instance, ribosomes are responsible for transcribing DNA, a vital function for protein synthesis and cell survival. Others, like the mitochondria, are responsible for producing energy. An appropriate analogy of an organelle is that of an organ within the body. Each organ is confined within the body and performs a specific function. In a similar manner, each organelle, confined within the cell, performs a particular function to help maintain the life of the cell. Most organelles are encompassed by individual membranes. These membranes, similar to the outer cell membrane, allow flow of material into and out of the organelle. A typical animal cell, with associated organelles, is shown in Fig. 1.3. Keep in mind that Fig. 1.3 is for a typical mammalian cell. Red blood cells in the human body do not contain organelles. This enables them to deliver a greater amount of oxygen to the body.

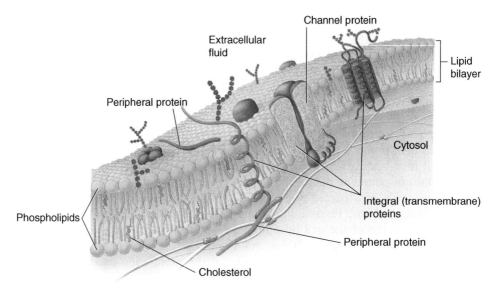

Figure 1.2 Current concept of the structure of the plasma membrane. Cholesterol is interspersed sporadically in one side of the phosopholipid bilayer, whereas proteins more commonly span both phosopholipid layers. From Tortora and Nielsen (2012), figure 2.2, p. 30.

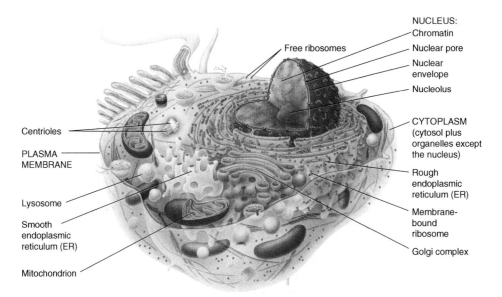

Figure 1.3 Diagram of a typical animal cell showing selected organelles and general organization within the cellular membrane. From Tortora and Nielsen (2012), figure 2.1, p. 29.

Another component of mammalian cells is genetic material. Genetic material, more commonly known as DNA, is located within the nucleus of each mammalian cell. Similar to other organelles, the nucleus is surrounded by a separate membrane, called the nuclear envelope. This membrane regulates the passage of substances into and out of the nucleus. It also localizes and protects the DNA within the cell. DNA is responsible for encoding messages for everything from the development of physical characteristics, such as hair and eye color, to when a cell should proliferate. The nucleus is the largest of the intercellular organelles and is often referred to as the control center of the cell. Although the nucleus controls the function of mammalian cells, red blood cells do not contain a nucleus. Since red blood cells do not divide once mature, there is no need for maintaining DNA and, hence, no need for a nucleus.

TISSUE GROUPS

Cells are organized into groups that have similar structure and function. Once these cells have gathered together, they become known as tissue. Individual tissues are arranged into characteristic patterns of cells that are specialized for particular functions. The human body consists of four main tissue groups. These tissue classifications are epithelial, connective, muscle, and nervous. The following descriptions of each tissue group will explain basic differences in structure and function.

Epithelial tissue is the covering or lining found on many body surfaces. If the epithelial tissue is a cover, it is located primarily on the outside of the body. The skin is the cover that assists in keeping the inside of the body safe from environmental hazards. When epithelial tissue is utilized as a lining, it is located inside the body. The respiratory system is lined with epithelial tissue that aids in the protection of the lungs. Within the primary classification of the epithelium, the cells are divided into three additional groups that differentiate between cell shapes and functions. These are squamous, cuboidal, and columnar.

Each of the three types of epithelial cells is specialized in both location and function. Squamous epithelial cells are flat and irregular in shape. Often, squamous epithelium is characterized as the most superficial covering. These cells are used in the formation of skin. Cuboidal and columnar cells are found in linings. Cuboidal cells, as their name implies, are cube-like in shape and found as a single layer. They are generally found as the lining of ducts throughout the body, such as the sweat glands. Columnar epithelial cells are more rectangular in shape. They line the digestive system and are used for absorption and secretion. Shown in Fig. 1.4 are the common epithelial cell arrangements.

Muscle tissue is found as elongated cells, called muscle fibers, throughout the body. The tissue is highly cellular and well vascularized. As the fibers contract, movement of either a body part, such as the arm, or an organ, such as the heart, is produced. There are three types of muscle tissue: skeletal, cardiac, and smooth.

Skeletal muscle is found as sheets of tissue, packaged by connective tissue, that attach to the skeleton. As the name implies, skeletal muscle is responsible for moving the skeleton. These muscles are the "flesh" of the body. Skeletal muscle cells are cylindrical, contain several nuclei per cell, and appear striated. The striations, or stripes, are created by precise arrangements of contracting proteins within the cell.

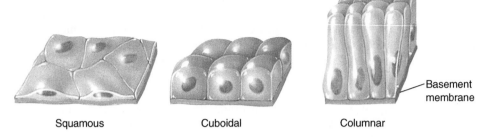

Squamous   Cuboidal   Columnar

Figure 1.4   Epithelium tissue types. Squamous cells are most commonly found in the skin, cuboidal cells are utilized as lining for glandular ducts, and columnar cells are used for absorption of nutrients. From Tortora and Nielsen (2012), figure 3.5, p. 68.

Striations are also found in cardiac muscle. However, the structure of the cardiac muscle is different from the skeletal muscle in two ways. Cardiac muscle cells contain only one nucleus, and the cells are branched to fit tightly together at specific junctions. Cardiac muscle is responsible for circulating blood throughout the body with each contraction of the heart. In order to do this, cardiac muscle contracts in a steady rhythm. Unlike skeletal and cardiac muscles, smooth muscle does not contain visible striations. The cells contain one centrally located nucleus and appear spindle shaped. The role of the smooth muscle is to squeeze substances through organs, such as the stomach, via alternating contraction and relaxation. The contractions and relaxations are like waves moving through the tissue. As the contraction wave moves through the stomach, food is pushed into the intestines. Relaxation allows time for the muscle to reset and prepare for the next round of contractions. The muscle types of the body are shown in Fig. 1.5.

Muscle can be further categorized into two distinct groups. These are voluntary and involuntary muscles. Voluntary muscle is muscle that contracts on conscious thought. All muscles that control the skeleton are voluntary muscles. If the body does not need to move, the muscles remain relaxed. However, climbing a case of stairs requires skeletal muscles to exert force to cause movement of the legs. Involuntary muscles, on the other hand, contract without conscious thought. The heart and stomach are examples of involuntary muscles. Cardiac muscle, for instance, contracts in a rhythm of its own and does not need to be prompted to beat. The steady beat of the heart keeps the body alive by circulating blood.

Connective tissue is the most abundant tissue in the body and is considered its supporting fabric. In one way or another, each part of the body has an underlying layer of connective tissue that provides a stable interface for survival. Connective tissue is composed of large amounts of nonliving material located between cells. This material could be anything from water to calcium, depending on tissue function. The intercellular background of connective tissue is called the matrix. Once the matrix has been defined, connective tissue can be divided into four classes. The simplest classification of connective tissue is to use the hardness of that tissue. This leads to soft, fibrous, hard, and liquid connective tissues. A visual comparison of connective tissue types is shown in Fig. 1.6.

Soft connective tissue is primarily located subcutaneously, or beneath the skin. The matrix of soft tissue is semiliquid, so it acts as a cushion around internal organs.

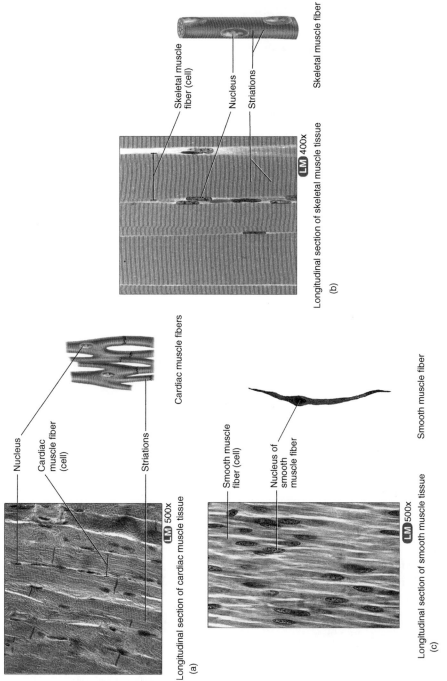

Figure 1.5 Muscle tissue types, including electron micrographs of each. Striated, or striped, cells are found in (b) skeletal and (a) cardiac muscle tissues. (c) Smooth muscle is found in the digestive system. From Tortora and Nielsen (2012), table 3.9, pp. 90–1, includes magnification factor for each electron micrograph.

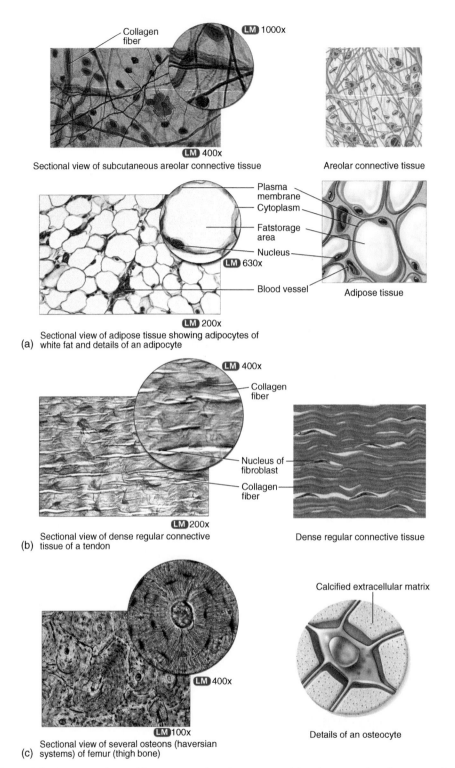

Figure 1.6 A comparison of four connective tissue types: (a) soft connective tissue, areolar, and adipose tissues; (b) collagen, or dense regular connective tissue; (c) hard connective tissue, or bone; and (d) liquid connective tissue, or blood. From Tortora and Nielsen (2012), tables 3.4, 3.5, 3.7, and 3.8, pp. 81, 83, and 87, include magnification factors.

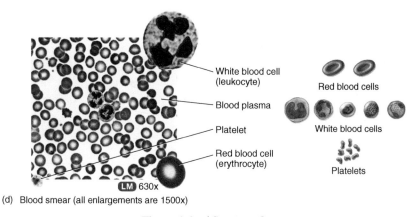

(d) Blood smear (all enlargements are 1500x)

Figure 1.6 (*Continued*)

Areolar and adipose tissues are the most common of the soft connective tissues. Areolar, or loose tissue, connects the skin to underlying muscle and also functions as mucous membranes, such as those in the digestive and respiratory systems. Adipose tissue, on the other hand, is a storage place for excess energy. Specialized adipose cells store energy as fat and release nutrients when the body requires more energy. Adipose also acts as a cushion around organs such as the eyes and kidneys.

The matrix of fibrous connective tissue contains a large amount of collagen. Collagen fibers are made mostly of protein and are arranged in a parallel fashion to give tissues strength and resilience. Tendons and ligaments are examples of fibrous connective tissue. Tendons, which attach muscle to bone, need to withstand exertion forces as the skeleton moves. If a runner did not have tendons, the muscles of the leg would tear away from the bones. Tendons allow great force to be applied to the bone by muscle without losing solid connections. In a somewhat similar way, ligaments hold bones together, as in the knee joint. Ligaments, again, need to withstand great force and be able to bounce back without injury. Sometimes the force exerted on a ligament is too great and a tear occurs. A common ligament tear is the ACL, anterior cruciate ligament, of the knee. Although fibrous tissue has a great amount of strength, it has poor blood supply. The lack of blood supply slows the repair time of the tissue. When injury occurs, such as an ACL tear, surgery is often required.

As the classification implies, hard connective tissue is strong and hard but not flexible. The matrix of hard connective tissue contains little to no water. Two types of hard connective tissue are cartilage and bone. Cartilage is most commonly found as a strong, flexible material throughout the body. It can act as a shock absorber, as seen between the vertebral segments, and to define structures such as the tip of the nose and the outer ear. Unlike cartilage, bone has no flexibility. The matrix of bone is made primarily of minerals, such as calcium, and very little water. Bones give the body its overall support and underlying structure.

The last connective tissue contains a liquid matrix. Cells are suspended in a liquid of some sort and circulate throughout the body. Included in this classification are lymph and blood. Lymph is excess fluid from tissues and organs that is not returned locally to the blood. The excess fluid is secreted by cells, collected by lymph vessels, and carried toward the heart. Lymph reenters the blood via ducts near the heart.

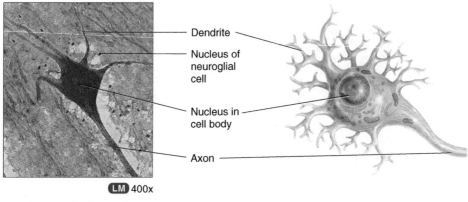

Dendrite

Nucleus of
neuroglial
cell

Nucleus in
cell body

Axon

LM 400x

Neuron of spinal cord

Figure 1.7 Electron micrograph and basic structure of a typical neuron. Unlike other tissues, neurons do not form sheets of tissue but long strands of tissue. The connections between cells occur between the dendrites and axons of neighboring cells. From Tortora and Nielsen (2012), table 3.10, p. 92.

As in other tissues, blood is made of two parts: blood cells and plasma. Plasma makes up approximately 55% of the blood volume and is composed mostly of water, about 92%. The plasma is the main medium for cell excretory products, such as dissipated proteins, glucose, and hormones, to leave the body. It also contains red blood cells. Red blood cells deliver oxygen from the lungs to tissue in the body. In the lungs, oxygen binds to hemoglobin in the red blood cells. The oxygen is released from the blood as it circulates throughout the body being replaced by absorption of carbon dioxide. The carbon dioxide is then transported to the lungs via plasma for exhalation.

Nerve tissue consists of many cells called neurons. Neurons are capable of both transmitting and generating electrical impulses. Individual neurons consist of a body, an axon, and dendrites. Shown in Fig. 1.7 is an electron micrograph of a single spinal cord neuron. The body of the cell contains the nucleus and is responsible for cell life. Each neuron contains one axon that transmits electrical impulses out of the cell and into a target cell. Target cells could be other neurons, where the electrical impulse continues, or muscle cells, where the impulse causes contraction. Dendrites receive impulses from other neurons and transmit the signal toward the cell body. The structure of the nerve tissue is similar to a wire. An electrical impulse travels from a neuron in the brain to a muscle cell in the leg. This is similar to turning on a light, the light switch being equivalent to the brain and the light bulb as the muscle. In essence, nerve tissue allows for the functions of feeling, initiation of movement, and regulation of basic body functions, such as breathing and heart rate.

TISSUE GROWTH

As cells become differentiated and begin to increase in number, they become united and begin forming the tissues previously described. Tissues need to know when to grow and when to stop growing. There are two pathways through which tissues grow, signal, or repair. Growth by signal occurs most commonly during embryonic development. At the end of gestation, all tissues are formed but remain highly mitotic and reproduce at an increased rate until adult body size is reached. A series of growth hormones influence growth of tissue and further development of physical characteristics. The most well-known growth hormone is the human growth hormone (HGH). HGH promotes growth in all tissues of the body. Under normal circumstances, HGH is produced by the pituitary gland. The amount of HGH is reduced and tissue growth ceases as children reach their adult size. In rare cases, some children do not produce enough HGH due to growth disorders. HGH can be supplemented to correct some conditions such as short stature and Turner syndrome. Additional hormones, such as testosterone and progesterone, have more specific roles in growth and development.

Growth by repair is different because there has generally been some sort of injury to a tissue or organ. Tissue repair occurs using regeneration, or replacement, of the injured tissue. However, the ability to regenerate is highly tissue dependent. Regeneration follows three main steps after an injury occurs. The first step is inflammation. Injured cells release inflammatory chemicals, which allow white blood cells and plasma to engorge the injured area. Once inflammation has occurred, the body begins to organize and restore the blood supply to the injured tissue via angiogenesis. Angiogenesis is a physiological process that stimulates new blood vessel growth from preexisting vessels. The reestablished blood supply brings necessary nutrients and growth factors to the injured tissue and the tissue begins to proliferate.

In some cases, the injury cannot be repaired by regeneration, and fibrosis is used. Fibrosis uses fibrous connective tissue to replace the damaged tissue. The repair steps are the same as above; however, the final outcome is different. When fibrosis is used, a scar, or white line, across the tissue is visible. Scarring is confluent fibrosis that obliterates the underlying tissue. The severity of the scar depends on the severity of the injury. Some surface epithelial injuries, such as a scratch, will have only a thin, or possibly no visible, scar. However, if the injury goes beyond the skin's surface, the scar will be more visible.

The majority of tissues in the body are able to grow, either by hormone signals or repair signals. However, nerve tissue does not recognize these signals. Nerve tissue ceases to divide at, or shortly before, birth. If a nerve is injured, electrical impulses cease resulting in possible loss of function. An injury to the spinal cord of Christopher Reeve is a well-known example of a severe nerve injury. The nerves were severed after a fall while riding a horse. Due to the injury, he lost most bodily functions from the neck down. If nerves had the ability to regenerate, the injury could have repaired itself, and Reeve would have regained the lost function.

During tissue growth, cells need to know when to stop dividing. When normal cells begin touching each other, they stop proliferating. This is known as contact inhibition, the primary stop pathway. Contact inhibition is a natural process that stops cell growth. This ensures cells have enough space to function properly. When cells lose the ability to recognize each other via contact, they can begin to proliferate uncontrollably and become dangerous to their host. Cancer cells commonly display a loss of contact inhibition. The cancerous cells continue to divide even when in contact with neighboring cells.

ORGANS AND ORGAN SYSTEMS

Organs contain tissues that are precisely arranged and joined together in structure to perform a common function. Two types of tissue generally make up an organ. These are main tissues, the parenchyma, and sporadic tissues, the stroma. As the name suggests, parenchyma is the primary tissue of the organ. The main tissue of each organ is unique to that organ and is not shared throughout the body. For instance, the main tissue of the heart is cardiac muscle. Cardiac muscle is not found in any other location in the body. Stroma, on the other hand, is spread sporadically throughout each organ and can be found throughout the body. An example is nervous tissue. Nerves are found throughout the body innervating each organ. In the case of the heart, nerves send signals from the brain to control the heart rate. Nerves also send signals from the heart to the brain to say everything is okay.

Functionally related organs are then grouped into organ systems. An organ system is defined as two or more functionally related organs working together. The organ system executes specific functions within the body. Although organ systems are grouped by overall function, individual organs can be shared among several systems. One example is the heart. The parenchyma of the heart is cardiac muscle, so it falls into the muscular system. However, the function of the heart is to circulate blood throughout the body. The functional system of the heart is the circulatory system. As can be seen, some organs have both tissue and functional system classifications. Table 1.1 shows a representative list of organs involved in each of the 11 organ systems but is not an all-inclusive list.

HOMEOSTASIS

The ultimate goal of the body is to maintain life. In order to do this, each system must act together to achieve homeostasis, a state of constancy. Homeostasis refers to keeping a steady state within an organism, "homeo" meaning the same and "stasis" meaning stable. There are three control mechanisms that assist the body in achieving homeostasis. They are receptors to sense change, a control center (the brain) to determine what action needs to be taken, and effectors that carry out the required action. Homeostasis in no way implies the body is a static or unchanging state. It simply refers to maintaining smooth function within the body at all times.

Thermoregulation is the ability of some organisms to self-regulate internal temperature. The internal temperature is maintained within set boundaries that do not rely on external temperatures. Humans are warm-blooded, meaning the internal temperature of the body is constant, usually between 98 and 100°F, and reliance on thermoregulation is vital. If internal body temperature rises significantly, over 113°F, for a prolonged amount of time, hyperthermia occurs. Proteins begin to denature and cellular processes cease. The other end of thermoregulation is hypothermia, when the body is not warm enough. Hypothermia sets in when core body temperature falls below 95°F, again for a long amount of time. Glucose levels rise due to decreases in both cellular consumption and insulin secretion. In both cases, death can occur if core temperature is not regained quickly.

TABLE 1.1   Brief Summary of the 11 Organ Systems, Including Some System Organs

System	Function	Organs[a]
Integumentary	• Contributes to thermoregulation through sweating • Provides protection from external pathogens and chemicals	Skin, subcutaneous tissue
Skeletal	• Provides internal framework for movement by muscles • Protects internal organs • Supports the body	Bones, ligaments
Muscular	• Moves the body • Produces heat	Muscles, tendons
Nervous	• Regulates body functions through electrochemical impulses • Interprets sensory information	Brain, nerves, eyes, ears
Endocrine	• Regulation of everyday metabolism through hormones • Regulates body functions, such as growth, by way of hormones	Pituitary gland, thyroid gland, pancreas
Circulatory	• Transportation of oxygen and nutrients to tissue and removes metabolic waste	Heart, blood
Lymphatic	• Drains excess tissue fluid and returns it to the blood • Initiates specific immune responses to pathogens	Thymus gland, lymph nodes
Respiratory	• Exchanges oxygen, from air, for carbon dioxide located in the blood	Lungs, trachea, diaphragm
Digestive	• Breaks down food into small molecules, through mechanical and chemical processes, for absorption and use by the body	Stomach, liver, pancreas
Urinary	• Regulates volume and pH of blood • Filters waste products from blood	Kidneys, urinary bladder
Reproductive	• Production of eggs (female) and sperm (male) • In females, provides site for growth and development of embryo–fetus	Female: ovaries, uterus Male: testes, prostate gland

[a]This is a representative list of organs, not an all-inclusive list.

Osmoregulation uses osmotic pressure of fluids to control the level of water and mineral salts within the blood. Osmotic pressure is a measure of how quickly water will move into one solution from another. An example is the flow of water from the kidneys into the bloodstream. If the mineral salt concentration in the blood is higher than normal, water is reabsorbed into the blood via the kidneys. In an opposite manner, if the mineral content of the blood is low, the kidneys absorb more water from the blood and urination increases. Osmoregulation ensures that the body fluids are held within a homeostatic range by regulating the water and salt content of the blood.

Since the blood is responsible for transporting water, mineral salts, glucose, and other nutrients throughout the body, maintaining a consistent level of sugar and proper pH balance is essential. Glucose, the primary energy source for all cells, must be held relatively constant. As blood glucose levels fall, after exercise for example, hormones such as glucagon are released into the blood and result in increased glucose levels. If the glucose concentration is above homeostatic limits, insulin is released from the pancreas causing glucose to be absorbed from the blood. In a similar fashion, blood pH is critical for proper functioning of the body. If the pH is too high or too low, proteins can become denatured and lose their functionality. Therefore, the body has strong mechanisms in place to maintain proper pH balance within a small window of tolerance.

Heart rate is essential for the delivery of blood to all parts of the body. It is measured in beats per minute and can change as the body's need to exchange carbon dioxide for oxygen increases. During exercise, heart rate increases to meet an increased demand for oxygen by the muscles. Heart rate decreases as the body enters a time of rest or sleep. Heart rate can be used as an indication of some underlying health issues. An increased heart rate, above 100 beats per minute and not caused by exercise, can indicate tachycardia. On the opposite end of the scale, a low heart rate implies bradycardia if the rate is less than 60 beats per minute. Associated with heart rate is respiration rate. Respiration allows blood to exchange carbon dioxide for oxygen in the lungs. Although respiration is vital to homeostasis, the main function is to oxygenate the blood.

To keep homeostasis working properly, three main organs are involved. They are the kidneys, liver, and brain. The kidneys are involved primarily with homeostatic maintenance of the blood. As mentioned previously, they are responsible for the water and mineral content, along with pH balance, of the blood. In addition to osmoregulation, the kidneys filter the blood to remove waste, such as urea, and channel it to the bladder for excretion. The liver stores much of the glycogen needed for energy throughout the body. As blood sugar levels drop, the liver releases glucose into the blood. The pancreas works in partnership with the liver by releasing glucagon to increase glucose release and insulin to encourage cellular glucose uptake. The brain is the ultimate control center of all homeostatic mechanisms. It monitors the levels of every salt molecule, glucose molecule, or waste product within the body. Without the brain, the kidneys could not determine if the mineral salt levels are high, and the liver would not know when to store glucose. The brain acts like an accountant at a business. It checks what is coming in, glucagon into the blood, and what is going out, cellular use of glucose out of the blood, to make sure the bottom line is beneficial for everyone involved.

Although the brain controls most of the homeostatic mechanisms within the body, two feedback loops are present to ensure a proper homeostatic state. The first, and most common, is the negative feedback loop. A negative feedback loop is triggered by some sort of action that lies outside of homeostatic limits. Once homeostasis has been restored, the loop is terminated. Internal body temperature is a good example of a negative feedback loop. When internal temperature rises, during exercise for example, the body attempts to cool itself. The most familiar method is sweating. As the body sweats, the water on the skin surface evaporates and cools the body. Once the core body temperature has returned to homeostatic levels, sweating ceases. The body has numerous negative feedback loops in place.

In addition to negative feedback loops, the body has a small group of positive feedback loops.

Positive feedback mechanisms do not allow reaction to a stimulus to stop the mechanism. The reaction continues to increase in magnitude. That is, the production of A increases the production of B, which in turn produces more A. This circular perturbation continues until an external stop occurs. An external stop is a force, or event, that terminates the production of A. The most well-known positive feedback signal is childbirth. As the cervix is stretched during labor contractions, the pituitary gland releases oxytocin into the bloodstream. The oxytocin stimulates the uterus to contract, which stretches the cervix, which signals for oxytocin release, hence more contractions. Once the baby is born and the placenta delivered, the external stop has occurred and the feedback loop terminates. Positive feedback mechanisms have their place within homeostasis, but since they have the potential to cause great harm, they are rare within the body.

SUMMARY

- Life is sustained through a compilation of chemicals, chemical reactions, and organization of these reactions.
- The basic functions of life are maintained and organized within a single cell.
- Each cell component is responsible for either directing chemical reactions within the cell, allowing passage of nutrients, or safeguarding DNA.
- Four tissue groups, epithelial, muscle, connective, and nerve, are made of cells with the same, or very similar, functions.
- As the human body grows, from childhood to adulthood, its tissue is stimulated to grow via hormones. Tissues can also grow in response to injury.
- As organs develop, organ systems are created by groups of organs that have the same final goal.
- Homeostasis ensures proper functioning of all organs and tissues in the human body by regulating its internal environment. Homeostasis maintains a stable, constant condition of properties like temperature and pH.

BIBLIOGRAPHY

Cohen BJ, Wood DL, Memmler RL. The structure and function of the human body. 7th ed. Philadelphia: Lippincott Williams & Wilkins; 2000.

Marieb EN, Hoehn K. Human anatomy and physiology. 7th ed. San Francisco, CA: Pearson Benjamin Cummings; 2007.

Scanlon VC, Sanders T. Essentials of anatomy and physiology. 6th ed. Philadelphia: F.A. Davis Co.; 2011.

Tortora GJ, Grabowski SR. Introduction to the human body: The essentials of anatomy and physiology. 6th ed. Hoboken, NJ: John Wiley & Sons; 2004.

Tortora GJ, Nielsen MT. Principles of human anatomy. 12th ed. Hoboken, NJ: John Wiley & Sons; 2012.

QUESTIONS

Chapter 1   Questions

1. The outer limit of a cell is the plasma membrane. Which of the following components are included in the membrane?
    i. Phospholipids
    ii. Cholesterol
    iii. Carbohydrates
    iv. Protein molecules
    a. i, ii, and iii
    b. i, iii, and iv
    c. i, ii, and iv
    d. i, ii, iii, and iv

2. All mammalian cells contain which of the following structures?
    i. Cell membrane
    ii. Genetic material
    iii. Cytoplasm
    iv. Organelles
    a. i, iii, iv
    b. i, ii
    c. i, ii, iii
    d. i, ii, iii, iv

3. The primary role of cellular organelles is
    a. metabolism.
    b. DNA replication.
    c. maintaining the life of the cell.
    d. confining enzymatic reactions.

4. The largest of all organelles is the
    a. nucleus.
    b. mitochondria.
    c. lysosome.
    d. ribosomes.

5. As cells become differentiated and gather together, they form tissues. These tissues are divided into four main groups. They are
    i. Epithelial
    ii. Blood
    iii. Nerve
    iv. Muscle
    v. Connective
    a. i, iii, iv, v
    b. ii, iii, iv, v
    c. i, ii, iii, v
    d. i, ii, iii, iv

6. Epithelial tissue can be described as a covering or a lining. Which of the three types of epithelial cells can be found as lining cells?
    i. Squamous cells
    ii. Columnar cells
    iii. Cuboidal cells
    a. i and ii
    b. ii and iii
    c. i and iii

7. Tissue that contains elongated cells, or fibers, is best classified as _____ tissue.
    a. nerve
    b. connective
    c. muscle
    d. epithelial

8. Muscle tissue is divided into three subclasses. Which of these subclasses are considered involuntary muscles?
    a. Skeletal and cardiac
    b. Cardiac only
    c. Smooth only
    d. Cardiac and smooth
    e. Smooth and skeletal

9. The body is made of four tissue types. Which tissue type is the most abundant?
    a. Muscle
    b. Nerve
    c. Epithelial
    d. Connective

10. Which of the connective tissue subclasses has the least amount of water in the extracellular matrix?

    a. Hard

    b. Fibrous

    c. Soft

    d. Liquid

11. The cells of nervous tissue contain which of the following components?

    i. Cell body

    ii. Nucleus

    iii. An axon

    iv. Extracellular matrix

    a. i, ii, and iv

    b. i, ii, and iii

    c. ii, iii, and iv

    d. i, ii, iii, and iv

12. A sporadic tissue is a tissue that is _____ in an organ.

    a. distributed evenly

    b. isolated as a line

    c. spread sporadically

    d. located in the center

13. Organ systems are groups of two or more organs that are

    a. unique in function.

    b. functionally related.

    c. isolated from other organs.

    d. completely dependent on each other to function properly.

14. Which of the following best describes homeostasis?

    a. Keeps heart and respiratory rates constant at all times

    b. Maintenance of body temperature

    c. Regulation of blood pH

    d. The ability to maintain a stable environment within the body

15. Homeostasis is most closely regulated by each of the following organs except

    a. liver.

    b. brain.

    c. kidneys.

    d. heart.

16. In which of the following homeostasis functions do the kidneys participate?

    a. Thermoregulation

    b. Osmoregulation

    c. Respiratory rate

    d. Negative feedback

CHAPTER 2

THE CELL

KEYWORDS

Cell cycle, organelles, cellular membrane, cellular transport, membrane junctions, p53, cellular replication

TOPICS

- General cell structure, including specific organelles and their main functions
- The key points of the cell cycle
- Location of cell cycle checkpoints and the role of p53
- Membrane transport and junctions
- Description of mitosis and meiosis
- Cell death

INTRODUCTION

The basic unit of living organisms is the cell. Cells were discovered by Robert Hooke in 1665 and described as the functional unit of life. Cells have been called many things, including the smallest unit of life and the building block of life. Unicellular organisms, such as bacteria, contain only one cell throughout their lifespan whereas multicellular organisms, including humans, contain many living cells. The human body contains about 100 trillion, or 10^{14}, cells at any given time.

Radiation Biology of Medical Imaging, First Edition. Charles A. Kelsey, Philip H. Heintz,
Daniel J. Sandoval, Gregory D. Chambers, Natalie L. Adolphi, and Kimberly S. Paffett.
© 2014 John Wiley & Sons, Inc. Published 2014 by John Wiley & Sons, Inc.

In 1839, the cell theory was developed by Matthias Jakob Schleiden, Rudolf Virchow, and Theodor Schwann. The cell theory states that organisms are composed of at least one cell, and these cells originate from preexisting cells. In addition to the implication of cell division, the theory states that vital functions within the organism occur in the cell and cells contain hereditary information.

This chapter discusses the basic structure of a cell. Cell structure not only includes construction of the cell itself but also the steps taken by the cell to proliferate.

CELL STRUCTURE

Cells are the basic unit of life. All organisms, whether unicellular or multicellular, begin with the function of a single cell. Cells, in general, can be divided into two types: prokaryotic, such as bacteria, and eukaryotic, such mammals. Two features separate these cell types. Prokaryotic cells contain a single external membrane to separate internal and external environments, whereas eukaryotic cells contain internal membranes in addition to their outer membrane. The internal membranes enable the cell to compartmentalize and isolate chemical reactions. In addition to internal membranes, eukaryotic cells have a cytoskeleton. The cytoskeleton provides internal structure and support for the cell. Prokaryotes lack a cytoskeleton.

As seen in Fig. 2.1, prokaryotic cells, or bacteria cells, do not contain a nucleus. The DNA is free to move in the cytoplasm. Eukaryotic cells, or mammalian cells, do contain a nucleus. The nucleus is a membrane-enclosed organelle that protects DNA from other organelles in the cytoplasm. Only mammalian cells will be discussed here.

Mammalian cells are generally split into two cell types. These are the somatic and gamete cells. Somatic cells form tissue and do not participate in reproduction. The tissue is ultimately used to provide life and movement to the organism. Gamete cells are only involved in reproduction. Formation of a gamete cells takes genetic material of the organism and packages it into specialized cells. These cells, when combined, are the beginnings of a new organism.

All mammalian cells contain cytoplasm. Cytoplasm is located between the outer plasma membrane and the nucleus. It is the aqueous phase of cells that contains a wide variety of solutes. The solutes consist of inorganic ions, building blocks of organic constituents, and intermediates of metabolic pathways, to name a few. The cytoplasm can be considered the gas station of the cell. When an organelle needs to refill its supply of a specific ion, that ion is transported from the cytoplasm into the organelle.

Located within the cytoplasm are the organelles of the cell, including the nucleus. The organelles have a wide range of functions from construction of proteins to energy production. Although the number of organelles is great and varies between tissue types, only a select few will be discussed here.

Ribosomes are the protein factory of the cell. The nucleus sends a sequence of messenger RNA (mRNA) to the ribosomes in one of two locations. If the protein sequence is for the endoplasmic reticulum (ER), the molecule travels to the rough ER where bound ribosomes directly insert the protein to the lumen of the ER. However, if the protein is for another purpose, free ribosomes perform protein

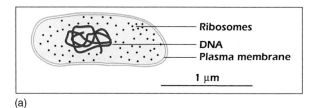

(a)

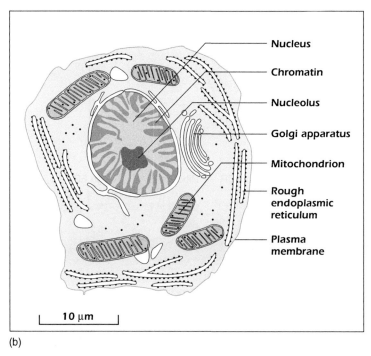

(b)

Figure 2.1   (a) Prokaryotic cells (bacterium), shown at the top, do not contain a nucleus. Genetic material is not isolated in the cell but free in the cytoplasm. (b) Eukaryotes (animal cell), on the other hand, isolate DNA within the nucleus, shown at the bottom. From Bolsover et al. (2011), figure 1.9, p. 10.

synthesis in the cytoplasm. In essence, mRNA is the blueprint for protein synthesis, and ribosomes are the general contractors that build from the blueprint.

The ER is the first stop for most proteins synthesized in the cell. It is a system of membrane-lined channels that stretch from the nucleus to the cell surface. Within the membrane convolutions, the ER is separated into three distinct regions: the rough ER, the smooth ER, and the transitional region. The rough ER is studded with ribosomes and is involved in the synthesis and folding of proteins. Ribosomes are not found on the smooth ER. It is dedicated to enzyme activity for metabolism of drugs, steroid synthesis, or calcium storage. The differences are shown in Fig. 2.2. Once the rough ER completes protein folding, proteins are transported to the transitional region. In the transitional region, vesicles used for protein transportation are formed. The transitional region is similar to a post office. It takes the folded

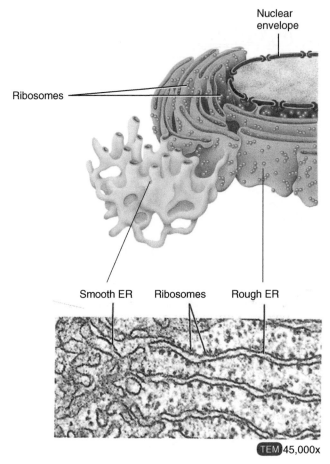

Nuclear envelope

Ribosomes

Smooth ER   Ribosomes   Rough ER

TEM 45,000x

Figure 2.2 The endoplasmic reticulum (ER) is found in two forms: the rough and smooth ER. Rough ER contains embedded ribosomes that assist with protein synthesis, seen on the right, while smooth ER lacks ribosome, seen on the left. The transitional region is not shown. An electron micrograph (bottom) shows a transverse section of the ER. From Tortora and Nielsen (2012), figure 2.10, p. 39.

proteins, packages them according to destination, and sends the package for delivery.

The abundance of ER varies between each cell type and function. Cells that specialize in the synthesis, storage, and secretion of proteins are historically richer in rough ER. For example, the pancreas is highly specialized in the synthesis and secretion of insulin and glucagon. Pancreatic cells will, on average, contain an area of ER that exceeds the surface area of the outer membrane.

Once the ER has completed protein folding, the protein is secreted to the Golgi apparatus. The Golgi complex is most commonly found within the cell as a stack of three, or more, compartments located near the nucleus. The stack looks similar to a stack of pancakes. Each compartment of the Golgi complex performs a primary function; however, enzymes located in the complex can translocate, which suggests that the compartments are not absolute in function. The Golgi apparatus is

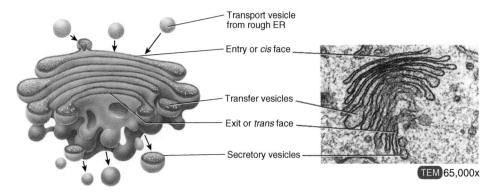

Transport vesicle
from rough ER

Entry or *cis* face

Transfer vesicles

Exit or *trans* face

Secretory vesicles

TEM 65,000x

Figure 2.3 Golgi apparatus is divided into separate compartments that appear as a stack of pancakes, each of which perform specific functions. One side of the Golgi receives the folded protein, the middle section processes the protein, and the opposite side ships the final protein to its destination. The general movement of protein from the ER through the Golgi from the receiving side through the secretory side. An electron micrograph (right) of a transverse section of the Golgi complex shows multiple layers of the organelle. From Tortora and Nielsen (2012), figure 2.11, p. 40.

responsible for modifying proteins before use by the cell. Some protein modifications are simply the addition or removal of sugar residues and proteolytic processing. Proteolytic processing involves cleaving full-length proteins into smaller, functional components. As seen with the ER, secretory cells have larger Golgi apparatus than nonsecretory cells.

In general, the Golgi apparatus contains a receiving side and a shipping side. The receiving side fuses with transport vesicles from the ER and begins protein modification. Once the modifications are complete, the Golgi complex packages the new protein and sends it into the cytoplasm via the shipping side. The basic structure of the Golgi complex is shown in Fig. 2.3. In addition to modifying proteins made by the ER, the Golgi apparatus synthesizes lipids and cholesterol to be used in plasma membranes.

Lysosomes are the digestive organelle of the cell. The lysosome contains specialized enzymes that break down proteins, DNA, and some carbohydrates. When lysosomes receive extracellular, or intracellular, particles and solutes, hydrolytic enzymes break the particles down. The constituents are transported across the lysosomal membrane to be reused through synthesis of other macromolecules. If the by-products are not needed, they are transported to the outer membrane and released into the extracellular space. Since cells are made of proteins and carbohydrates, the lysosome could potentially digest the cell itself. However, the membrane surrounding the lysosome is constructed to withstand the inner hydrolytic enzymes and prevent degradation of the cell itself.

The power house of the cell is localized in the mitochondria. Mitochondria produce energy for all cellular functions through catabolizing, or breaking down, nutrients taken into the cell. The elliptically shaped mitochondria contain a second inner membrane that folds into the central cavity. Specific enzymes necessary for energy production are located, and specifically arranged, within the folds of the inner membrane. Figure 2.4 shows the numerous folds of the mitochondrial inner

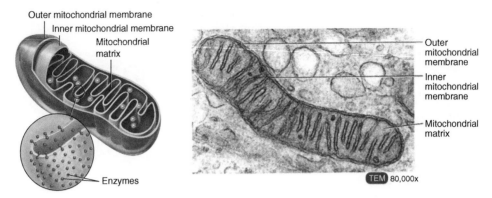

Outer mitochondrial membrane
Inner mitochondrial membrane
Mitochondrial matrix
Enzymes

Outer mitochondrial membrane
Inner mitochondrial membrane
Mitochondrial matrix
TEM 80,000x

Figure 2.4   The mitochondria contain two clearly separate membranes. The inner membrane is highly convoluted and responsible for energy production. Enzymes are specifically located within the mitochondrial matrix for efficient production of energy. An electron micrograph (right) of a transverse section of the mitochondria clearly shows the folds of the inner membrane. From Tortora and Nielsen (2012), figure 2.14, p. 43.

membrane. The specific enzyme arrangement facilitates an efficient sequence of catabolic reactions needed for energy production. As seen with the ER and Golgi complex, the number of mitochondria per cell greatly depends on the energy requirements of that cell. Cardiac muscle, for example, requires high levels of energy to function properly and many mitochondria are present to fulfill that need. On the other hand, the low energy requirements of lymphocytes can be met with only a few mitochondria.

Most of the proteins and enzymes found within mitochondria are transported from the cytoplasm. However, mitochondria do contain some DNA and ribosomes to produce proteins. DNA found within the mitochondria contains the sequence for proteins that contribute to the assembly of the organelle itself. Although DNA can be found within the mitochondria, it is not involved in cellular replication. Mitochondrial DNA is solely maternal in origin.

The nucleus is the most complicated of all organelles found within mammalian cells. It is the control center of the cell and contains the genetic material, or DNA, of the cell. Along with DNA, the nucleus contains machinery required for DNA replication and RNA transcription and processing. The nucleus is enveloped in a double membrane to effectively separate the DNA, RNA, and replication machinery. The outer nuclear membrane is fused with the outer membrane of the ER. The inner membrane of the nucleus is used to separate immature RNA from the translation apparatus. Figure 2.5 shows both nuclear membranes along with the connection between the ER and the nucleus.

Within the nucleus lies the nucleolus. The nucleolus is responsible for surrounding transcriptionally active regions of RNA, specifically, RNA that contains the sequence used to form ribosomal bodies. Recall from earlier discussion that ribosomes are used to interpret mRNA from the nucleus and synthesize proteins for use in the cell. The nucleolus also processes other stable RNA.

The nucleus houses DNA molecules, which are extremely long and called chromosomes. Chromosomes contain all the genetic material needed for life.

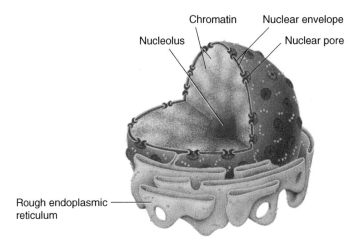

Figure 2.5   Nuclear envelope showing the nuclear membranes and the connection between the ER and the nucleus. From Tortora and Nielsen (2012), figure 2.15, p. 44.

Transcription of DNA leads to the production of mRNA. The mRNA then delivers a sequence of nucleotides to the rough ER, and synthesis of a protein begins in the ribosomes.

Located just outside the nucleus are two centrioles. Centrioles are rod-shaped structures that are perpendicular to each other. During cell division, the centrioles migrate to opposing ends of the cell. Centrioles organize spindle fibers that are involved in chromosome separation during cellular division, discussed later.

CELL MEMBRANES

Cellular membranes, or plasma membranes, separate the interior of cells from the external environment. The membrane is selectively permeable, meaning that only certain ions and molecules can enter the cell. Movement into and out of the cell is closely regulated by the plasma membrane. The basic structure of the plasma membrane is a phospholipid bilayer that is embedded with cholesterol and protein. The cholesterol acts as a stabilizer for the membrane by reducing the phospholipid fluidity. Proteins are mostly utilized for cellular transport and junction formation. The fluid mosaic model is the best model for plasma membranes.

In 1972, S.J. Singer and Garth Nicolson came up with the idea of treating plasma membranes as two-dimensional entities. In their model, lipid and protein molecules are able to diffuse more or less easily across the membrane. In Fig. 2.6, the fluid mosaic model of a cellular membrane is shown. What has been discovered since 1972 are three basic domains within the membrane, each with a specific function. These are protein–protein complexes, lipid rafts, and pickets and fences.

Protein–protein complexes are used mainly for transportation across the plasma membrane. The protein complexes can be located across the membrane, on one side of the bilayer or peripheral. These complexes act as ion channels, proton pumps, or cellular receptors. Lipid rafts are tightly packed, highly organized, groups of lipids

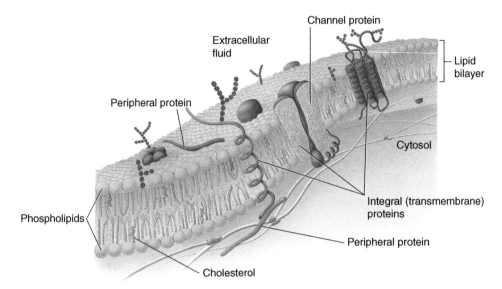

Figure 2.6   A typical plasma membrane demonstrating the phospholipid bilayer, with associated cholesterol and protein complexes. From Tortora and Nielsen (2012), figure 2.2, p. 30.

that float freely within the plasma membrane. The lipid rafts serve as organization centers for molecule assembly and protein trafficking, among other duties. Pickets and fences, the last domain, are the scaffolding of the cell. They are made of cytoskeleton proteins and maintain the overall structure and shape of the cell.

In addition to the outer plasma membrane, each organelle is surrounded by a membrane. Organelle membranes separate the functional cavities of the organelle from the cytoplasm of the cell. The composition of each organelle membrane depends on the function of the organelle. Lysosomes, as mentioned previously, are responsible for breaking down proteins and carbohydrates. The acidic nature of lysosomal enzymes requires a specialized membrane to prevent leakage into the cytoplasm.

The most specialized membrane is the nuclear envelope. The nuclear envelope is a selectively permeable membrane that separates the nucleus from the cytoplasm. Nuclear pores fuse the two membranes together. These pores control movement of macromolecules into and out of the nucleus. One purpose of the nuclear pores is to ensure that only fully processed mRNA is delivered to ribosomes for protein synthesis.

The inner membrane primarily acts as support for the nucleus. Support comes from the nuclear lamina, a dense fibrillar network. Along with structural support, the lamina assists in the organization of chromosomes. Chromosomes attach to the lamina and await signals for DNA transcription and replication. Lamina can also act as an anchor for external proteins or protein complexes, such as nuclear pore proteins.

The outer membrane of the nucleus is continuous with the outer membrane of the rough ER. It is not uncommon to have proteins, folded by the rough ER, accumulate between the two nuclear membranes until needed. The primary role of the outer membrane is to separate the cytoplasm from the nucleolus.

MEMBRANE TRANSPORT

Although the plasma membrane is impermeable to ions and other molecules, transport mechanisms are incorporated into the membrane. Membrane transport allows the cells to take in necessary molecules, such as water. There are two transport systems used by the cell: passive and active.

As the name implies, passive transport does not require energy. Proteins embedded within the membrane allow molecules and ions to move, more or less freely, across the membrane. Three examples of passive transport will be discussed here. They are osmosis, diffusion, and facilitated diffusion.

Osmosis is the most simplistic method of passive transport. It is described as a diffusion of water across selectively permeable membranes. As the definition implies, osmosis is solely responsible for water movement. Water moving through a paper towel is an example of osmosis. When the paper towel comes into contact with water, the water can be seen moving through the paper towel causing the towel to become wet.

Diffusion, in a similar fashion to osmosis, moves molecules from a high concentration area to a lower concentration area. Molecules outside the cell are generally more concentrated than inside the cell. This concentration gradient allows diffusion to proceed without hindrance. An example of diffusion occurs in the lungs with each breath. The cells of the lungs have a high oxygen concentration and a low carbon dioxide concentration. Blood returning from the body, on the other hand, has low oxygen and high carbon dioxide. The carbon dioxide of the blood diffuses into the lungs for exhalation as the oxygen diffuses across cellular membranes into the blood for circulation.

Facilitated diffusion requires help from transporters. Energy is still not required; however, molecules, such as glucose, are too large to diffuse freely. Transporters, located in the membrane, assist diffusion by attaching to the molecule and changing shape. This shape change propels molecules from outside the cell into the cytoplasm.

Active transport requires energy, or adenosine triphosphate (ATP), for the movement of molecules from one area to another. In an opposite manner to passive transport, active transport moves molecules from a low concentration region to an area of higher concentration. So, active transport moves against concentration gradients. The use of ATP activates pumps that transport molecules into the cells. An example is a muscle cell releasing sodium from the cytoplasm to the extracellular space. The external environment contains a higher concentration of sodium than the cell itself, so an energy-driven pump is necessary to rid the cell of excess sodium.

CELLULAR JUNCTIONS

Mammalian cells require external support to enable the formation of tissue and, ultimately, functional organs. Extracellular support can be found within the plasma membrane as cellular junctions. These junctions allow cells to communicate with each other and anchor themselves to impart mechanical strength to tissue. Four types of cellular junctions connect the plasma membranes of cells, each in a distinct way. These junctions are tight, gap, adherens, and desmosomes.

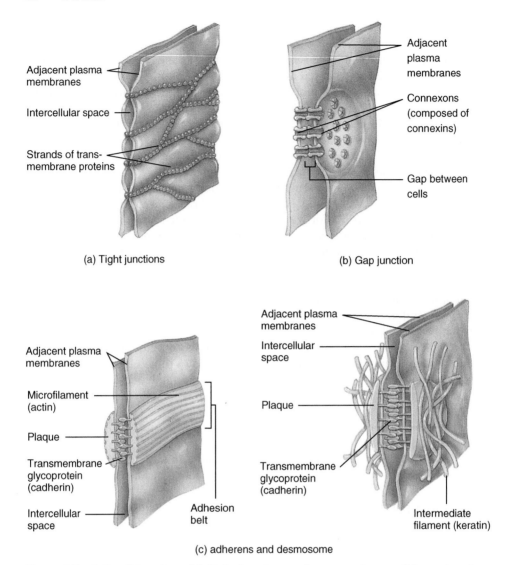

Adjacent plasma membranes

Intercellular space

Strands of trans-membrane proteins

(a) Tight junctions

Adjacent plasma membranes

Connexons (composed of connexins)

Gap between cells

(b) Gap junction

Adjacent plasma membranes

Microfilament (actin)

Plaque

Transmembrane glycoprotein (cadherin)

Intercellular space

Adhesion belt

Adjacent plasma membranes

Intercellular space

Plaque

Transmembrane glycoprotein (cadherin)

Intermediate filament (keratin)

(c) adherens and desmosome

Figure 2.7   Cell–cell junctions. (a) Tight junctions seal two membranes, (b) gap junctions allow for some movement between membranes, and (c) adherens (left) and desmosomes (right) form localized spot connections between cells. From Tortora and Nielsen (2012), figure 3.2, p. 64.

Tight junctions occlude any extracellular space between cells. They act as a seal between the membranes. As seen in Fig. 2.7a, tight junctions appear as two membranes fused into one. This seal greatly limits the diffusion of water, ions, and large solutes. Cellular migration is also inhibited by tight junctions. The most common location of tight junctions is in the epithelial tissue. Since the epithelial tissue is a covering or lining for the body, tight junctions help prevent the extracellular components, such as stomach acid, from seeping into and damaging the underlying tissue.

Gap junctions, like tight junctions, connect cells together. However, gap junctions form channels between neighboring cells, not tight seals, and do not occlude the extracellular space between cells. In Fig. 2.7b, gap junctions appear as staples holding two pieces of paper together. Gap junction channels facilitate the flow of small molecules between neighboring cells. This flow of molecules allows the cells to communicate readily with each other. In a sense, gap junctions are similar to streets in a city. Streets connect neighborhoods together while allowing for some space between houses.

Unlike tight junctions that seal cells together and gap junctions that form channels between cells, cellular adhesion also utilizes adheren and desmosome junctions. Adheren junctions are found primarily in the epithelial tissue. They are belt-like junctions that encircle the cells in a continuous manner. The continuity of an adheren junction helps maintain the physical integrity of the epithelial tissue. In a similar manner, desmosomes provide strong connections between epithelial and muscles tissues. These junctions are disk-like connections, similar to weld spots holding two pieces of metal together. Figure 2.7c shows adherens and desmosomes in a similar fashion.

CELL CYCLE

Patterns of cellular growth and behavior are manifestations of the cell cycle. The cell cycle describes the growth and division of cells throughout their lifetime. The goal of the cell cycle is to produce two daughter cells that maintain the accuracy of the parent cell. The cell cycle incorporates a continuous growth cycle with a discontinuous chromosome cycle. Through four stages of the cell cycle, cellular growth and division are integrated with relative smoothness. The cell cycle is shown in Fig. 2.8.

The G1, or growth, phase is the longest and most varied of the cell cycle phases. During the G1 phase, the cell increases in mass and synthesizes new organelles. Cells require structural proteins and enzymes during the G1 phase, which results in increased protein synthesis. If nutrient supply is poor, or the temperature is too hot or cold, this phase can be delayed. The cell enters a dormant phase, or G0 phase, until conditions improve. The cell reenters the G1 growth phase once nutrients are restored. At this point, the cell completes G1 and enters the S phase.

Occurring between growth phases G1 and G2, DNA is replicated in the S phase portion of the cell cycle. The goal is to take the chromatin of the nucleus and create two semiconserved copies. Each copy contains one original, or parental, chromatin paired with one new, or daughter, chromatin. These copies must be precise and accurate replications of parent DNA. DNA synthesis occurs rapidly, approximately 100 nucleotides/s, but must maintain an incredible accuracy of only 1 incorrect base in 10^9 nucleotide additions. In addition to DNA replication, the S phase detects and repairs DNA damage. When replication apparatus comes into contact with damage, a pause signal is sent downstream to halt replication and initiate repair. After the damage is repaired, replication continues.

Once S phase is complete, the cell enters a second growth phase, or G2, of the cell cycle. The G2 phase consists of rapid cell growth and protein synthesis in preparation for mitosis. G2 is also used for proofreading replicated DNA. As in S phase, if DNA damage or mis-replication is found, the cell is halted from proceeding until

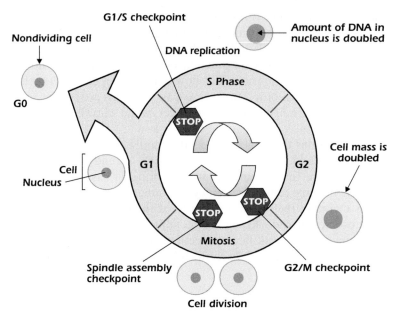

Figure 2.8   Phases of the cell cycle, giving a brief outline and main characteristic of each phase. From Bolsover et al. (2011), figure 18.6, p. 304.

the damage is repaired. Once DNA damage has been repaired, or the cell found to be without damage, the cell enters the mitosis phase of the cell cycle. If the damage cannot be repaired, apoptosis, or death, of the cell occurs.

M phase, or mitosis, equally partitions the parent cell into two daughter cells. The ultimate goal of mitosis is to divide the chromosomes of the cell into two identical sets. Once the chromosomes are separated, the cell is divided by cytokinesis. Cytokinesis divides the cytoplasm and all cellular organelles between two cells. Each daughter cell contains approximately an equal share of each cellular component from the parent cell. As can be seen, mitosis is a fast and highly complex process. Mitosis is further divided into five distinct phases, which will be discussed later.

Throughout the cell cycle, there are strategically placed checkpoints. Cell cycle checkpoints monitor cell growth and DNA replication. Three checkpoints will be discussed here. They are the G1, G2, and metaphase checkpoints. The G1 checkpoint has a twofold purpose. To begin, cellular growth and environmental conditions are taken into consideration. The cell must reach a particular size to continue onto the S phase. Without proper nutrients, the cell is unable to complete required growth and protein synthesis, and cell cycle progression is ceased. The G1 checkpoint also checks DNA for damage prior to replication. When DNA damage is present, progression of the cell cycle is halted until repairs have been completed. Once the cell is of appropriate size and DNA damage has been repaired, the cell cycle continues.

At the end of the G2 phase, the cell enters a second checkpoint, the G2 checkpoint. DNA has been completely replicated by this point in the cell cycle. Cells begin proofreading the DNA to check for unreplicated DNA, replication errors, and damage within the DNA. Similar to the G1 checkpoint, cell cycle progression can be halted at the G2 checkpoint to allow time for repair. The cell is allowed to continue to M phase when repairs are complete. However, if damage is too extensive, the cell is sent into apoptosis.

The metaphase checkpoint occurs during the M phase and assures that the mitotic spindle has completely formed and chromosomes have properly aligned within the cell. Another name for this checkpoint is the spindle checkpoint. The spindle assembly is the attachment point within the cell for chromosomes prior to cell separation. If the spindles are not completely or properly formed, or the chromosomes have improperly attached, additional time is allowed for the cell to complete spindle formation or align the chromosomes. The cell continues and finishes cell division once the chromosomes are aligned.

Having just discussed the role of checkpoints within the cell cycle, it is now necessary to discuss the role of p53. p53, also known as protein 53, is a protein that has been shown to suppress tumor formation. p53 is crucial in multicellular organisms, such as humans, where it is involved in regulation of the cell cycle. In general, the level of *p53* found in a normal cell is kept low. When p53 is not needed, the protein is continuously degraded to prevent protein activation. However, there are two reasons for the cell to activate p53, and they are DNA damage and apoptosis.

As discussed earlier, the cell cycle contains two DNA checkpoints: one checkpoint prior to DNA replication, G1, and a second afterward, G2. DNA damage signals trigger an increase of p53 within the cell. This increase is a result of lengthening the time prior to p53 degradation. When DNA damage is encountered, damaged DNA is bound by p53, which activates expression of several proteins, such as p21, that halt the progression of the cell cycle. p21 halts cell cycle progression by inhibiting the activity of downstream cell cycle proteins. This inhibition prevents the G1/S transition. While the cell cycle is paused, p53 initiates synthesis of DNA repair proteins. p53 prevents damaged DNA from being replicated, thus suppressing potential tumor formation. The cell reenters the cell cycle after repairs have been completed. At this time, excessive p53 protein is rapidly degraded and levels return to normal.

However, if DNA damage is beyond repair, p53 initiates the pathway to apoptosis. Apoptosis is a regulated form of cell death, which is discussed later. The way in which p53 triggers cell death is not well understood. p53 is thought to initiate synthesis of proteins that interfere with apoptotic suppressing proteins. Proteins, such as BCL-2, prevent the cell from entering an apoptotic pathway. If the protein is transformed from its suppressing mode, apoptosis occurs. One way p53 causes apoptosis is by initiating the synthesis of Bax proteins. Bax proteins antagonize BCL-2 and send the cell into an apoptotic pathway. By initiating cell death, p53 prevents the replication of severely damaged DNA.

In order for p53 to function fully, two intact and functional genes are required. If one copy of the gene is nonfunctional or mutated, tumor suppression is reduced. The p53 gene can be damaged in the cells from replication errors or mutagens, including radiation. If p53 damage goes unrepaired, the cell could begin uncontrolled division that can potentially lead to a tumor. Humans that have only one fully functional copy of p53 tend to develop cancer early in adulthood, a disease known as Li–Fraumeni syndrome. Li–Fraumeni syndrome is a rare heredity disorder that greatly increases susceptibility to cancers linked to mutations of the p53 gene.

As seen with p53 gene mutations, tumor cells take on a new and uncontrolled form of cell division. The overall phase progression remains the same, but the checkpoints become unreliable or bypassed altogether. As mentioned previously, checkpoints help ensure the normal growth of a cell. Normal growth involves checking DNA for damage and repairing that damage. Damage repair allows the cell to divide into new normal daughter cells. If the DNA damage is overly extensive or unrepairable, the cell initiates apoptosis to prevent mutations from proliferating. The damage is not allowed to continue on to future cellular generations. Loss of these checkpoints, such as seen with a damaged p53 gene, increases replication of damaged DNA and potential for uncontrolled growth. Figure 2.9 compares normal

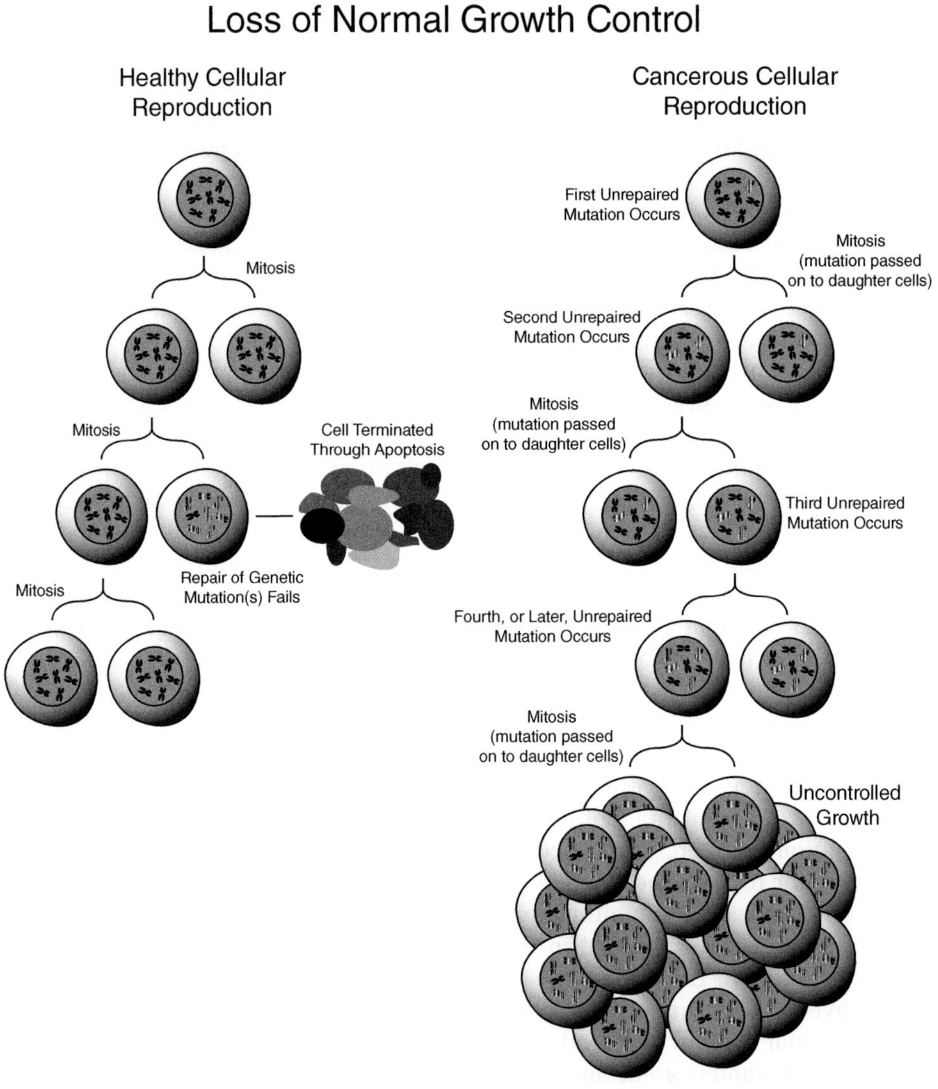

Loss of Normal Growth Control

Healthy Cellular Reproduction

Cancerous Cellular Reproduction

Mitosis

First Unrepaired Mutation Occurs

Mitosis (mutation passed on to daughter cells)

Second Unrepaired Mutation Occurs

Mitosis

Cell Terminated Through Apoptosis

Mitosis (mutation passed on to daughter cells)

Mitosis

Repair of Genetic Mutation(s) Fails

Third Unrepaired Mutation Occurs

Fourth, or Later, Unrepaired Mutation Occurs

Mitosis (mutation passed on to daughter cells)

Uncontrolled Growth

Figure 2.9   Tumor cell division. DNA damage is detected in normal cells are either repaired or the cell is sent into an apoptotic pathway. Cancerous cells do not repair DNA damage, and incorrect DNA is replicated as the cell begins proliferation.

cell growth against cancerous cell growth. Cells that have lost growth control continue to divide, replicating the mutation and passing it on to future cell generations. DNA damage continues to accumulate within the cell during uncontrolled growth and eventually forms a tumor.

CELLULAR DIVISION

Cell division is a process by which cells multiply. The overall idea of cell division is DNA replication followed by cytokinesis. As mentioned earlier, each cell replicates through four specific steps. Interphase includes phases G1, S, and G2. Metaphase is separated because it involves a series of steps specific to somatic or gamete cells. As metaphase is detailed further, it becomes divided into mitosis and meiosis. Mitosis is the final cell division steps taken by somatic cells, whereas meiosis is for gamete cells.

Cell division by mitosis goes through five distinct phases. A brief overview of each step is shown in Fig. 2.10. During the first phase, prophase, the cell condenses the chromatin of the nucleus. Chromatin becomes highly structured and known as chromosomes. Sister chromatids, from DNA replication in S phase, are attached to each other at a central point, the centromere. The centromere is a region of DNA in which sister chromatids come into contact most closely. It is also used for mitotic spindle attachment, discussed later. In addition to chromatid condensation, the two centrioles begin migration to each pole of the cell. The final piece of prophase is the beginning of nuclear envelope degradation. In order for the chromosomes to separate, the nuclear membrane must be degraded.

Following the complete disintegration of the nuclear membrane, the sister chromatids are spilled into the cytoplasm and begin migration toward the mitotic spindle. The cell enters metaphase once chromosomes attach completely to the mitotic spindle. The mitotic spindle is fully formed once the centrioles completely migrate to opposite poles of the cell. Chromosomes align across the center of the cell and form a "metaphase plate." The phrase "metaphase plate" comes from the appearance the chromosomes take on as a plate viewed from the side.

Chromatid separation begins during anaphase. Anaphase is characterized by shortening of the mitotic spindle. As some of the spindle microfibrils shorten, the sister chromatids are pulled apart. The separation is abrupt and results from centromere degradation. This separates the duplicated chromatids into two identical, but distinct, sets. The spindles also contain microfibrils that push the centromeres apart. Further separation of the centromeres ensures complete division of DNA.

Once the sister chromatids have completely separated, the cell enters telophase. The nuclear envelope reforms around each set of chromatids and creates two identical nuclei at opposite poles of the mother cell. Once the nuclear envelopes have reformed, the cell begins cytokinesis. Cytokinesis is the relatively equal division of cytoplasm and cellular organelles. It is characterized by the formation of a cellular furrow, or indentation, in the center of the mother cell. As the furrow enlarges, two daughter cells begin to form. Two new and completely functional cells are formed at the end of cytokinesis.

Gamete cells, in a similar fashion to somatic cells, go through cellular division. However, gamete cells undergo a division process known at meiosis. There are

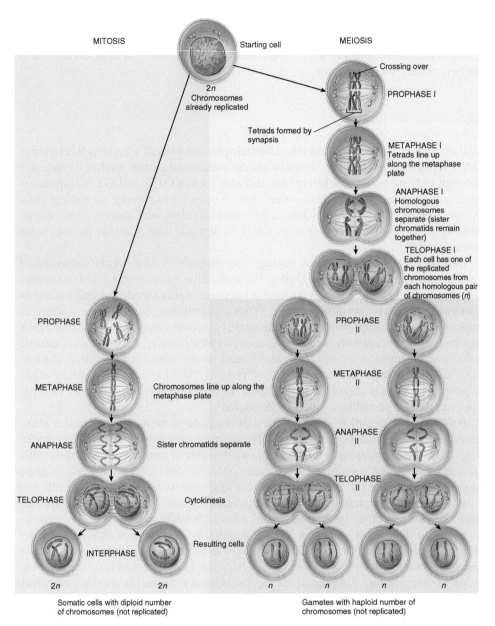

Figure 2.10   Stages of mitosis and meiosis, beginning with interphase and continuing through telophase. In each phase, a basic drawing and explanation is given to display the main features and differences between mitosis and meiosis. From Tortora and Nielsen (2012), figure 2.21, p. 53.

several distinct differences between mitosis and meiosis. The main difference is that cells divide once in mitosis and twice in meiosis. Mitosis maintains the number of chromosomes through each division whereas meiosis takes a diploid cell (46 chromosomes in humans) and forms four haploid gamete cells (23 chromosomes).

The overall phases of the meiosis cell cycle remain the same as in mitosis. However, the M phase of meiosis is split into two differing phases. These phases are meiosis I and meiosis II. Meiosis I is referred to as the reduction division since it takes the diploid cell and reduces the chromosome number to that of a haploid cell. Meiosis II is the equational division. The chromosomes are not replicated but partitioned equally among the daughter cells. Within each phase of meiosis, beginning with meiosis I, the cell goes through similar M phase steps of mitosis: prophase, metaphase, anaphase, and telophase.

During prophase I of meiosis, the replicated chromosomes, from S phase, seek their homologous partners, similar to mitosis. This paring occurs through the entire length of the chromatid, not just the centromere as in mitosis. Alignment of the chromatids occurs at discrete spots down the length of the homologs, similar to buttoning a shirt. Groups of four chromatids, called tetrads, are formed. Crossover events occur within the tetrads between sister chromatids and are unique to prophase I. This allows exchange of genetic material between maternal and paternal chromosomes. Shown in Fig. 2.10 are all the stages of meiosis, beginning with meiosis I and ending with meiosis II.

The tetrads formed in prophase I align at the spindle equator. Alignment is completely random, meaning either the maternal or paternal chromosome will be on one side of the equator. Once alignment is complete, the cell enters anaphase I and the spindle begins to pull and push the chromatids apart. The homologous chromatids act as a unit, as if replication had not occurred. As the sister chromatids are distributed to opposite ends of the cell, two nuclear membranes reform around individual sets of chromatid and the cell enters telophase. The final step of meiosis I is cytokinesis, and the daughter cells become completely independent of each other.

Meiosis II mirrors mitosis in every way except that chromatin is not replicated before prophase II begins. The outcome of meiosis II is the formation of four haploid cells (23 chromosomes in humans) that result from the two diploid cells formed in meiosis I. The progression of meiosis II is shown in Fig. 2.10. As with meiosis I, there are four steps in meiosis II.

During prophase II, the nuclear envelope disappears and the chromatin thickens and shortens. Centrioles migrate to polar ends of the cell and form the spindle. As the cell enters metaphase II, the spindle fibers attach to the centrioles at each pole and the chromatid themselves. Migration of the centrosomes establishes a new equatorial plane. The chromatids are then aligned along the new plane, and anaphase II begins once proper alignment and attachment occur. During anaphase II, the sister chromatids are pulled apart. Separation of the chromatids occurs by cleaving the centromeres and once separated, chromatids are called chromosomes. The spindle fibers pull sister chromosomes to opposite poles of the cell. As seen previously, meiosis II ends with telophase II and cytokinesis. During telophase II, the spindle disappears, and nuclear envelopes are formed around the chromosomes. Cytokinesis, as describe previously, begins once the nuclei have migrated completely to opposite poles of the cell.

CELL DEATH

As in life, all good things must come to an end. Cells are no different. The life cycle of a cell depends on numerous factors. The function of the tissue and cell damage are factors to be considered. Cell death occurs through three processes, each occurring in response to specific stimuli. Cell death can be classified as autophagy, necrosis, or apoptosis.

Autophagy is the process of self-degradation. It is a highly regulated process to maintain proper balance between protein synthesis and degradation within the cell. Autophagy is the main mechanism used by starving cells. The starving cell breaks down nonessential components and uses the constituents as temporary nutrient sources. These nutrients are reallocated and used for essential processes. Autophagy is a last attempt for survival by a starving cell.

Necrosis is death by injury, or accident. Factors that cause necrosis are external to the cell or tissue and include traumatic and chemical insults. Essentially, necrosis is premature cell death. Traumatic insults result in damage to the plasma membrane. The loss of membrane integrity allows water to engorge the cell. As the cell swells, the plasma and organelle membranes burst, resulting in necrotic death. Necrotic cells do not undergo the same chemical reaction as normally dying cells and have the potential of releasing harmful chemicals into surrounding tissue. As an example, the hydrolytic enzymes contained within lysosomes can worsen tissue damage. If not treated quickly, the damage can lead to gangrene in which a significant amount of contiguous necrotic death is seen in the surrounding tissue. Chemical insults, such as those from a rattle snake bite, also cause necrosis surrounding the wound site. Again, if the wound is not treated, gangrene has the potential of setting in.

Programmed cell death, or apoptosis, is the body's ability to decide when a cell dies. Apoptosis is a latent ability possessed in all multicellular organisms and involves a series of events to reduce the cell into its basic constituents for reuse without releasing harmful substances into the surrounding tissue. Apoptosis is extremely important throughout life beginning with embryonic development, maintaining tissue homeostasis and regulating cell viability through hormones. These are just a few examples of apoptosis. In addition to the importance of apoptosis, there are several classes of cells that are more prone to apoptosis. Some of these classes are harmful and unnecessary cells. An example of a harmful cell is a T cell that attacks the body. The main function of a T cell is to find foreign cells within the body and destroy them. When T cells attack the body, they are considered harmful and commonly die by apoptosis. Unnecessary cells undergo apoptosis when their function serves no purpose. During embryonic development, webbing forms between the digits of the fingers and toes. As the fetus develops, the webbing becomes nonfunctional and apoptosis is used to eliminate the cells.

SUMMARY

- Mammalian cells are classified as either somatic or gamete cells.
- General cell organization begins with the cytoplasm, which houses a number of organelles.

- Organelles, such as the ribosomes and mitochondria, have specific functions that are not shared with each other.
- The abundance of certain organelles, such as the ER, depends on the requirements of the particular cell.
- The nucleus is the brain of the cell. It signals cellular division and is responsible for DNA replication.
- Cellular membranes are found surrounding not only the cell itself, but also the individual organelles.
- Membrane transport is a vital series of processes for acquiring needed nutrients for cell function.
- Cell junctions allow cells to communicate and provide strength to tissue.
- The cell cycle incorporates a continuous growth cycle with a discontinuous chromosomal cycle is a relatively seamless manner.
- Checkpoints are located at specific points within the cell cycle.
- p53 is involved in cell cycle checkpoints and with suppression of tumor development.
- Cell division occurs through the four phases of mitosis: prophase, metaphase, anaphase, and telophase.
- Cell division differs between somatic (mitosis) and gamete (meiosis) cells.
- Cell death can be separated into three distinct categories: autophagy, necrosis, and apoptosis.

BIBLIOGRAPHY

Bolsover SR, Shephard EA, White HA, Hyams JS. Cell biology: A short course. 3rd ed. Chichester, UK: Wiley-Blackwell; 2011.

Cohen BJ, Wood DL, Memmler RL. The structure and function of the human body. 7th ed. Philadelphia: Lippincott Williams & Wilkins; 2000.

Pollard TD, Earnshaw WC. Cell biology. Philadelphia: Saunders; 2002.

Scanlon VC, Sanders T. Essentials of anatomy and physiology. 6th ed. Philadelphia: F.A. Davis Co.; 2011.

Tortora GJ, Nielsen MT. Principles of human anatomy. 12th ed. Hoboken, NJ: John Wiley & Sons; 2012.

QUESTIONS

Chapter 2   Questions

1. Eukaryotic and prokaryotic cells differ by the presence of
   a. an external membrane.
   b. cytoplasm.
   c. a nucleus.
   d. a, b, and c

2. The stages of mitotic growth for mammalian cells have been divided into four phases: G1, S, G2, and M. During which phase of the cell cycle would you expect DNA to be most easily damaged by X-rays?
   a. Early S phase
   b. G1/S phase
   c. G1 phase
   d. G2/M phase

3. Which of the following organelles can be found either bound to another organelle or free in the cytoplasm?
   a. Ribosome
   b. Golgi apparatus
   c. Endoplasmic reticulum
   d. Mitochondria

4. Which of these organelles is involved in both drug metabolism and in protein synthesis?
   a. Golgi apparatus
   b. Ribosome
   c. Endoplasmic reticulum
   d. Mitochondria

5. Which of the following transport systems requires cellular energy?
   a. Facilitated diffusion
   b. Active
   c. Passive
   d. a and c

6. Which of the following organelles contains hydrolytic enzymes responsible for digestion?
   a. Mitochondria
   b. Nucleus
   c. Lysosome
   d. Golgi apparatus

7. Although DNA is found primarily in the nucleus, it is also located in which other organelle?
   a. Endoplasmic reticulum
   b. Lysosome
   c. Mitochondria
   d. Golgi apparatus

8. Which organelle houses genetic material?

   a. Mitochondria

   b. Endoplasmic reticulum

   c. Nucleus

   d. Ribosome

9. In which mitotic phase does the spindle shorten?

   a. Metaphase

   b. Telophase

   c. Prophase

   d. Anaphase

10. Cellular junctions can be separated into four subclasses. Which of the four junctions provide strong connections between cells in a spot-like fashion?

   a. Tight and adheren junctions

   b. Gap and desmosome junctions

   c. Tight and desmosome junctions

   d. Adheren and desmosome junctions

11. If the total cell cycle time is 24 hours, G2 is found to be 6 hours, M phase is determined to be 1 hour, and S phase is measured at 8 hours, how long should G1 be?

   a. 3 hours

   b. 6 hours

   c. 9 hours

   d. 12 hours

12. Generally speaking, the most variable stage of the cell cycle is

   a. M phase.

   b. G1 phase.

   c. G2 phase.

   d. S phase.

13. An increased level of p53 gene protein is involved in

   a. arresting cell in the G1 phase of the cell cycle.

   b. stimulating repair of DNA damage.

   c. apoptosis.

   d. a, b, and c

14. Mitosis and meiosis are different in which of the following ways?

   a. They both have only one single cell division.

   b. The chromosome number remains unchanged.

   c. Meiosis has two cell divisions.

   d. There is no difference.

15. How is apoptosis different from autophagy and necrosis?
    a. Cells die in each, so they are the same
    b. Self-degradation
    c. Programmed death
    d. Accidental death

16. Overexpressed levels of the p53 gene
    a. arrests cells in S phase of the cell cycle.
    b. can increase levels of p21 that causes G1 cell arrest.
    c. can stimulate the apoptotic pathway.
    d. Both b and c.

CHAPTER 3

RADIATION CHARACTERISTICS AND UNITS

KEYWORDS

Ionizing radiation, electromagnetic spectrum, X-ray, gamma ray, alpha particle, beta particle, exposure, dose, effective dose, equivalent dose, half-life, activity, radiation units, gray, sievert, roentgen, rad, rem, becquerel, curie

TOPICS

- Basic physics of ionizing radiation
- Types of ionizing radiation and their characteristics
- Units for quantifying radiation, including traditional and Système International (SI) units
- The purpose and use of each radiation unit

INTRODUCTION

Radiation is energy transmitted through a medium as either electromagnetic (EM) waves or subatomic particles. Larger particles (e.g., molecules, pollen, raindrops, bowling balls) may be capable of transmitting energy, but they do not qualify as radiation. The medium through which radiation is transmitted may be vacuum, air, tissue, or some other material. In this course, we are especially concerned with what happens when radiation is transmitted through the cells and tissues of living organisms.

Radiation Biology of Medical Imaging, First Edition. Charles A. Kelsey, Philip H. Heintz,
Daniel J. Sandoval, Gregory D. Chambers, Natalie L. Adolphi, and Kimberly S. Paffett.
© 2014 John Wiley & Sons, Inc. Published 2014 by John Wiley & Sons, Inc.

Ionizing radiation is radiation with sufficient energy that it can knock some of the electrons out of the atoms or molecules in a material that it passes through. The process of changing the number of electrons in an atom (adding or removing) is referred to as *ionization*; an atom with unequal numbers of protons and electrons is an *ion*.

When ionization occurs in living tissue, the electron may quickly recombine with its atom, and little damage may occur; but in some cases, significant damage at the cell, organ, or organism level may occur. A fundamental process caused by ionizing radiation is the splitting of atoms or molecules into positively and negatively charged fragments. These ions may then participate in chemical reactions, resulting in chemical changes that can lead to disruptions of cellular function in living tissue. Ionizing radiation comes from a variety of sources, including cosmic rays, natural radioactivity in the soil and in building materials, industrial sources (e.g., airport scanners), and medical devices (e.g., diagnostic X-ray or radiation therapy machines).

Many people fear radiation for several reasons: it cannot be seen, smelled, heard, or felt; it can cause biological damage; journalists like to write about the potential dangers of radiation (with a frequency and fervor that is often out of proportion to the harm it actually causes). In many ways, radiation is similar to electricity, but we have become accustomed to living with electricity in our homes and offices. Although electricity and automobiles (not to mention tobacco and ethanol) cause *many* more injuries and deaths each year than radiation, we tend to fear the unknown. Most people have no experience with radiation, beyond UV exposure from the sun and the occasional medical X-ray. Therefore, the average person is more frightened of radiation than electricity, because the average person knows something about how electricity is used and controlled (e.g., it can be shut off with a switch, "live" wires can be insulated with a plastic coating). Some sources of radiation (nuclear reactors, X-ray machines) can also be shut off, but the radiation we most fear comes from radioactive materials (radioactive waste generated in nuclear power plants, nuclear materials in weapons). Although radioactive materials cannot be turned off, simple measures, such as the use of shielding materials and maintaining a safe distance, are very effective at avoiding harmful radiation exposure.

One good property of radiation is that it is very easy to detect. Ionizing radiation passing through air creates an electrical charge that is easy to measure. Many of our medical colleagues wish there were a meter or detector for common diseases, such as cancer or Alzheimer's, which was as sensitive and readily available as radiation detectors.

The details of how radiation interacts with matter in general and biological matter in particular, will be the topic of later chapters. In this chapter, we will introduce the types of ionizing radiation and discuss their characteristics. We will also introduce the units of measurement used to quantify radiation.

TYPES OF IONIZING RADIATION

There are two basic types of ionizing radiation: EM radiation and particulate radiation. Briefly, EM radiation involves the transmission of energy, but not mass. In contrast, particulate radiation consists of subatomic particles having both mass and

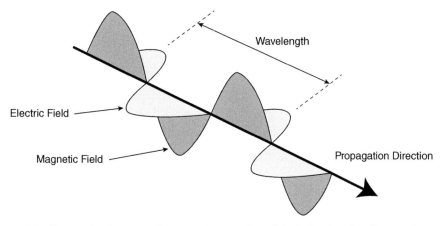

Figure 3.1   For an electromagnetic wave, the wavelength is defined as the distance between adjacent peaks.

energy. Importantly, both EM and particulate radiation with sufficient energy are capable of tearing electrons out of atoms or molecular bonds in matter.

EM RADIATION

EM energy has both wave- and particle-like characteristics. The wave description is more useful for describing EM energy propagating through space or a medium. Figure 3.1 illustrates the wave-like properties of radiation. Like any traveling wave, a traveling EM wave will have a propagation speed (v, in units of m/s), a wavelength (λ, in units of m), and a frequency (f, in units of s^{-1}). In a given medium, the speed is constant, so a wave with higher wavelength will have a lower frequency, where $v = \lambda f$.

On the other hand, when EM energy interacts with matter, it is absorbed or emitted in discrete amounts (i.e., quanta), as if it were a particle. The quantum of EM energy is called a *photon*. Calling a photon a "particle" is somewhat misleading, since photons have no mass. Because EM radiation possesses both wave- and particle-like properties simultaneously, the energy E of an absorbed or emitted photon is related to the wavelength in a simple way:

$$E = hf/(2\pi), \tag{3.1}$$

where h is Planck's constant ($h = 6.626 \times 10^{-34}$ J-s). The Système International (SI) unit of energy is the joule (J), but radiation energies are more conveniently expressed in electron volts (eV), where 1.602×10^{-19} J = 1 eV. An electron volt is the amount of kinetic energy gained or lost when a single electron moves through a potential difference of 1 V. As an example, an electron moving from the positive to the negative terminal of a 9-V battery will gain 9 eV of energy. An electron volt is an extremely small unit of energy, compared with energy scales used to describe ordinary objects and processes. A donut contains about 60 mJ or 3.7×10^{17} eV of stored energy. A 60-W lightbulb is expending more than 3×10^{20} eV (300 trillion MeV) per

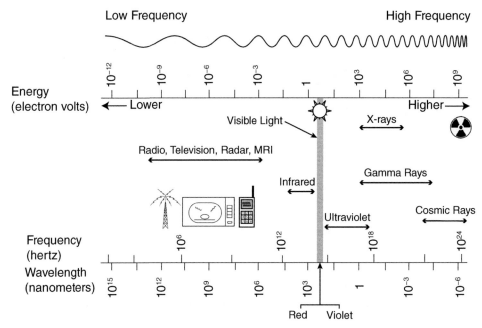

Figure 3.2   The electromagnetic (EM) spectrum, showing the corresponding wavelength, frequency, and energy scales. Note that shorter wavelengths correspond to higher frequencies and energies. Visible light occupies only a small portion of the EM spectrum and is near the upper end of the nonionizing energy range.

second. Nevertheless, the energy of a few dozen electron volts, deposited in an atom in tissue, is a potentially significant event in radiation biology. The energy of EM radiation extends from lower-energy radio waves to high-energy gamma rays. Figure 3.2 presents portions of the EM spectrum from the low-energy, long wavelength end to the high-energy, short wavelength end.

Infrared and visible light are forms of EM radiation, encountered every day, which cause some biological effects. We feel heat (mainly due to photons in the infrared energy range), and we see using visible light, both of which are biological effects. However, infrared and visible photons are not energetic enough to cause ionization (i.e., eject orbital electrons from atoms). Ionizing EM radiation includes photons with energies of about *10 eV or higher* (including the far UV, X-rays, and gamma rays). Ionizing radiation can cause chemical changes that may result in significant biological effects, including cell death or cancer. Figure 3.3 illustrates the ionization of an atom by an incident X-ray.

Ionization is a *quantum effect*—understanding this concept is very important to understanding the biological effects of EM radiation. If an electron requires a 12-eV energy gain in order to be ejected from an atom in some material, then the atom must absorb a *single* photon of energy 12 eV or greater. To produce ionization, the photon energy must be greater than the energy required to remove an electron from the material. It must be greater than the electron's binding energy. If there are many 4-eV photons striking the material, one might think that three of them together could eject an electron. But ejecting an electron is not like lifting a

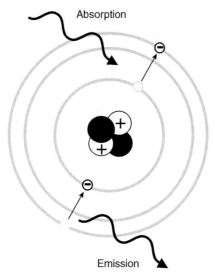

Figure 3.3 Absorption of a photon of EM radiation by an atom results in the sudden transition of an electron to a higher energy level. Emission of a photon involves the transition of an electron to a lower energy level.

Volkswagen—even though one person cannot lift a Volkswagen, several people working together can. Ionization is more like trying to throw a rock across a wide river. If one person cannot throw a rock far enough, and none of his friends can throw a rock far enough, then the whole group can throw rocks at a furious rate, and not a single rock will make it across the river. In the same way, multiple nonionizing photons do not add together to eject an electron from an atom or split a molecule into fragments. While a very high intensity of nonionizing radiation (i.e., many low-energy photons) can cause significant heating, leading to burns or even death, a certain level of nonionizing radiation exposure (i.e., heat) is *absolutely necessary* for the survival of living organisms. Ionizing radiation is different: it results in fundamentally different mechanisms of biological harm, it appears one can live without it, and it is not clear whether *any* amount of ionizing radiation is actually good for you.

Note that radiation emitted from cell phones is nonionizing. The energy of photons emitted from a cell phone is lower than the energy of many of the photons coming from a toaster (which emits significant energy in the infrared and even the lower end of the visible spectrum). In the consumer realm, it makes sense to fear tanning beds, which do emit *ionizing* radiation that will increase one's risk of melanoma, the most serious type of skin cancer. However, there is no conclusive experimental evidence at this point (2011) that cell phones (or any other devices that emit low-energy photons—such as hair dryers or FM radios) cause cancer. Nonetheless, worrying about cell phone radiation has been a popular topic in the press in the first decade of the 21st century. Similarly, there is no conclusive evidence that living near power lines or power substations causes cancer (a popular topic in the latter decades of the 20th century), for all the same reasons mentioned earlier.

X-rays and gamma rays are the forms of ionizing EM radiation that are the most important to consider for a course in radiobiology applied to medicine. X-rays and gamma rays lie at the high-energy part of the EM spectrum as shown in Fig. 3.3. Note that gamma rays and high-energy X-rays are physically identical. The reason for the different names arises from differences in their origin (inside vs. outside the nucleus). X-rays are produced in the orbital electronic shells of an atom or by interactions between charged particles and the nucleus, whereas gamma rays are emitted from an unstable nucleus after rearrangement of the particles inside the nucleus, as described in more detail later.

As noted earlier, gamma rays and X-rays are photons, which possess zero electrical charge and zero mass, and therefore have a relatively low probability of interacting in matter. As a result, photons can penetrate deeply into matter, because the interactions required to dissipate their energy are infrequent. Photons do carry energy and can ionize atoms or molecules via direct interactions with orbital electrons. They do not have a well-defined maximum penetration depth in matter, but we can define an average penetration depth for a given material. To effectively shield gamma rays and X-rays requires electron-dense materials, for example, steel or lead.

ATOMS AND ISOTOPES

The atom is the smallest unit of matter possessing a unique chemical identity. Atoms consist of subatomic particles: positively charged protons and uncharged neutrons occupy a dense nucleus, which is surrounded by a "cloud" of negatively charged electrons.

Atomic nuclei are denoted by the atomic number Z, which is the number of protons in the nucleus, and the atomic mass number A, which is the total number of nucleons (protons and neutrons) in the nucleus. To label nuclei, Z is written to the lower left of the chemical symbol, and A is written to the upper left of the chemical symbol. The nucleus of an element with chemical symbol X would be written ^A_ZX. As an example, the carbon-12 nucleus, which has six protons and six neutrons, is written as

$$^{12}_{6}C.$$

The chemical characteristics of an atom are defined by its electron configuration, which is the basis for the assignment of elements to particular columns in the periodic table, shown in Fig. 3.4. Recall that elements in the same column of the periodic table have similar chemical properties. In the neutral atom, the number of electrons equals the number of protons. Therefore, all atoms with the same number of protons in their nuclei have the same chemical characteristics. By definition, atoms with the same number of protons are the same element and are denoted by the same chemical name and chemical symbol (e.g., six protons = carbon = C). Thus, the chemical symbol and the atomic number (Z) are actually redundant, and Z is often omitted when specifying a nucleus (e.g., carbon-12 or ^{12}C). The simplest atom is hydrogen (^{1}H) with one proton in the nucleus and one electron. The most abundant isotope of helium (^{4}He) has two protons and two neutrons in the nucleus.

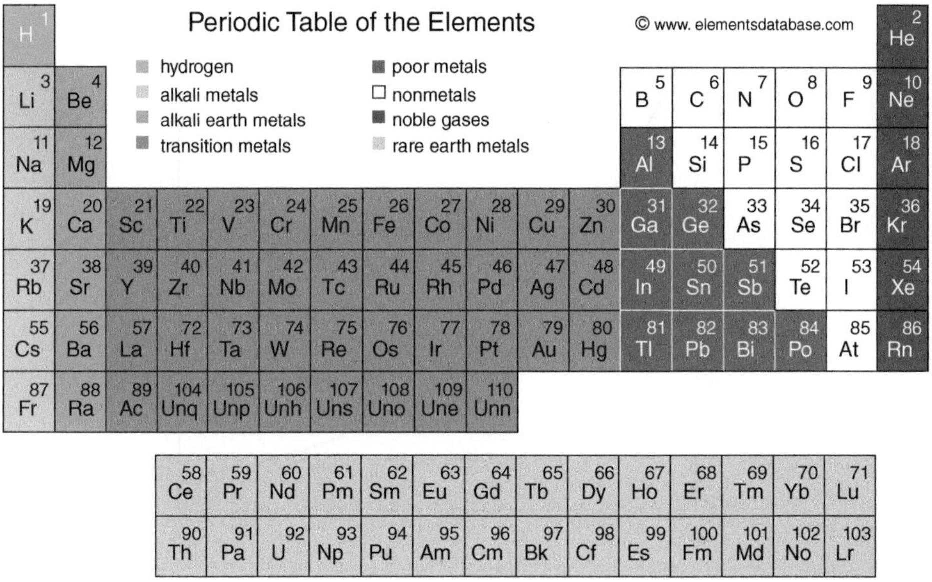

Figure 3.4 The periodic table of the elements organizes the elements according to their electronic structure. The number in the upper right corner is the number of protons in the nucleus. From Halliday et al. (1994), Appendix E.

Isotopes have the same number of protons but may have different numbers of neutrons, and therefore different mass numbers. For example, the different isotopes of carbon are written as

$$ {}_{6}^{11}\text{C}, {}_{6}^{12}\text{C}, {}_{6}^{13}\text{C}, \text{ and } {}_{6}^{14}\text{C}. $$

${}_{6}^{13}\text{C}$ means this isotope of carbon has 13 nucleons, which includes six protons, in the nucleus. By subtraction, the number of neutrons (N) in the ${}_{6}^{13}\text{C}$ nucleus is seven (i.e., $13 - 6 = 7$).

The two important forces in the nucleus are ordinary electrostatic repulsion (i.e., the Coulomb force between the positively charged protons) and the strong nuclear force, which is attractive and holds the nucleus together. (Note that there are only four fundamental forces; the other two are the weak nuclear force and gravity.) In order for a nucleus to remain in existence indefinitely, there must be a balance between the repulsive and attractive forces. Such a nucleus is referred to as "stable." Unstable nuclei will give up energy until they achieve a more energetically stable configuration; energy given up by an unstable nucleus is emitted in the form of particles with high kinetic energies (e.g., a fast-moving electron). Generally, the energies are high enough to cause ionization, which is why we are concerned with nuclear stability in this course.

Energetically stable nuclei tend to have roughly the same number of protons and neutrons. If a nucleus is unstable (too many neutrons or too many protons), it transforms into a new, more stable nucleus by a radioactive decay process. There are many different decay processes, but the ones most relevant to radiobiology involve

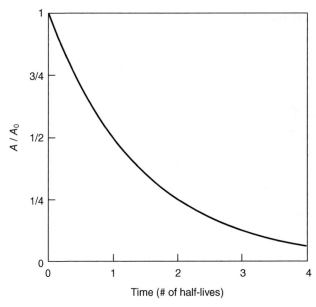

Figure 3.5   The activity of a radioisotope decays exponentially as a function of time with a rate constant λ according to the equation $A/A_0 = \exp(-\lambda t)$. The half-life $T_{1/2}$, defined to be the time required for half of the radioactive nuclei to decay, equals $(\ln 2)/\lambda$.

the emission of particles (alphas, betas, positrons, or neutrons), or the emission of high-energy photons (gamma rays).

Given one unstable nucleus, it is impossible to predict when it will decay. However, given a huge group of identical unstable nuclei, then, statistically, one can predict with high precision how long it will take for a given fraction of the group to decay. Every radioactive isotope decays with a half-life that is constant and unique to that isotope. The half-life is simply the time required for half of the nuclei (no matter how many you have) to decay into another type of nucleus. (So, if the half-life is 1 hour, one can reliably say that half of the nuclei will decay in 1 hour, but one cannot say which particular individual nuclei will be the ones to decay.) The time dependence of the activity of an isotope undergoing radioactive decay is shown in Fig. 3.5. The half-life cannot be altered by any ordinary physical means, for example, by freezing or compressing the substance. As stated earlier, the radiation emitted from radioactive materials cannot be "turned off." Note that the half-life does not depend on the number of nuclei present.

In a radiation biology course, it is useful to distinguish between the half-life of a radioactive isotope and the biological half-life of a foreign substance introduced into an organism. When physicists and biologists say "half-life," they may be talking about different concepts entirely:

- *Physical Half-Life.* The time statistically required for half of a group of unstable nuclei of a particular isotope to decay. This number is a constant (no external effects). For example, iodine-131 has a physical half-life of about 8 days.

TABLE 3.1 Half-Life Values (Physical and Biological) for Various Isotopes

Isotope	Half-Life in Days		
	T (Physical)	T (Biological)	T (Total)
^{3}H	4.5×10^3	12	12
^{14}C	2.1×10^6	40	40
^{90}Sr	1.1×10^4	1.8×10^4	6.8×10^3
^{99m}Tc	0.25	1	0.20
^{137}Cs	1.1×10^4	70	70
^{210}Po	138	60	42
^{235}U	2.6×10^{11}	15	15

- *Biological Half-Life.* The time required for an organism to "flush out" half of a contaminant (through exhalation, urination, etc.). The biological half-life can be affected by various conditions (respiration rate, fluid intake, etc.). The biological half-life reduces the effective lifetime of a radioactive source in an organism—the radioactive source is decaying, while it is also simultaneously being eliminated by the organism. Rates are given by the inverse of the time (i.e., second is a unit of time, per second or s^{-1} is the unit describing the rate), and rates add in the normal arithmetic sense. Therefore, the effective half-life of a radioactive source in an organism is given as follows:

$$\frac{1}{T_{\text{Total}}} = \frac{1}{T_{\text{Physical}}} + \frac{1}{T_{\text{Biological}}}.$$

- *Total (or Effective) Half-Life.* The time required for the radioactivity in a patient to be reduced to half through the combined effects of the physical decay of the isotope and the biological elimination of the isotope. *The total or effective half-life is always shorter than either the physical half-life or the biological half-life (Table 3.1).*

PARTICULATE RADIATION

The primary types of ionizing radiation of concern in radiobiology are alpha particles, beta particles, X- and gamma rays, and neutrons. In the discussion that follows, keep in mind that the masses of the proton and neutron are similar, with $m_p = 1.673 \times 10^{-27}$ kg and $m_n = 1.693 \times 10^{-27}$ kg, whereas the electron mass is about 2000 times smaller ($m_e = 9.11 \times 10^{-31}$ kg). The electric charges of the proton, neutron, and electron are +1, 0, and −1, respectively. The positron β^+ has the same mass as an electron but the opposite charge (i.e., β^+ charge is +1).

Alpha Particles

As described earlier, alpha particles are emitted during the decay of radioactive nuclei. The alpha particle is comprised of two protons and two neutrons (with a net positive charge of +2). The positively charged alpha particles (++) interact with electrons (–) in a material to efficiently ionize atoms along the alpha particle path. As a result of these interactions, the alpha particle loses a large amount of energy over a short distance, which limits the penetration depth of alpha particles to only a few centimeters in air or less than a millimeter in human skin.

Electrons (Beta Particles) and Positrons

Electrons may be emitted by an unstable nucleus, as described earlier, in which case they are called beta particles. Electrons may also be produced from photon interactions with matter, the product of ionization by an X-ray, for example. High-energy electrons may also be produced by acceleration by a high voltage in a linear accelerator for the purposes of radiation therapy, that is, to treat tumors. Regardless of their source, basic electron characteristics are the same. Positrons are just electrons with the opposite charge, and they have similar interaction characteristics as electrons, so we mention them here. At the end of its path through a material, a positron interacts with an electron, fully converting its mass into energy as two gamma photons.

Beta particles (electrons and positrons) are nearly 8000 times less massive than alpha particles, and they have a charge of 1 (–1 for electron, +1 for positron). Like alpha particles, beta particles interact with the electrons in a material via Coulomb interactions, resulting in ionization. Compared with alpha particles, beta particles are more easily scattered due to their much lower mass. Thus, they have zigzag paths in matter, as shown in Fig. 3.6. Because of their lower charge, beta particles are not as effective at causing ionization. Therefore, a beta particle travels further before giving up all its energy (several centimeters in human tissue) compared with an alpha particle of the same energy.

Neutrons

Neutron radiation consists of neutrons that are not contained in a nucleus and are instead moving through a medium. Neutron radiation can be complicated, because

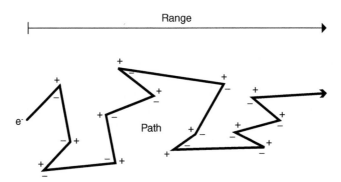

Figure 3.6 The range of an electron is defined to be the penetration depth, while the electron path is the total distance traveled. The path is much greater than the range for electrons due to multiple scattering events.

when a neutron has lost enough energy, it can be absorbed by a target nucleus, which causes the nucleus to become radioactive. The radioactive nucleus will then emit an alpha particle, a beta particle, or a gamma ray in order to become more energetically stable.

Neutrons are about 2000 times more massive than electrons, but less massive (by a factor of 4) than alpha particles. They interact with charged particles only by colliding with them, because neutrons are not charged. Collisions lead to multiple scattering events as they travel through a material, with some energy lost during each scattering event. Because they are not slowed by Coulomb interactions, they can penetrate deeply into a material and are relatively difficult to stop. The neutron interactions that lead to the greatest energy loss are collisions between neutrons and hydrogen nuclei in hydrogenous materials. Therefore, materials such as water or plastic are usually effective for stopping neutrons. For very high-energy neutrons, more dense materials such as steel or lead may be required. In general, the penetration of neutrons is greater than electrons but smaller than X-rays of the same energy.

Protons

Proton ionizing radiation is not a product of natural radioactive decay and is therefore encountered only very infrequently. High-energy protons can be produced in particle accelerators (by ionizing hydrogen and then exposing it to a high voltage). In the United States, protons are used for radiation therapy at only a few highly specialized facilities with accelerators specifically designed for proton therapy. Protons are more penetrating than alpha particles due to having half the charge and are scattered less than electrons due to their greater mass (Table 3.2).

RADIATION UNITS: TRADITIONAL AND MODERN

If a subject is exposed to ionizing radiation, energy may be deposited in the subject's tissue, which may result in various types of chemical or physical damage. However, absorbing radiation energy generally does not cause the subject to become

---

TABLE 3.2 Characteristics of 2-MeV Radiations and Their Approximate Range in Tissue

Radiation	Mass (kg)	Mass (AMU)	Charge	Range in Tissue for 2-MeV Radiation (cm)
X- or gamma rays	0	0	0	14 (= 1 HVL)[a]
Electrons	9.1×10^{-31}	5.5×10^{-4}	−1	1
Protons	1.672×10^{-27}	1.0073	1	0.01
Neutrons	1.675×10^{-27}	1.0087	0	5.5
Alpha particles	6.64×10^{-27}	4.001	2	0.001

[a]X- and gamma ray photons do not have a definite range because their attenuation is exponential. To indicate their penetrating ability, the half-value layer, HVL, is introduced. The HVL is the amount of material required to reduce the intensity to one-half the incident value.

radioactive. Similarly, if a body is exposed to light, it generally does not begin to glow (unless the body contains fluorescent proteins, such as those found in jellyfish). On the other hand, if a person is exposed to radioactive dust (i.e., actual chunks of radioactive material that stick to the skin or enter the lungs) or a person is injected with a radioactive isotope, then this person would become a radiation source. Thus, it is important to be able to properly quantify radiation, the energy imparted by radiation, and the effect of this imparted energy on human subjects.

Two quantities of interest are exposure and dose. As the name implies, exposure quantifies the amount of radiation that a subject is exposed to. Dose, on the other hand, is a measure of the energy that is actually absorbed after an exposure. Furthermore, the dose that is absorbed has different biological effects depending on the radiation type and which part of the body absorbs the dose, as described in more detail later.

Exposure

The precise definition of exposure is the number of ion pairs formed in a given volume of air when it is exposed to radiation. The modern SI unit of exposure is the C/kg, which is defined as the amount of charge produced in 1 kg of air. In practice, exposure is the number of X-rays incident on a body. The old unit, still in common use, is the roentgen (R, where 1 R = 2.58×10^{-4} C/kg, in air). One mR is 1/1000 of 1 R. The roentgen has many limitations but is useful in describing the amount of radiation striking a body.

Note that exposure measures the total amount of radiation received, without regard to whether the exposure occurred over a short time period or a long time period. Thus, another important quantity is the exposure *rate*. The exposure rate is a measure of radiation intensity and is usually expressed in units of R/h or mR/h.

Absorbed Dose

Since exposure applies only to quantifying X-ray and gamma radiation in air, a different unit is needed to quantify the radiation energy absorbed in materials, particularly when considering other types of radiation, such as alpha or beta particles. Dose is a measure of the amount of energy deposited per unit amount of matter. It is more important than counting the number of X-rays, because the amount of energy deposited depends on the energy and type of radiation, not just the number of photons. Furthermore, the energy absorbed by different materials may differ, even if they receive exactly the same exposure. For example, the dose to a person will be slightly different than the dose to an equivalent mass of air.

The SI unit measuring dose is the gray (Gy). One gray is equal to 1 J deposited per kilogram of material (1 Gy = 1 J/kg). The older (cgs) unit, still common in the literature, is the rad. One rad is equal to 100 ergs deposited per gram of material. The conversion from rad to gray is 100 rad = 1 Gy.

Dose can be used to quantify the energy absorbed by a medium for any type of radiation (photon or particulate). However, dose, by itself, is not sufficient for specifying the biological consequences of radiation exposure. In other words, dose can be used to quantify the energy absorbed by a body, but it does not quantify the harm or risk to the body.

Equivalent Dose

The biological consequences of radiation exposure depend not just on the amount of energy deposited but also the type of radiation the subject is exposed to. Some types of radiation produce more significant biological effects than others for the same absorbed dose. The equivalent dose accounts for factors that modify the biological effects of the absorbed radiation energy. The equivalent dose relates the amount of a particular type of radiation (e.g., alpha particles) to the same amount of a standard radiation. The standard radiation is usually taken to be 250 keV X-rays.

To obtain the equivalent dose, the absorbed dose (in gray) of a given type of radiation is multiplied by a weighting factor, w_R, which is related to the relative biological effectiveness (RBE) of different types of radiation. (We will discuss the RBE in more detail in a later chapter.) The unit for the equivalent dose is the sievert. For alpha particles, the weighting factor may be as high as 20, so that 1 Gy is equivalent to 20 Sv. In other words, a given dose of alpha particles is 20 times as effective ($w_R = 20$) as the same dose of 250-keV X-rays in producing tissue damage. For X-rays and gamma rays, the weighting factor is 1 so that the gray and sievert are equivalent for those radiation sources:

$$H_T = \sum_R w_R D_{T,R}.$$

- T is some tissue (or organ).
- R is the radiation type.
- H_T is the equivalent dose to tissue T (Sv).
- $D_{T,R}$ is absorbed dose to tissue T from radiation R.
- w_R is radiation weighting factor for radiation of type R.

The old unit of equivalent dose is the rem (roentgen equivalent man), and the old name for the quantity "equivalent dose" is "dose equivalent." The dose equivalent used quality factors Q, instead of weighting factors w_R. In the context of comparing the effects of different types of radiation, the rem has the same function as the sievert, and 1 Sv = 100 rem. For example, from a chest X-ray exam, the (old) dose equivalent would be of order 5 mrem. In modern terms, we would say the equivalent dose is of order 0.05 mSv. Roughly the same equivalent dose (i.e., same biological harm) is received during an intercontinental plane flight (due to cosmic radiation in the upper atmosphere). A much larger dose (>100 mSv) is required in order to observe biological effects in a person after a single exposure (Table 3.3).

In summary, the equivalent dose accounts for both the energy absorbed per unit mass (dose) and the RBE of the radiation type (quantified by the weighting factor). Equivalent dose enables the relative harm (or risk) of a given dose of radiation to be estimated and compared with any other dose of any type of radiation.

Note that in older literature, the units R, rad, and rem are used somewhat interchangeably. For photon radiation, which is the type most commonly encountered in the clinical setting, an *exposure* of 1 R leads to an *absorbed dose* of about 1 rad and a *dose equivalent* of about 1 rem. This convenient equivalence follows from the definitions of the units and the RBE of photon radiation. However, one must remember that 1 R = 1 rad = 1 rem only applies to photon radiation. An absorbed

TABLE 3.3   Quality (Q) and Radiation Weighting Factors (W) for Various Radiations Specified in the International Commission on Radiological Protection (ICRP) Publications 20 and 60

Radiation	Q (ICRP 20)	W (ICRP 60)
X-ray, gamma ray, beta	1	1
Neutrons		
Thermal	2	5
0.01 MeV	2.5	10
0.1 MeV	7.5	10
0.5 MeV	11	20
>0.1–2 MeV		20
2–20 MeV		5
Unknown energy	10	
High-energy protons	10	5
Alpha, fission fragments, heavy nuclei	20	20

dose of 1 rad from fast neutrons would have a greater biological effect (dose equivalent = 10 rem).

Effective Dose

The effective dose relates the biological harm of a partial body exposure to the harm of total body irradiation. It should not be surprising that irradiation of an arm results in less overall harm than irradiation of an entire torso. The effective dose is equal to the dose to the entire body that would produce the same level of harm as a dose to the part of the body actually exposed. The effective dose is obtained by first multiplying the equivalent dose to each critical organ by the tissue weighting factor, w_T, and then adding up all the weighted doses. Table 3.4 presents the tissue weighting factors for important organs as defined for the United States and internationally:

$$H_E = \sum_T w_T H_T.$$

- H_E is the effective dose.
- H_T is the equivalent dose to tissue T.
- w_T is the tissue weighting factor.

For example, the gonads are one of the critical organs (i.e., they have a high weighting factor), but during a head computed tomography (CT) exam, they are not exposed. The contribution to the effective dose from exposure to the gonads is therefore zero because H_E is zero for that tissue. Although the equivalent dose (energy deposited in the exposed tissues, multiplied by the radiation weighting factor w_R) from a chest X-ray is about 0.05 mSv, the effective dose is less than half of this value (approximately 0.020 mSv for patients with breasts or approximately 0.013 mSv for patients without breasts), because the chest X-ray does not expose the gonads or colon and exposes only a small fraction of the bone marrow, tissues that are heavily weighted in calculating the effective whole body dose.

TABLE 3.4 Tissue Weighting Factors Specified by the Nuclear Regulatory Commission and Used in the U.S. (a) and the Tissue Weighting Factors Recently Recommended by the International Commission on Radiological Protection (b) (By Definition, the Sum of All Wt Values Is 1)

(a)

Organ or Tissue	Wt
Gonads	0.25
Breast	0.15
Red bone marrow	0.12
Lung	0.12
Thyroid	0.03
Bone surfaces	0.03
Remainder tissues	0.30
Whole body	1.00

In the United States, the calculation of effective dose is performed according to Nuclear Regulatory Commission Regulations, using tissue weighting factors published in the Code of Federal Register 10.20.1003.

(b)

Organ or Tissue	Wt	Sum of Wt Values
Bone marrow, colon, lung, stomach, breast	0.12	0.60
Gonads	0.08	0.08
Bladder, esophagus, liver, thyroid	0.04	0.16
Bone surface, brain, salivary glands, skin	0.01	0.04
Remainder tissues[a]	0.12	0.12
Whole body		1.00

These tissue weighting factors were recommended by the International Commission on Radiological Protection in 2007 (ICRP Publication 103, Ann. ICRP 37 [2–4]).

[a]Includes adrenals, extrathoracic region, gallbladder, heart, kidney, lymph nodes, muscle, oral mucosa, pancreas, prostate, small intestine, spleen, thymus, and uterus/cervix.

Activity

The level of radioactivity of a radioactive source can be understood by considering all of the unstable atoms in the source. These atoms are continuously decaying, so the greater the number of unstable atoms, the greater the number of disintegrations per second (dps). One disintegration per second (dps) is defined to be 1 becquerel (Bq), the SI unit of activity. The older unit of activity is the curie (Ci), which is still in use in most medical facilities. One Ci is equal to 37 GBq. The strange conversion factor originates in the fact that the curie was originally defined as the number of disintegrations per second produced by 1 g of radium, about 3.7×10^{10} dps. Since the curie is a very large number, relative to the activity of radioisotopes used in medical procedures, the microcurie (μCi) or millicurie (mCi) is typically used in quantifying clinical doses.

Like exposure rate, which is a measure of the number of X-rays or gamma rays incident per unit time, activity is a measure of the number of disintegrations per unit time. During exposure to a radioactive source, the dose to a nearby object will be proportional to the activity, but it will also depend on many other factors (the amount of energy associated with each disintegration, the distance from the source, the absorption characteristics of the object). Similarly, the activity does not indicate the level of biological damage due to the radioactive material, which would require consideration of the type of radiation emitted and its biological effectiveness. Figure 3.7, Table 3.5, and Table 3.6 summarize the radiation quantities discussed in this chapter.

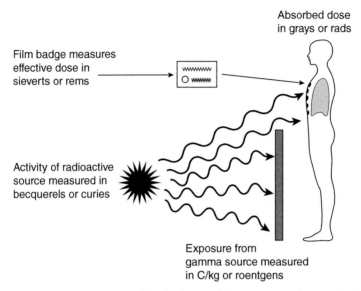

Figure 3.7 Important radiation quantities include activity, exposure, dose, and effective dose.

TABLE 3.5   Summary of New and Old Radiation Units

	Activity of Source	Absorbed Dose	Equivalent or Effective Dose	Exposure
Old standard unit	Curie	Rad	Rem	Roentgen
SI unit	Becquerel	Gray	Sievert	Coulomb/kilogram

TABLE 3.6   Conversion Factors Relating New and Old Radiation Units

To Convert from	To	Multiply by
Rad	Gray	0.01
Gray	Rad	100
Rem	Sievert	0.01
Sievert	Rem	100
Curie	Becquerel	3.7×10^{10}
Becquerel	Curie	$1/(3.7 \times 10^{10})$

SUMMARY

- Radiation is energy transmitted through a medium as photons (electromagnetic energy) or subatomic particles.
- Ionizing radiation is radiation with sufficient energy to remove electrons from atoms or molecules in the medium through which it travels.
- The most important types of ionizing radiation are high-energy photons (X-rays and gamma rays), alpha particles, beta particles, neutrons, and positrons.
- Each type of radiation is characterized by its mass, energy, and electric charge.
- Radioactive isotopes are characterized by their physical half-life (time for half of the radioactivity to decay), biological half-life (time for half of the isotope to be eliminated from the body), and the effective half-life (time for the activity in a body to be reduced by half through physical and biological processes).
- Exposure is a measure of how many ion pairs are formed in a given amount of air when exposed to high-energy photons. The SI unit of exposure is the C/kg (charge produced in 1 kg of air); the old unit is the roentgen (R).
- Dose is a measure of the amount of energy absorbed per unit mass of material. The SI unit of dose is the gray (1 Gy = 1 J/kg); the old unit is the rad.
- Equivalent dose is obtained by multiplying the dose by a weighting factor corresponding to the relative biological effect on the body due to the radiation type.
- Effective dose is equal to the dose to the entire body that would produce the same level of harm as the dose to the part of the body actually exposed. The effective dose is obtained by first multiplying the equivalent dose to each critical organ by a tissue weighting factor and then adding up all the weighted doses.
- Remember that equivalent dose is weighted by radiation type, while effective dose is further weighted by tissue type. The SI unit of equivalent dose and effective dose is the sievert (Sv); the old unit is the rem.
- Activity is a measure of the number of radioactive decays per unit time from a radioactive source. The SI unit of activity is the becquerel (1 Bq = 1 disintegration/s); the old unit of activity is the curie (Ci).

BIBLIOGRAPHY

Bushberg JT. The essential physics of medical imaging. 2nd ed. Philadelphia: Lippincott Williams & Wilkins; 2002.

Friedberg W, Copeland K, Duke FE, O'Brien K 3rd, Darden EB Jr. Radiation exposure during air travel: Guidance provided by the Federal Aviation Administration for air carrier crews. Health Phys. 2000 November;79(5):591–5.

Halliday D, Resnick R, Walker J. Fundamentals of physics. 4th ed. New York: Wiley; 1994.

Hendee WR, Ibbott GS. Radiation therapy physics. 2nd ed. St. Louis, MO: Mosby; 1996.

Mettler FA Jr., Huda W, Yoshizumi TT, Mahesh M. Effective doses in radiology and diagnostic nuclear medicine: A catalog. Radiology. 2008 July;248(1):254–63.

Saha GB. Physics and radiobiology of nuclear medicine. 3rd ed. New York: Springer; 2006.

Chapter 3   Questions

1. Which part of the electromagnetic spectrum can produce ionization?
   a. Electrons
   b. Infrared
   c. Gamma radiation
   d. Microwaves

2. Nonionizing radiation
   a. has no biological effects.
   b. includes radio frequencies, cell phone frequencies, and infrared radiation.
   c. may cause effects such as the excitation of electrons to a higher energy level or an increase in molecular vibrational energies, which results in tissue heating.
   d. Both b and c

3. Isotopes of the same element are nuclei with
   a. the same number of neutrons.
   b. the same number of protons.
   c. the same mass number.
   d. the same number of electrons.

4. High-energy photons have _____ wavelengths and _____ frequencies compared with low-energy photons.
   a. longer, higher
   b. longer, lower
   c. shorter, higher
   d. shorter, lower

5. Photons are
   a. quantized electromagnetic energy.
   b. massless.
   c. electrically neutral.
   d. a, b, c.

6. In order to ionize an atom, a particle or photon must have an energy greater than
   a. 1 MeV.
   b. 1 keV.
   c. the binding energy of an electron in the atom (of order 10 eV).
   d. 0 eV. The energy of a single particle does not matter, because the energy from many particles or photons can combine to ionize an atom.

7. Ionization is an important concept in radiation biology, because
    a. it is the basis for the damaging biological effects caused by radiation, and it provides a mechanism for detecting and measuring radiation.
    b. it describes how protons are ejected from the nucleus of an atom, causing biological damage to a cell.
    c. it is the process by which alpha, beta, and gamma radiation are produced.
    d. it selectively damages DNA.

8. The most deeply penetrating radiation is the
    a. gamma ray.
    b. alpha particle.
    c. electron.
    d. proton.

9. A particle with a mass number of 4 and a charge of +2 is
    a. an alpha particle.
    b. a proton.
    c. a neutron.
    d. an electron.

10. Although they have nearly the same mass, a neutron will penetrate more deeply than a proton with the same energy, because
    a. neutrons are scattered more easily.
    b. neutrons do not experience electrostatic forces.
    c. protons are easily absorbed by atomic nuclei.
    d. protons cause ionization, but neutrons are nonionizing.

11. The three most common types of radiation produced by unstable nuclei are
    a. microwave, X-ray, and gamma.
    b. alpha, gamma, and neutron.
    c. beta, gamma, and neutron.
    d. alpha, beta, and gamma.

12. If an isotope has a physical half-life of 10 days and its biological half-life is also 10 days, then its total half-life is
    a. >10 days.
    b. 10 days.
    c. <10 days.
    d. There is not enough information to determine.

13. If you were exposed to a beta-gamma source such as iodine-131, which units could be used to quantify the amount of radiation energy absorbed by your body?

   a. roentgen, C/kg

   b. rad, gray, J/kg

   c. rem, sievert, J/kg

   d. curie, becquerel

14. 1.0 mSv is equivalent to

   a. 1.0 mrem.

   b. 10 mrad.

   c. 10 mCi.

   d. 100 mrem.

15. The difference between the absorbed dose and the equivalent dose is

   a. the absorbed dose depends on the energy of the radiation.

   b. the equivalent dose is more ambiguous as to biological effects.

   c. the equivalent dose weights the absorbed dose according to the energy and type of radiation to account for the biological effects.

   d. There is no difference in practice.

16. Which statement best describes the difference between the equivalent dose and the effective dose?

   a. Because the units are the same, there is no actual difference.

   b. The equivalent dose is proportional to the absorbed dose, but the effective dose is not related to the absorbed dose.

   c. The effective dose weights the equivalent dose to account for the radiation sensitivity of particular tissues.

   d. The equivalent dose enables the comparison of the biological effects of a dose to a particular organ to the biological effects of a whole body dose.

CHAPTER 4

RADIATION INTERACTIONS WITH TISSUE

KEYWORDS

Radiation interactions, direct interactions, indirect interactions, charged particles, neutrons, photons, linear energy transfer, half-value layer, relative biological effectiveness

TOPICS

- Interaction of charged and uncharged particles with matter
- Interactions between photons and matter
- Quantities used in characterizing radiation interactions with tissue
- Linear energy transfer (LET) and relative biological effectiveness (RBE) of different types of radiation
- Direct and indirect interactions in tissue

INTRODUCTION

This chapter is concerned with the deposition of energetic radiation into living tissues. Before discussing the biological effects of radiation, we will consider ionizing radiation interactions in tissue. This includes the processes through which radiation interacts with tissue and how these interactions affect biological systems. Finally, damage produced by different types of radiation will be discussed.

CHARGED PARTICLE INTERACTIONS

Charged particles interact with the tissue through electrostatic interactions. These interactions result in slowing of the charged particle and a loss of kinetic energy (KE). The lost energy is transferred to the surrounding tissue by excitation and ionization. Excitation occurs when a particle interacts with and excites an atom. The excited atom may then de-excite and emit radiation. Ionization occurs when a charged particle removes an orbital electron from an atom. The result of ionization is a free electron and a positively charged ion. The negative electron and positive ionized atom are called an ion pair. For air and tissue, the average energy per ion pair is approximately 34 eV. Roughly, a third of this energy goes into removing the electron from the atom, and the rest goes into excitation and KE. Ionization in water and organic material is very important in radiation biology due to the formation of free radicals, which is an important cause of radiation damage.

The electrostatic interaction of a charged particle is proportional to the charge of the particle. Particles with multiple charges such as alpha particles (+2 charge) have stronger electrostatic interactions with the medium than singly charged particles such as electrons (−1 charge). As a result, alpha particles lose energy more rapidly in matter than do electrons.

Another mechanism of energy loss by charged particles is radiative emission. In this case, a charged particle interacts with the electromagnetic (EM) field of an atom and the resulting electrostatic force changes the direction of the charged particle. This abrupt change in direction results in the emission of EM energy. The emitted photons are referred to as "bremsstrahlung," a German word for "braking radiation." Bremsstrahlung emission is only of importance for light charged particles, namely electrons and positrons, which are readily deflected from a straight path.

EM RADIATION INTERACTIONS

X-rays and gamma rays are high-energy EM radiations with zero mass and zero electrical charge. The basic unit or "packet" of EM radiation is the photon. As discussed in the previous chapter, high-energy photons have higher frequencies and shorter wavelengths, and they penetrate more deeply in tissue than low-energy photons.

Ionizing photons have three main interaction mechanisms—(1) the photoelectric effect, (2) Compton scattering, and (3) pair production—each of which is prevalent over a different energy range. The photoelectric interaction and Compton scattering are dominant for the lower energies used in diagnostic imaging. The total likelihood of a photon interacting with a medium *decreases* with increasing photon energy.

Photoelectric Effect

The photoelectric effect is the dominant process at low photon energies (tens of electron volts up to 100 keV). In a photoelectric interaction, the incident photon is completely absorbed by the atom, and the photon energy is transferred to an orbital electron. For the photoelectric interaction to occur, the orbital electron must have

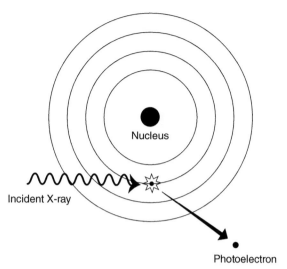

Figure 4.1 Photoelectric effect. The net result of the photoelectric effect is the complete absorption of the incident X-ray and the ejection of a photoelectron.

a binding energy (BE) that is less than the energy of the photon. Figure 4.1 illustrates the photoelectric effect. The atom is ionized when this electron, which gains enough energy from the photon to overcome its BE, is ejected from the atom. The ejected electron is called a photoelectron. Thus, the photoelectron's KE differs from the photon energy by its BE:

$$KE_e = E_{ph} - BE_e. \tag{4.1}$$

At energies encountered in diagnostic imaging, the photoelectron travels less than a few millimeters in tissue. If an inner shell electron is ejected, then an outer shell electron will fill the inner shell vacancy. The inner shell has a stronger BE, and the excess energy is usually released as a characteristic X-ray. Characteristic X-rays from tissue elements (i.e., carbon, nitrogen, and oxygen) have very low energies and do not exit the patient because of their low energies.

Compton Scattering

The Compton interaction typically involves an interaction between an incident photon and an outer shell electron, resulting in a scattered photon and a scattered electron. The incident photon loses a portion of its energy in the collision and changes direction (which causes blurring of diagnostic X-ray images). Outer shells of an atom are lightly bound, so removal of the electron from the atom does not require much energy. The incident photon energy is shared between the scattered photon and the scattered electron. Figure 4.2 shows the essentials of a Compton interaction. Compton scattering is the dominant process at intermediate photon energies (100 keV to 10 MeV).

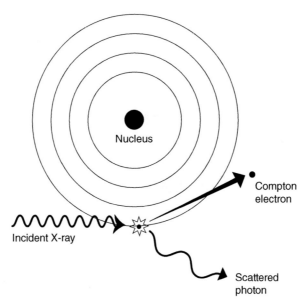

Figure 4.2   Compton scattering. The energy of the incident photon is shared between the scattered photon and the Compton (recoil) electron.

Unlike the photoelectric effect, Compton scattering results in a recoil electron and a scattered photon, both of which are capable of producing further ionization. Recall that the net result of the photoelectric interaction is complete absorption of the photon and emission of an energetic electron. The major contribution of the Compton interaction in medical imaging is an increase in patient dose and loss of contrast in the image.

Pair Production

Pair production occurs when the incident photon interacts with a nearby nucleus, creating an electron–positron pair. A positron is the antiparticle of the electron. The positron has the same mass as an electron but opposite charge. From Einstein's equation for mass–energy equivalence ($E = mc^2$), the mass of an electron or positron is equivalent to an energy of 0.511 MeV. For pair production to occur, the incident photon must therefore have an energy of at least 1.022 MeV, because the mass of the electron–positron pair is formed from the incident photon energy. Any energy above the threshold is shared as KE between the electron–positron pair. Figure 4.3 illustrates the pair production reaction.

The photoelectric effect and Compton scattering are the most important modes of interaction for photons in the diagnostic energy range. As summarized in Fig. 4.4, below approximately 100 keV, the photoelectric effect is the most frequent mode of interaction between photons and tissue. Compton scattering is the dominant mode of interaction in the 100 keV to 10 MeV range. Above approximately 10 MeV, pair production becomes the most common mode of interaction for photons in tissue. It is important to keep in mind that in all three processes, energy is transferred from a photon to electrons.

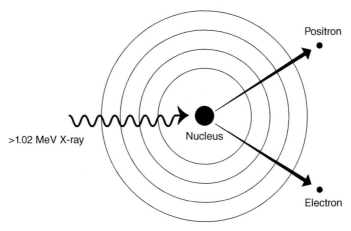

Figure 4.3   Pair production. An incident photon with energy greater than 1.022 MeV can generate a positron/electron pair. The positron and electron have rest masses of 0.511 MeV and share the excess kinetic energy.

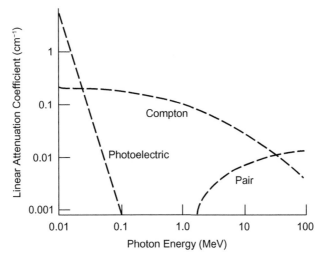

Figure 4.4   Probability of interaction versus photon energy for (1) the photoelectric effect, (2) Compton scattering, and (3) pair production.

NEUTRONS

Neutrons are indirectly ionizing particles that cannot interact by the Coulomb force due to their neutral charge. Instead, neutrons lose energy by collisions that transfer KE to the tissue.

Neutron interactions are complex and depend on the neutron KE. A discussion of all types of neutron interactions is beyond the scope of this book. The majority of the energy lost by neutrons in a hydrogen-containing medium (such as living tissue) is through collisions with hydrogen nuclei producing recoil protons. These

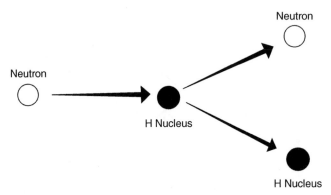

Figure 4.5 Neutrons experience scattering, particularly in hydrogenous materials. The target nucleus is typically a single proton (hydrogen nucleus), which gains kinetic energy from the incident neutron.

energetic protons, like energetic electrons, then go on to damage biological systems via ionization of atoms/molecules along the particle path. Figure 4.5 shows how an uncharged neutron can transfer energy through a collision with a charged nucleus producing subsequent ionizations.

SPECIFIC IONIZATION

For charged particles, we can define the specific ionization as the number of ion pairs formed per unit path length. Alpha particles can produce several thousand ion pairs per millimeter. For beta particles (electrons), the specific ionization is 50–100 ion pairs per millimeter. Energetic neutral particles, such as neutrons and photons, can liberate charged particles (e.g., protons, electrons) for which the specific ionization can then be defined. Specific ionization differs for different materials and tissues.

LINEAR ENERGY TRANSFER (LET)

LET is the energy transferred by radiation per unit path length in soft tissue. LET is the product of the average energy transferred per ion pair and the specific ionization (number of ion pairs per unit length). LET is usually expressed in units of keV/μm. The specific ionization (ion pairs per path length) is greatest for heavy charged particles such as the alphas. Alphas leave a densely ionized particle track (high specific ionization) *and* deposit a relatively large amount of energy per unit length. Alphas and neutrons (which produce recoil protons) are considered high-LET radiations. On the other hand, betas and photons (which liberate electrons) leave a sparsely ionized particle track. The amount of energy deposited per unit path length is relatively low, so beta particles and X-rays/gamma rays are considered low-LET radiations.

Although photons do not carry charge, they set electrons in motion and thus produce ionization. Once a photon transfers energy to an electron, the LET is that

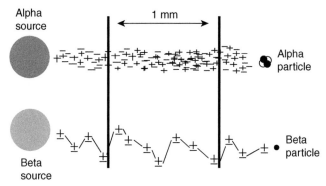

Figure 4.6   Alpha particles have high specific ionization and a relatively straight path as they interact with matter. Electrons have a lower specific ionization and more contorted path.

of electrons. Likewise, neutrons do not carry charge, but they set protons in motion. The LET for neutrons is therefore similar to that of protons.

The LET depends on the type of radiation and its energy. Lower-energy particles interact more strongly and have a higher LET, compared with higher-energy particles of the same type.

PATH AND RANGE OF CHARGED PARTICLES

Charged particles undergo electrostatic interactions, attractive or repulsive, that may deflect the particle from a straight path. Charged particles with low mass such as the electron are easily deflected. The *path* of an electron is therefore a series of random scatters that appears as a contorted path as shown in Fig. 4.6. Heavy charged particles, such as alphas, which are over 7000 times more massive than an electron and have twice the charge, are not as easily deflected. These particles tend to take relatively straight paths as they lose energy in matter. The path length of a particle is a measure of the actual distance that the particle has traveled, not the distance "as the crow flies."

As particles slow, the rate of energy transfer increases. Heavy ions therefore exhaust most of their KE at the end of the particle track. As shown in Fig. 4.7, the specific ionization as a function of distance traveled for heavy ions rises to a maximum, called the Bragg peak, and then drops to zero once the particle's KE is spent.

The *range* of a particle is a measure of the penetration depth in the medium. (The range *is* measured "as the crow flies.") For beta particles, the path length, because it is contorted, is usually much longer than the range (see Fig. 4.6). By contrast, the range of an alpha particle is nearly the same as the path length, because the path is relatively straight. The range of a particle is inversely proportional to the amount of energy lost by the particle per unit distance traveled. Particles that produce a large amount of ionization in a relatively short distance, such as the alpha particle, lose energy rapidly and have relatively short ranges. On the other hand, particles that sparsely ionize atoms along their path lengths have relatively long ranges. In other words, *range is inversely proportional to LET.*

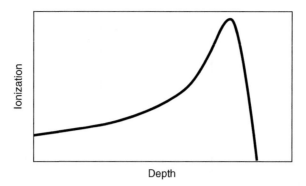

Figure 4.7 For heavy charged particles, such as protons, the specific ionization increases as the particle loses energy moving through the material, resulting in a Bragg peak.

The range also depends on the energy of the incident particle, with a more energetic incident particle of a given type having a greater range than a less energetic particle of the same type. For example, the relatively energetic beta particles from phosphorus-32 have a maximum range of 7 m in air and 8 mm in tissue. The low-energy betas from hydrogen-3, on the other hand, are stopped by only 6 mm of air or 6 μm of tissue.

HALF-VALUE LAYER (HVL) (PHOTONS)

A photon traveling in matter tends to lose its energy all at once in a chance encounter (in contrast to multiple interactions that are involved in slowing a charged particle). Therefore, statistically speaking (i.e., considering the behavior of a large group of identical photons) energy deposition by photons in matter does not have a well-defined range and does not exhibit a Bragg peak.

Because photons undergo only chance encounters with matter, their penetration drops off exponentially and is better characterized by the HVL. The HVL is expressed as a thickness of a specified material—for example, 5 mm of aluminum, or 5 in. of concrete. It is defined as the thickness of a particular material that will attenuate the flux of photons of a particular energy by a factor of 2. For example, for a 100-keV X-ray beam, the HVL for aluminum is approximately 3.5 mm. You can only measure the HVL if you have many photons, because it is a statistical quantity. (In other words, any *individual* photon either deposits its energy at a well-defined location or passes through the medium, but it is not practical, or useful, in radiobiology to measure the range of individual photons.)

Figure 4.8 shows how the attenuation of X-rays or gamma rays exponentially decreases as the radiation passes deeper into the material, so there is no definite cutoff. Therefore, a given gamma ray has a finite probability of passing through any medium of any depth. The minority of diagnostic X-rays that pass through the body (and strike the detector) are used to form a radiographic image. Because the HVLs of bone, tissue, and gold are different, the amount of attenuation due to each material is different, resulting in the image contrast you see in the X-ray image (Fig. 4.9).

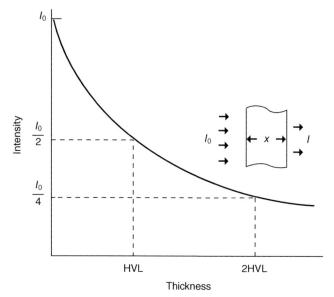

Figure 4.8 The intensity of an X-ray beam is attenuated exponentially as a function of the thickness of an absorbing medium. The half-value layer (HVL) is the thickness of material required to attenuate the beam by a factor of 2.

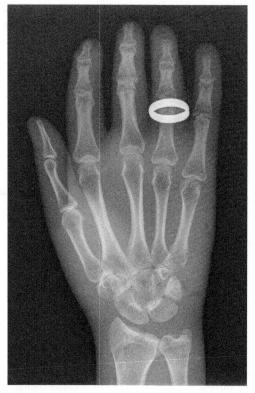

Figure 4.9 An X-ray image demonstrates differential attenuation of X-rays by different materials (muscle, bone, gold ring).

Like the range of charged particles, which depends on energy, the HVL also depends on the energy of the incident photons. A greater thickness of shielding material is required to attenuate higher-energy photons by a factor of 2 compared with lower-energy photons. Recall that the probability of photon interaction with matter *decreases* with increasing photon energy, so one must provide a greater thickness of material to make up for the reduced probability of interaction per unit thickness.

EFFECTS ON TISSUE

Direct Action

When energetic charged particles interact directly with the critical targets in cells (e.g., DNA molecules), the process is referred to as *direct action*. For example, an incident alpha particle may directly break the chemical bonds in a DNA molecule. Direct action is the dominant damage-inducing process of high-LET radiations (neutrons and alpha particles). Figure 4.10 shows a photoelectron being ejected and directly interacting with a DNA strand.

Indirect Action

When radiation interacts with other molecules/atoms (e.g., water) in the cell to produce free radicals, and the free radicals then diffuse and damage critical targets in the cell, the damage is said to occur by *indirect action*, as illustrated in Fig. 4.10.

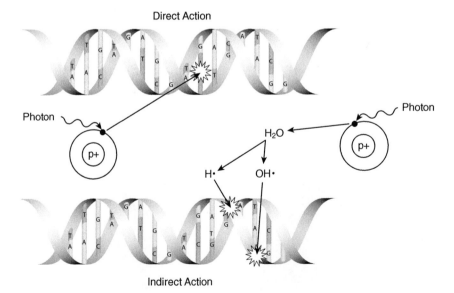

Figure 4.10   In the case of indirect action, the incident photon ejects an electron, which creates a free radical; the diffusing free radical can then cause damage to the target (here, a DNA molecule). In the case of direct action, the ejected electron directly interacts with the target.

Indirect action is the dominant process of low-LET radiations (photons, beta particles).

When radiation ionizes an atom, an ion pair could be formed. For example,

$$H_2O + X\text{-ray} \rightarrow H^+ + OH^-.$$

An ion pair can simply recombine, or it could chemically react and damage biomolecules in cells. In general, ion pairs are a minor source of radiation damage.

Alternatively, radiation damage can lead to the formation of free radicals, which can lead to damaging chemical reactions. A free radical is an atom or molecule carrying an unpaired orbital electron in the outer shell. Atoms and molecules with an unpaired electron are associated with a high degree of chemical reactivity. (Note that a neutral molecule can have an unpaired electron in the outer shell. An ion can also have an unpaired electron in the outer shell. So you can have a free radical, or an ion radical, depending on the net charge.) Free radicals interact strongly with biomolecules and are therefore a major source of radiation damage.

As just one example of free radical formation, we can look at X-ray interaction with a water molecule. If an X-ray interacts with a water molecule, it could knock out one of the outer shell electrons in the oxygen atom, thus producing H_2O^+, which is referred to as an ion radical, since it is charged and has an unpaired electron:

$$H_2O + X\text{-ray} \rightarrow H_2O^+ + e^-.$$

The lifetime for the ion radical is approximately 10^{-10} seconds, in which time it may react with another water molecule to form hydronium (an acid) and the highly reactive hydroxyl radical:

$$H_2O^+ + H_2O \rightarrow H_3O^+ + OH^{\bullet}.$$

The hydroxyl radical ($OH\cdot$) has nine electrons (eight form a closed shell, leaving one unpaired). Taking into account the hydroxyl radical lifetime and the diffusion coefficient at body temperature, the average range of the hydroxyl radical is about twice the diameter of DNA. It is estimated that two-thirds of the X-ray damage to DNA is caused by hydroxyl radicals. Figure 4.11 shows how neutrons (uncharged) can also produce hydroxyl radicals. An exhaustive description of radiation–tissue interactions resulting in free radical formation is beyond the scope of this book:

- Direct action:
  - involves direct interaction of an energetic particle (proton, neutron, electron, alpha) with a biological target, such as DNA;
  - dominant process of high-LET radiations (neutrons and alpha particles).
- Indirect action:
  - involves the creation of a free radical by an energetic particle; the free radical then interacts with the biological target;
  - dominant process for sparsely ionizing radiations (X-rays and beta particles).

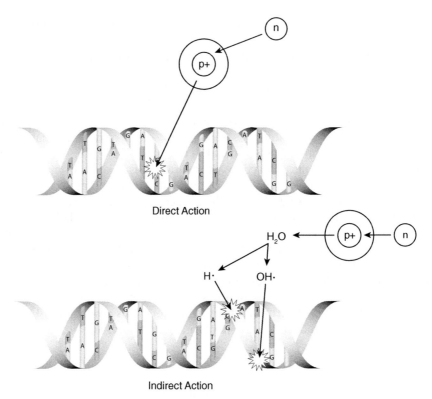

Direct Action

Indirect Action

Figure 4.11 Neutrons cause damage by either indirect or direct action, but direct action (caused by a recoil proton directly interacting with the target) is more common for neutrons, and other high-LET radiations, such as alpha particles.

THE RELATIVE BIOLOGICAL EFFECTIVENESS (RBE) OF HIGH- VERSUS LOW-LET RADIATIONS

The RBE is a commonly used method of quantifying the biological damage produced by a given type of radiation. The RBE is the ratio of the dose of some reference radiation required to produce a certain amount of damage to the dose of test radiation required to produce the same amount of damage (Eq. 4.2). In the literature, the reference radiation varies, but a common choice is 250-kVp X-rays. (Note that kVp denotes the voltage used to produce an X-ray beam in a standard X-ray tube—the X-rays in the beam will actually have a range of energies up to a maximum of 250 keV.)

$$\text{RBE} = \frac{\substack{\text{Dose of reference radiation required} \\ \text{to produce a certain amount of damage}}}{\substack{\text{Dose of test radiation required} \\ \text{to produce the same amount of damage}}}. \tag{4.2}$$

For example, if we wished to measure the RBE of 14.7-MeV neutrons, we could irradiate one population of cells with 250-kVp X-rays and another identical population of cells with 14.7-MeV neutrons. We would then carefully determine the respective doses that produce the same amount of cell death. If we found that 150 mGy of neutrons produced the same amount of cell death as 650 mGy of 250-kVp X-rays, the RBE would be calculated as follows:

$$RBE = \frac{\text{Absorbed dose of 250-kVp X-rays}}{\text{Absorbed dose of 14.7-MeV neutrons}} \qquad (4.3)$$

$$RBE = \frac{650\ \text{mGy of 250-kVp X-rays}}{150\ \text{mGy of 14.7-MeV neutrons}} = 4.3. \qquad (4.4)$$

The RBE is an index of radiation quality with respect to biological damage. In the case discussed, it can be said that the 14.7-MeV neutrons are 4.3 times more damaging to cells than 250-kVp X-rays. Note that the RBE is a dimensionless quantity because it is the ratio of an absorbed dose divided by another absorbed dose in the same units.

Generally, the RBE increases with increasing LET. For a given dose, high-LET radiations are usually more efficient at producing biological damage than low-LET radiations. Remember that higher LET means that a given amount of energy is deposited over a shorter distance. It turns out that depositing a little energy in each of many cells is often not as effective at damaging cells as depositing a lot of energy in just a few cells. However, the RBE increases with increasing LET only up to some maximum value. The maximum RBE occurs when the LET is approximately 100 keV/μm. Beyond this value, higher LET does not contribute to more cell damage. LET values greater than 100 keV/μm are said to produce "overkill."

As an analogy, imagine that you are stuck in quicksand, and poison darts are being fired at you (one per second) by a passing enemy who is being chased by a tiger. Assume the enemy has 20 darts. If the enemy is running very quickly, the darts will be far apart (say, 0.5 m), so in all likelihood you will be hit by only one dart, and perhaps your friend, who is also stuck in the quicksand, will also be hit by one dart. If two darts are required for a lethal dose, the one dart you each receive will be no problem, unless another enemy is also firing at you and you are unlucky enough to be hit a second time. (This is like the situation with low-LET radiation.) If the first enemy is able to slow down, perhaps because the tiger is distracted by a gazelle, then the darts might end up arriving with a closer spacing, for example, at 15-cm intervals. In this case, you are guaranteed to be hit by two or more darts, and so is your friend, so you will both die. (This is like optimal-LET radiation.) If the enemy stands still (because the tiger is actually eating the gazelle) and unloads all 20 darts into you, then only you will die, and your friend will actually survive. (This is "overkill," and it is a bad strategy for administering poison darts or radiation therapy.) In this last case, the biological effect is actually reduced (only one of you dies) even though the LET is very high, because all the darts were wasted on one target. Figure 4.12 illustrates how the effectiveness of radiation, as measured by the RBE, first increases, reaches a peak, and then decreases as the LET of the radiation increases.

Killing a cell generally requires damage to more than one site. Thus, low-LET radiations, which create sparse ionization, require more than one radiation track to

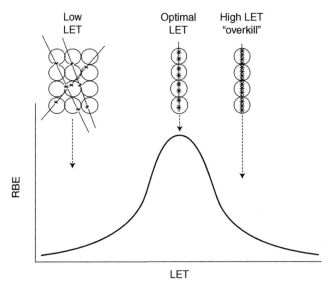

Figure 4.12 Typical RBE versus LET variation. The dose is proportional to the number of asterisks (*). If we assume two "hits" are required to kill a cell, then twice the dose of "high-LET" radiation is required to kill four cells, compared with the dose of "optimal-LET" radiation required to kill four cells. The high-LET radiation is less efficient because more radiation is deposited per cell than is necessary for killing. A similar dose of "low-LET radiation" kills only one cell.

pass through the same cell to induce cell death. With an optimal-LET radiation, one radiation track passing through a cell will be sufficient to produce death. On the other hand, overly ionizing radiation results in overkill; more energy than is needed to induce death is deposited into a single cell. In medical physics (if one thinks about radiation therapy), overkill would lead to both excessive and potentially ineffective patient doses—excessive in the sense of causing extra damage to surrounding healthy tissue and ineffective in the sense of having a reduced RBE for the cancer cells that you actually want to kill.

Historically, the RBE has been used to determine the "quality factors" for dose equivalent (the traditional quantity) and the "weighting factors" (w_E) used to determine the equivalent dose (the modern quantity). Dose equivalent and equivalent dose were discussed previously in Chapter 3. The equivalent dose is a measurement used by various regulatory agencies and others in an attempt to relate the dose a person has received to the possible biological consequences of the received dose. Details of the biological consequences of radiation exposure will be discussed in later chapters.

In this chapter, we have discussed how ionizing radiation interacts with matter and many of the descriptors that define these interactions. Each descriptor has a relationship to the biological effect of the radiations. Table 4.1 summarizes some of these key parameters and gives examples of typical values for various types of radiations.

TABLE 4.1 Summary of Radiation Properties for Various Radiations

Type of Radiation	LET (keV/μm) in Tissue	Approximate Range in Tissue (cm)	RBE
Diagnostic X-rays	~3	4 (HVL)	1
250-keV X-rays	2	6.5 (HVL)	1
3-MeV electrons	0.2	1.5	1
20-MeV protons	4.7	1	2
2.5-MeV alpha particles	166	0.001	20

For comparison with the LET, the diameter of a DNA helix is about 0.0024 μm, and a cell is of order 10 μm in diameter.

SUMMARY

- Charged particles interact with matter via electrostatic interactions, resulting in the slowing of the charged particle and a loss of KE. The energy is transferred to the surrounding medium, resulting in excitation or ionization of atoms in the medium.

- Photons interact with matter primarily by the photoelectric effect, Compton scattering, or pair production. The photoelectric effect is the dominant interaction below 100 keV. Compton scattering is the dominant process at intermediate photon energies of 100 keV to 10 MeV (the relevant energy range for many diagnostic and therapeutic medical procedures), and pair production dominates above 10 MeV.

- The primary interaction of neutrons with biological matter is scattering, resulting in the recoil protons, which go on to damage biological systems via ionization of atoms/molecules along the proton path.

- Specific ionization is the number of ion pairs formed per unit path length. LET is the energy transferred per unit path length. The LET is the product of the specific ionization and the average energy transferred per ion pair.

- The penetration of charged particles in matter is characterized by their range, which is the depth of maximum energy deposition. Photons do not deposit their energy at a specific depth, but rather interact at random points in a medium. Statistically, the intensity of many photons interacting with matter decays exponentially with depth. The HVL is the depth at which the photon intensity is reduced to half of the incident value.

- Range and LET are inversely related. High-LET radiation will quickly deposit its energy over a short range, while low-LET radiation will deposit its energy more slowly as it traverses a medium, resulting in a longer range.

- Direct action involves the interaction of an energetic particle (proton, neutron, electron, alpha) with a biological target, such as DNA. Direct action is the dominant process of high-LET radiations (neutrons and alpha particles).

- Indirect action involves the creation of a free radical by an energetic particle; the free radical then interacts with the biological target. Indirect action is the dominant process for sparsely ionizing radiations (X-rays and beta particles).
- The RBE is used to quantify the biological damage produced by a given type of radiation. The RBE of a given type of radiation is defined as the ratio of the dose of a standard radiation (e.g., 250-kV X-rays) to the dose of the radiation type of interest, such that the doses compared produce the same amount of biological damage.
- Generally, the RBE increases with increasing LET. For a given dose, high-LET radiations are usually more efficient at producing biological damage than low-LET radiations. However, the maximum RBE occurs at a LET of approximately 100 keV/μm. Above this value, higher LET does not contribute to more cell damage, and RBE decreases.
- Photons, electrons, and positrons are considered low-LET radiations with low RBE. Neutrons and alpha particles are considered high-LET radiations with high RBE.

BIBLIOGRAPHY

Fajardo LF, Berthrong M, Anderson RE. Radiation pathology. New York: Oxford University Press; 2001.

Hall EJ, Giaccia AJ. Radiobiology for the radiologist. 6th ed. Philadelphia: Lippincott Williams & Wilkins; 2006.

Protection ICoR. Relative biological effectiveness (RBE), quality factor (Q), and radiation weighting factor (w(R)). A report of the International Commission on Radiological Protection. Ann ICRP. 2003;33(4):1–117.

Saha GB. Physics and radiobiology of nuclear medicine. 3rd ed. New York: Springer; 2006.

Shapiro J. Radiation protection: A guide for scientists, regulators, and physicians. 4th ed. Cambridge, MA: Harvard University Press; 2002.

Turkington TG, Zalutsky MR, Jaszczak RJ, Garg PK, Vaidyanathan G, Coleman RE. Measuring astatine-211 distributions with SPECT. Phys Med Biol. 1993 August;38(8):1121–30.

Turner JE. Atoms, radiation, and radiation protection. 2nd ed. New York: Wiley; 1995.

QUESTIONS

Chapter 4   Questions

1. Charged particles of radiation interact with matter mainly by
   a. the photoelectric effect.
   b. coulomb interactions.
   c. Compton scattering.
   d. a and c.

2. Hydroxyl radicals damage biological targets by
  a. causing chemical reactions, resulting in changes in the structure and/or function of important biomolecules.
  b. knocking protons out of atoms.
  c. causing excessive heating.
  d. being absorbed by nuclei, resulting in the emission of high-energy photons.

3. In the photoelectric effect, the photon is
  a. scattered and the atom is excited.
  b. absorbed and the atom is excited.
  c. absorbed and the atom is ionized.
  d. scattered and the atom is ionized.

4. Pair production requires incident photons with energies greater than 1 MeV because
  a. the rest mass of the proton is greater than 1 MeV.
  b. the rest masses of the positron and electron are each approximately 0.5 MeV.
  c. the binding energy of the nucleons must be overcome.
  d. None of the above.

5. The dominant process by which sparsely ionizing radiations damage tissue is
  a. indirect action.
  b. direct action.
  c. direct ionization.
  d. recoil protons.

6. Which of the following sequences is correctly ordered in terms of increasing LET if the incident particles have the same energy?
  a. Alpha particles, electrons, protons
  b. Protons, electrons, alpha particles
  c. Electrons, alpha particles, protons
  d. Electrons, protons, alpha particles

7. Mechanisms by which ionizing radiation damages human cells include direct damage to DNA in the nucleus and
  a. heating.
  b. cytoplasm leakage.
  c. production of free radicals.
  d. electrical current imbalance.

8. Which of these best describes beta radiation?
  a. Sparsely ionizing, straight path, large HVL
  b. Sparsely ionizing, jagged path, moderate range
  c. Densely ionizing, straight path, very short range
  d. Densely ionizing, jagged path, long range

9. Which photon processes are dominant in the context of diagnostic radiology?
    a. Compton scattering and photoelectric effect
    b. Photoelectric effect and pair production
    c. Compton scattering and pair production
    d. Compton scattering and photodisintegration

10. A free radical is
    a. any charged particle.
    b. an atom or molecule with an unpaired electron in the outer shell.
    c. an atom with an even number of electrons.
    d. a chemically stable atom.

11. The main interaction process of neutrons in biological matter is
    a. Compton scattering.
    b. coulomb interactions with orbital electrons.
    c. absorption resulting in the fission of heavy nuclei.
    d. scattering by hydrogen nuclei, resulting in recoil protons.

12. In tissue, alpha particles have
    a. a short range and high specific ionization.
    b. a short range and low specific ionization.
    c. a long range and high specific ionization.
    d. a long range and low specific ionization.

13. The half-value layer is the thickness of a medium that
    a. reduces the biological damage to half the value of some reference radiation.
    b. attenuates half of the incident photon beam, for a particular beam energy.
    c. reduces the energy of incident charged particles by a factor of 2.
    d. attenuates half the incident photon beam, independent of energy.

14. A new type of ionizing radiation has been discovered called Q-rays. In a test of 1-MeV Q-rays, a dose of 800 mGy will produce the same degree of cell killing as a 200-mGy dose of 250-kVp X-rays. The relative biological effectiveness of 1-MeV Q-rays
    a. cannot be determined, because it depends on several additional factors that are not given.
    b. is 0.25.
    c. is 4.
    d. is 16.

15. Overkill occurs when
    a. the RBE is so high that all the cells die.
    b. the range of the ionizing radiation is so great that even cells at very large depths are killed.
    c. the ionizing radiation dose is too large.
    d. the LET is so high that more energy is deposited into each cell on the particle track than is required for killing a single cell.

16. The RBE _____ with increasing LET.
    a. increases to a maximum, and then decreases
    b. increases
    c. decreases
    d. does not vary

CHAPTER 5

CELL SURVIVAL CURVES

KEYWORDS

Cell survival curve, shoulder region, cell repair, radiosensitizers, radioprotectors, linear–quadratic model, single-target model, multitarget model, sublethal damage, linear energy transfer, oxygen enhancement ratio, surviving fraction

TOPICS

- Cell survival curves and how they are obtained
- The significance of the two portions of the survival curve
- Effects of different radiation conditions, type, and oxygen on the shape of the survival curve
- The relationship between cell repair and the shoulder region of a survival curve
- Common mathematical models used in analyzing cell survival curves and the key parameters associated with each model
- Clinically important radiosensitizers and radioprotectors

INTRODUCTION

A cell survival curve is a plot of the number of cells that survive to form colonies as a function of radiation dose. Thus, cell survival curves measure *reproductive* cell

Radiation Biology of Medical Imaging, First Edition. Charles A. Kelsey, Philip H. Heintz,
Daniel J. Sandoval, Gregory D. Chambers, Natalie L. Adolphi, and Kimberly S. Paffett.
© 2014 John Wiley & Sons, Inc. Published 2014 by John Wiley & Sons, Inc.

death. Some damaged cells may continue to function for a time, but if they do not reproduce, they are not counted as survivors.

In a cell survival experiment, cells are seeded onto petri dishes and exposed to various doses of radiation. The number of cell colonies that subsequently grow is determined. Each colony is assumed to be derived from a single surviving cell. A cell survival curve is a plot of the fraction of cells that survive (normalized by the fraction of cells that survive with no radiation exposure) versus the radiation dose; each point on a cell survival curve corresponds to a single dose of radiation. Usually, the log of the surviving fraction is plotted on the vertical axis versus dose on the horizontal axis. Mammalian cell survival curves generally show an exponential response to high doses of radiation with a "shoulder" of varying widths in the low-dose range. The effect of radiation on cells can be observed by noting how the cell survival curve changes under different conditions. These changes in condition include using different types of radiation, changing the environment, adding or subtracting oxygen, or delivering the radiation at different times or during different parts of the cell cycle. The study of survival curves revealed many aspects of radiation damage long before the structure of DNA was elucidated.

THE *IN VITRO* SURVIVAL CURVE

"*In vitro*" means outside a living organism—for example, in a test tube or petri dish. Cell survival can be defined in terms of the reproductive ability of the cells; that is, cells that cannot reproduce are effectively dead. This definition makes sense in the context of common laboratory experiments used to study the effects of radiation on cells prior to the 1980s, when DNA probes began to be available. Cells that continue to reproduce (in petri dishes in the lab) form colonies that are visible to the naked eye, and it is easy to count the surviving colonies after irradiation. This experimental design made it possible to establish many basic facts regarding radiation effects on cells in the early days of radiobiology. By varying the conditions during and after exposure, the factors influencing cell response to radiation can be isolated and studied. The shape of the survival curve contains information regarding the overall sensitivity of the cells, as well as the ability of the cells to repair and recover from radiation damage. Theoretical models have been developed to explain the shapes of the resulting survival curves in terms of cell survival characteristics.

Although reproductive capacity is a good way of defining "cell survival" in the context of *in vitro* radiobiology experiments, it is not applicable to all cell types. Some cells such as nerve, muscle, and secretory gland cells are nonproliferating. For these cell types, what matters to an organism exposed to radiation is whether the nonproliferating cells maintain function. For proliferating cells (e.g., intestinal lining, stem cells, cells in a cancerous tumor), the reproductive capacity is important, in both the organism and in the laboratory. Reproductive capacity is also referred to as "clonogenic potential."

The loss of clonogenic potential is a very narrow definition of cell death. A cell that is exposed to radiation may be apparently intact, it may synthesize protein/DNA, and it may even carry out several cycles of mitosis; but if it cannot carry out *sustained replication*, then it has not survived, according to the definition here.

CELL SURVIVAL CURVES: DESCRIPTION OF EXPERIMENTAL METHOD

Cell cultures are generated by extracting live cells from various species of mammals such as mice, rats, or humans. The cell population is first grown in a tissue culture flask. The cells are then released from the flask by adding trypsin, the cells are counted, and then a known number of cells is plated onto growth medium in a petri dish and maintained under appropriate conditions (correct temperature, atmosphere, nutrient levels) to survive and grow.

In order to study radiation effects on the cells, many petri dishes are plated under the same conditions using genetically identical cells. Some dishes are not irradiated and are maintained as controls, and the rest of the dishes are exposed to various doses of radiation. The irradiated cells and control cells are then incubated for some time (e.g., a few days up to a couple of weeks) to allow colonies to arise from the surviving cells. A colony is assumed to form by the sustained proliferation of a single cell. Figure 5.1 illustrates a typical cell survival experiment. Here, populations of identical cells are irradiated with increasing doses of radiation.

Figure 5.1 shows a plot of the surviving fraction of cells as measured by the number of colonies formed by the surviving cells relative to the control. If a cell forms a colony, as shown in the photographs in Fig. 5.2, it is assumed to have survived irradiation and to have maintained its reproductive ability. This type of procedure is called a clonogenic assay or a survival assay.

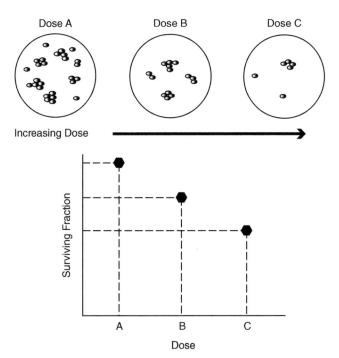

Figure 5.1   Survival curves are generated by irradiating populations of genetically homogeneous cells with increasing doses of radiation. A plot of the surviving fraction as a function of dose is known as the cell survival curve.

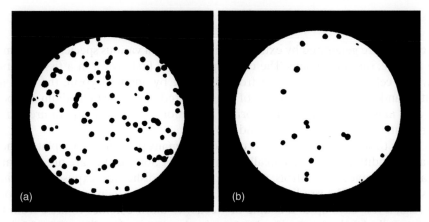

Figure 5.2 Comparison of petri dishes containing (a) unirradiated and (b) irradiated cells. The difference in the number of surviving colonies is apparent to the naked eye. *Source*: Nias (1998), figure 6.6.

CELL SURVIVAL CURVES: QUANTIFICATION

In order to quantitatively interpret the results of cell survival assays, it is important to define two quantities: the plating efficiency and the surviving fraction.

Plating Efficiency

The plating efficiency is simply the percentage of seeded cells that survive to form colonies under control conditions (i.e., no radiation or other modifying factors):

$$PE = 100 \times (\text{\# of colonies counted/ \# of cells seeded}). \qquad (5.1)$$

Knowing the plating efficiency allows one to normalize out effects that lead to cell death but are not attributable to radiation. For example, assume the plating efficiency is found to be 50%. Then, in a later experiment using the same cells and the same incubation conditions, half of the cells irradiated with a 1 Gy dose of X-rays survive. In this particular case, the 1 Gy dose had *no* measureable effect (i.e., the cells died at the same rate, with or without X-ray irradiation).

Surviving Fraction

Once the plating efficiency is determined, then a meaningful determination of the surviving fraction can be made, that is, the fraction of cells that survive or die due to the radiation that one is testing:

$$SF = \text{\# of colonies counted}/(\text{\# of cells seeded} \times [PE/100]). \qquad (5.2)$$

Another way to compute the surviving fraction (equivalent to the above) is

$$SF = (\text{\# of colonies counted/ \# of cells seeded})_{\text{test}} /$$
$$(\text{\# of colonies counted/ \# of cells seeded})_{\text{control}} \qquad (5.3)$$

where "test" denotes the test condition (some radiation dose) and "control" denotes identical cells not treated with radiation.

Whichever equation is used, the important thing is to ensure that the surviving fraction is computed *relative to the survival of a control population*, in order to account for uninteresting factors that might influence cell survival (temperature, adequacy of the growth medium). This ensures that the effect of the radiation dose can be separated from the other factors.

SURVIVING FRACTION VERSUS DOSE: THE CELL SURVIVAL CURVE

A plot of the surviving fraction of cells as a function of the radiation dose is called *the cell survival curve*. The survival curve is usually plotted on a log-linear graph (also referred to as a semilog plot) for reasons explained in detail later. The surviving fraction is plotted on the logarithmic axis (vertical) against dose, which is plotted on the linear axis (horizontal). Representative survival curves for high- linear energy transfer (LET) particles and low-LET radiation (X-rays) are shown in Fig. 5.3.

The shape of the high-LET curve is typical for mammalian cells irradiated by neutrons or alpha particles. The shape of the low-LET curve is typical for mammalian cells irradiated by X-rays, gamma rays, or beta particles. The low-LET curve is therefore the response that is expected when irradiating cells in conventional

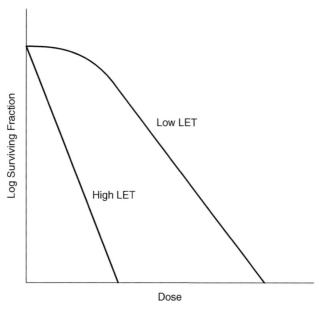

Figure 5.3 Representative cell survival curves for high-LET particles and low-LET X-rays. High-LET radiations produce curves that are steeper with little or no shoulder.

radiotherapy and diagnostic imaging. Survival curves for mammalian cells usually have a shoulder (curved section) in the lower-dose region, as shown in the low-LET curve. Models have been developed to account for survival curves with different shapes obtained under different conditions.

MODELING THE SHAPE OF THE SURVIVAL CURVE

There are three models used to mathematically describe cell survival curves: the single-target/single-hit model, the multitarget model (also known as the two-component model), and the linear–quadratic (LQ) model. Each model has its own advantages and disadvantages. The models are based on the idea of a "target" within the cell. The target is often viewed as a sensitive region on the DNA molecule that when hit by radiation may cause cell death.

The single-target/single-hit model has little practical application, but is useful in explaining the multitarget and LQ models. In the single-target/single-hit model, it is assumed that a cell has a single target that when hit causes the cell to die. In this case, the cell has no opportunity to repair the radiation damage. The single-target/single-hit model is inadequate to explain most cell survival data from mammalian cells, because it does not account for the shoulder portion of the curve at low doses.

The multitarget (two-component) and LQ models are both considered multiple-target models. Both models assume that each cell contains two or more targets that must be hit before the cell is killed. In order to be killed, the cell must accumulate enough hits in a short amount of time, such that the enzyme repair mechanisms are not capable of repairing all of the damage in between hits. However, after the first target is hit, the cell may have enough time to repair the damage before the next target is hit. In this case, the first hit is an example of sublethal damage. Sublethal damage occurs at a dose that is not sufficient to cause very much cell death. Thus, there are two dose regimes (low dose causing mostly sublethal damage, and high dose, causing lethal damage) that explain the shoulder (i.e., the change in slope) of the survival curve. Importantly, the multiple-target models provide a way to account for the presence of the shoulder region observed in mammalian cell survival curves. The multiple-target models fit the experimental data well, but still have limitations. Regardless of the underlying mechanisms, the major interest in survival curves data is in predicting radiation effects on humans.

SINGLE-TARGET/SINGLE-HIT MODEL

The simplest mathematical model to explain the radiation killing of cells is the single-target/single-hit model. In this model, a single hit on a single cellular target results in cell death. The curve from this model is shown in Fig. 5.4. The survival curve is exponential and can be fit by Equation 5.4:

$$SF = e^{-D/D_0}. \tag{5.4}$$

In this model, D is the dose delivered and D_0 is a constant, defined as the dose that gives on average one hit per target. If there is one hit per cell *on average*, then

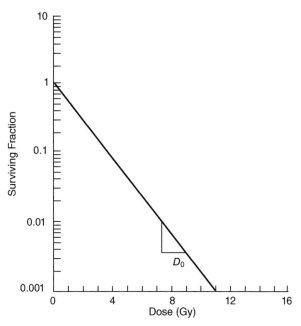

Figure 5.4 Schematic representation of the single-target/single-hit survival curve. The survival curve is linear on a log-linear plot, with a slope of $1/D_0$.

statistically, some cells receive more than one hit, some receive exactly one hit, and some receive zero hits. In this case, Poisson statistics are used to describe the statistics of small numbers of random events—for example, $0, 1, 2$. A dose $D = D_0$ reduces the surviving number of cells to 37% of the initial population. Therefore, D_0 is sometimes called D_{37}. Note that D/D_0 is the average number of hits per cell.

Taking the natural log (ln or $\log_e$) of both sides of the equation, one obtains

$$\ln SF = -D/D_0. \tag{5.5}$$

By plotting the quantity (ln SF) versus D, one obtains a straight line with slope $-1/D_0$. Equivalently, one can plot the SF versus D on a log-linear scale, as shown in Fig. 5.4, and one will also obtain a straight line. The single-target/single-hit model can be used to describe data resulting from experiments involving viruses and bacteria, but is generally a poor model for describing mammalian cell survival.

MULTITARGET MODEL (ALSO "TWO-COMPONENT MODEL" OR "D_q, D_0, AND N MODEL")

Figure 5.5 shows typical survival curves for densely (high-LET) and sparsely ionizing (low-LET) radiations, along with definitions of the key parameters of the multitarget model, namely the parameters n, D_q, and D_0.

The simplest equation for the multitarget model is

$$SF = 1 - (1 - e^{-D/D_0})^n. \tag{5.6}$$

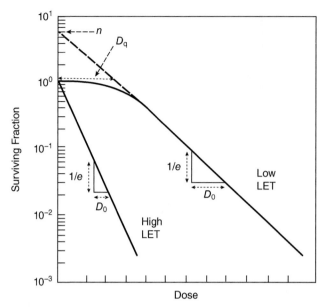

Figure 5.5 Typical cell survival curves for high-LET (densely ionizing) and low-LET (sparsely ionizing) radiations. The parameter D_0 characterizes the final slope of the curve. The parameter n or D_q characterizes the shoulder region of the low-LET curve.

The parameter n was originally understood to be the number of targets in the cell. Notice that if $n = 1$, then Equation 5.6 reduces to Equation 5.4. In other words, the multitarget model reduces to the single-target/single-hit model for $n = 1$, as expected. This is illustrated in Fig. 5.6, which shows the results of Equation 5.6 evaluated for $D_0 = 2$ Gy and $n = 1$ or 4. Notice that both curves have the same limiting slope at high dose, which turns out to be $1/D_0$, the same as in the single-target/single-hit model.

Thus, the multitarget model can be used to fit cell survival curves from either high-LET (no shoulder) or low-LET (shoulder) radiations by using different values of n (see Fig. 5.6). However, assuming that n is the number of critical targets leads to a logical inconsistency, because different values of n can be obtained for different types of radiation using the *same* cell type. If the cells are the same, but n changes with radiation type, n must depend on more than just the number of targets in the cell.

The multitarget model may be further modified (to improve the shape of the curve in the low-dose region) by multiplying the multitarget term by a single-target term:

$$SF = e^{-D/D_1}(1-[1-e^{-D/D_0}]^n).\qquad(5.7)$$

Equation 5.7 is the version of the multitarget model sometimes called the two-component model, because it has both a single-target and a multiple-target component. Multiplication by the single-target factor gives the curve a finite slope (of $1/D_1$) at $D = 0$. Equation 5.6 results in a curve with zero slope at $D = 0$.

The multitarget models do a reasonably good job of fitting real mammalian cell survival curve data, particularly in the high-dose region. Furthermore, the

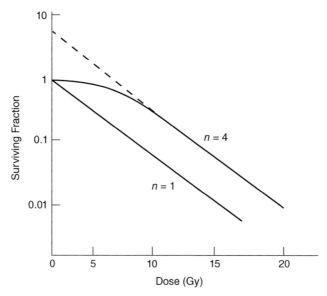

Figure 5.6 Multitarget model (Eq. 5.6) evaluated for $D_0 = 2$ Gy and $n = 1$ or 4 shows the effect of different n values on the resulting survival curves.

multitarget models give us a small number of parameters (D_0, D_q, n), which are easy to determine graphically, as described later. By determining the parameters graphically, one avoids tedious calculations to obtain nonlinear least squares fits of Equation 5.6 or Equation 5.7. This was undoubtedly an advantage of these models before personal computers became ubiquitous.

For the densely ionizing radiation curve (labeled high LET in Fig. 5.5), there is no shoulder (i.e., the slope is constant), so n and D_q turn out to be uninteresting in this case. The high-LET curve is completely characterized by the *slope* of the semilog plot, which is proportional to $1/D_0$. As is seen from the graph, D_0 is the increase in dose required to decrease survival by a factor of e. (Recall that $e = 2.7183$.) If the dose is increased additively by D_0, then the surviving fraction will be decreased by a factor of 2.72 (i.e., the surviving fraction will be about $1/e$, or 37%, of what it was at the lower dose). As an example, assume $D_0 = 5$ Gy for a particular cell type. If one gives the cells a 5 Gy dose, the surviving fraction will therefore be about 0.37 $(=2.7183^{-1})$. If the dose is increased to 10 Gy, then the surviving fraction will be $(0.37)^2 = 0.14$. Every additional 5 Gy of dose results in a multiplicative factor of 0.37 in the surviving fraction.

Note that the slope $(1/D_0)$ can also be defined for the linear portion of the low-LET curve in Fig. 5.5, in exactly the same way. In general, if D_0 is small, the slope is large, and the cells are said to be radiosensitive—that is, a small additional dose of radiation results in significantly more cell killing. If D_0 is a relatively large number, the slope is relatively low, and the cells are said to be radioresistant; that is, a large additional dose is required to produce a significant increase in cell killing.

Large $D_0 \Rightarrow$ small slope $\Rightarrow$ radioresistant

Small $D_0 \Rightarrow$ large slope $\Rightarrow$ radiosensitive

The exponential relationship at high dose has been found for all mammalian tissues in which it has been possible to test the cells. The reason for the difference in shape between the high-LET and low-LET curves at low doses is discussed in more detail later.

For the sparsely ionizing radiation curve (on a semilog plot), there is a bending "shoulder" region at low dose, before the curve reaches the limiting slope of $1/D_0$ at high dose. In this case either the parameter n or D_q is used to characterize the shoulder. D_q characterizes the width of the shoulder and has units of dose. For $D > D_q$, the dependence of survival on dose is exponential (straight-line on semilog plot, with slope $1/D_0$). Graphically, D_q and n are obtained by extrapolating the exponential (straight) portion of the curve back to $D = 0$. The extrapolation number n is the dimensionless number, greater than 1, where the extrapolated line intercepts the vertical axis. D_q is the dose at which the extrapolated line intersects the horizontal line corresponding to $SF = 1$. In the low-LET curve (Fig. 5.5), $n = 6$ and $D_q = 2.5$ Gy. For the high-LET curve (Fig. 5.5), which shows no shoulder, the intersection is at one so $n = 1$ and $D_q = 0$, which is the minimum possible value.

Using the multitarget model, the shapes of cell survival curves can be compared using the parameter D_0 to describe the exponential slope, and either n or D_q to describe the size of the shoulder. All of these parameters are easy to determine using a graph of the data and a straight edge. Most mammalian cells have D_0 values between 1 and 2 Gy, extrapolation numbers between 1 and 5, and D_q values between 0.5 and 2.5 Gy. Figure 5.5 represents typical values for human cancer cells *in vitro*. For example, D_0 is about 1 Gy (100 rad) for the high-LET curve and 1.5 Gy (150 rad) for the low-LET curve.

The Significance of the Multitarget Parameters

In the past, D_q was understood to be the quasi-threshold value, the dose at which significant radiation effects appear, which is true observationally, but does not really address the underlying mechanisms. Originally, n was viewed as the number of targets in the cell. This interpretation came about, in part, because in early experiments, the observed values of n tended to fall around 2, which correlates with the idea that two hits are required to break both strands of the DNA molecule. However, later experiments yielded n values as high as 12. Currently, n is simply viewed as a measure of the shoulder width. Higher values of D_q and higher values of n correspond to a wider shoulder. Cellular repair of radiation damage is discussed in greater detail in Chapter 7.

The values for D_0 in Table 5.1 fall in a fairly narrow range, mostly between 1 and 2 Gy. The D_0 values only provide information regarding radiosensitivity over the dose range beyond the shoulder region, and there is simply not much variation. There are much larger variations in values for D_q and n, which reflect the size of the shoulder portion of the curves. The variation in the size of the shoulder region reflects the *clinically useful* difference in the radiosensitivity of different cell lines. Smaller shoulders indicate more radiation-sensitive cells. Fractionated radiation therapy exploits these differences. Medical imaging doses are nearly always in the shoulder region of the survival curve.

TABLE 5.1 List of Survival Curve Parameters Using the Multitarget Model

Cell Population	Assay	D_0 (Gy)	D_q (Gy)	n
HeLa	*In vitro*	1	0.65	2
Chinese hamster (ovary)	*In vitro*	2	2.1	3
Chinese hamster (lung)	*In vitro*	1.7	4	10
Chinese hamster	*In vitro* spheroid	1.7	9	200
Mouse leukemia	*In vivo*	1	1.15	3
Rat rhabdomyosarcoma	*In vitro*	1.2	3	10
Mouse sarcoma	*In vivo*	1.34	2.9	9.5

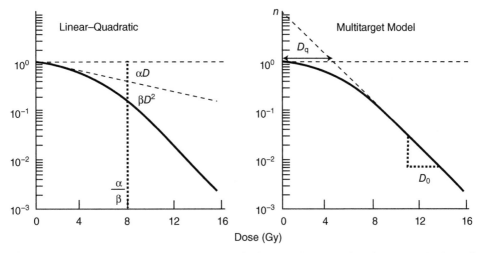

Figure 5.7 Schematic representation of survival curve data showing linear–quadratic and multitarget models applied to the same data. Notice the difference in the parameters used in the models.

LQ OR α/β MODEL

The LQ or α/β model provides a better fit of the initial shoulder region of the survival curve. Figure 5.7 shows a comparison of the multitarget and LQ model parameters. Assume that the data being modeled in Fig. 5.7 is the same in both cases; just the mathematical model differs. The LQ model uses two parameters, α and β, to describe the curved portion of the survival curve. The survival curve is viewed as being composed of a linear and a quadratic portion. The linear component is considered the "single-hit" portion and is described by coefficient α. The quadratic component is the "multiple-hit" portion of the curve, which is described by coefficient β. Note that α and β are coefficients; they do not refer to alpha particles or beta particles.

The linear component of the curve is represented by α, which has units of inverse dose. The argument of the exponential is dimensionless. The linear component accounts for cell killing due to single hits. Single-hit survival is given by

$$SF_1 = \exp(-\alpha D). \tag{5.8}$$

The term β characterizes the curving component and has units of inverse dose squared. The quadratic component of the curve is used to account for two-hit cell killing (or "dual action"). Note that the probability of two-hit killing is proportional to D^2. The two-hit survival component is given by

$$SF_2 = \exp(-\beta D^2). \tag{5.9}$$

Assuming that the single-hit and two-hit mechanisms are independent, the overall expression for the curve is

$$SF = SF_1 \cdot SF_2 = \exp{-(\alpha D + \beta D^2)}. \tag{5.10}$$

This equation results in a survival curve that fits the low-dose data very well, but it continuously curves downward in the high-dose regime on a semilog plot. However, the high-dose portion of the survival curve is well described by a *straight* line on a semilog plot. Thus, the LQ curve does not fit high-dose survival data very well, but this region is not in the dose range of medical applications.

The ratio α/β has units of dose. α/β is equal to the dose D at which the linear and quadratic contributions to the survival curve are equal (8 Gy in Fig. 5.7):

$$\text{when } \alpha D = \beta D^2$$

$$\text{then } D = \alpha/\beta.$$

The α/β ratio is another way of characterizing the shoulder width. In particular, a higher α/β ratio indicates a narrower shoulder. A lower α/β ratio indicates a wider shoulder, as shown in Fig. 5.8.

Although the LQ (α/β) model does not predict the complete survival curve, it is valuable because it is applicable in the dose ranges used for clinical radiotherapy. An advantage of this model is that it has two adjustable coefficients that can be used to model low-dose survival curves under different external conditions.

APPLICATION OF THE MULTITARGET AND LQ MODELS IN RADIOBIOLOGY

For more than 50 years, the multitarget model was the more commonly used model to describe mammalian cell survival curves. This model works well in the high-dose region in describing the basic response of cells to ionizing radiation. It can be used to characterize the sensitivity of cells to different types of radiation. It can also be used to characterize the effects of the environment on cell sensitivity. However, it does not work as well in the low-dose shoulder region. The LQ model is better suited to describe the cellular response in the low-dose, clinically relevant region.

The LQ model is often used to describe the radiation sensitivity of mammalian cells. The value of the α/β model is that it is more accurate than the multitarget model in the low-dose region (0–3 Gy) of the cell survival curve. The LQ model is often used in radiation therapy biology to explain the differences in early- and

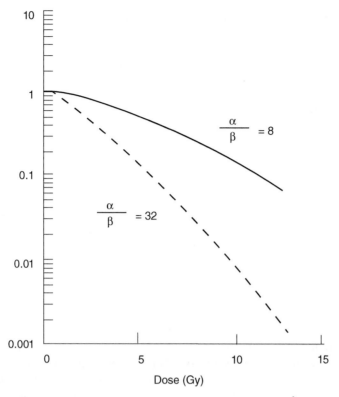

Figure 5.8 The linear–quadratic model evaluated with β = 0.0125 Gy^{-2} and α/β = 8 or 32 Gy shows the effect of two different α/β ratios on the resulting survival curve.

late-responding tissues. Low values of α/β (1–5 Gy) indicate the cells are radioresistant or late responders, and high values of α/β (6–12 Gy) indicate they are radiosensitive or early responders.

Survival curves are useful when comparing the sensitivities of two or more cell types (as in Table 5.1). However, survival data are obtained under controlled laboratory conditions much different than *in vivo* conditions. Experiments show a difference in the *in vivo* versus *in vitro* radiosensitivity of genetically identical cell lines. Therefore, the information obtained from *in vitro* survival curves should be applied with care.

Summary of models:

- High-LET, densely ionizing radiation shows little or no shoulder in cell survival curves.
- Low-LET, sparsely ionizing radiation shows a shoulder in cell survival curves.
- For both densely and sparsely ionizing radiation, $1/D_0$ defines the high-dose slope, which is a measure of the radiosensitivity in the high-dose region.
- D_q or n defines the shoulder width, which is a measure of repair and radiosensitivity in the low-dose (clinical) region.
- α/β characterizes the width of the shoulder region in the LQ model. A large α/β ratio indicates a narrow shoulder.

- The LQ model does not fit the high-dose region of the curve, but is superior in the low-dose region of the curve, applicable to clinical medicine.

FACTORS AFFECTING THE SHAPE OF SURVIVAL CURVES

The Shoulder Region: Multihit Cell Killing Mechanisms and Cell Repair

The shoulder region is perhaps the most important and interesting portion of the cell survival curve, because it is relevant to clinical medicine and can possibly be used to predict the effect of low doses on humans. This is the dose region of most exposures from medical and industrial sources of radiation including diagnostic and therapeutic radiology. The shape of the shoulder region is different for different cell lines under the same external conditions. The shoulder region can also be different for the same cell line under different external conditions (e.g., different O_2 concentrations).

When modeling cell survival curves, *two assumptions* are usually made to explain the shoulder region. These assumptions are as follows:

- Radiation interactions which are not individually fatal may be collectively fatal.
  - In some cases, the two "hits" required to kill the cell may be the result of a single radiation event (e.g., one alpha particle can damage many sites in the same cell). In other cases, the two "hits" may be the accumulated result of two separate radiation hits. If an X-ray causes only one hit, a second X-ray will be required to produce the second hit. Mathematically, the two independent events necessitate the higher-order factors, which produce the shoulder in the survival curve.
- Individual damage sites, which are reparable at lower doses, become fatal at higher doses, because the efficiency of the cellular repair mechanisms decreases with increasing dose.
  - A cell may repair a few damaged sites quickly to keep the cell on schedule to complete the cell proliferation cycle. However, there are physiological limits on the rate of DNA repair. Hence, a large radiation dose may overwhelm the repair process.

These two assumptions are not mutually exclusive. In the case of two-hit lethal damage, there may be a delay between the first and second hit. If repair to the first hit can be completed before the second hit occurs, the shoulder will be broader. If the probability of the second hit is high, and the first hit repair is typically not completed before the second hit, the shoulder will be narrow.

SURVIVAL CURVE SHAPE AND LET

The shape difference between high- and low-LET survival curves is explained by the difference in the density of radiation damage due to the two types of radiations. High-LET damaging events occur so densely along the particle track that virtually no cells experience just a single hit. Nearly all cells on the particle track immediately experience two or more hits. If each cell on the particle track receives two hits on average, the LET is ideal, and the relative biological effectiveness (RBE) is high. Because multiple hits occur nearly simultaneously (as a *single event*), the cell is unable to repair one hit before a second (lethal) hit occurs. The high-LET survival curve is therefore expected to show *little or no shoulder*, which is what is observed for high-LET radiations.

With sparsely ionizing radiation (low LET), the density of damaging events is not high enough to ensure that all cells along an ionization track experience two damaging hits. Therefore, the RBE of low LET radiation is low. In this case, damage must be accumulated via interaction with two photons or beta particles (two separate events). If the dose is low, then most cells will experience zero or one damaging hit (which turns out to be nonlethal), and virtually no cells are likely to be in the path of two different photons or betas, so there is little cell death. Since the events leading to cell death are separate, they may be well separated in time, allowing the possibility of repair of one hit to occur prior to a second hit. Once the radiation dose is increased to a particular threshold level, then the majority of cells will be "hit" at least once. At that point (the transition between the low- and high-dose regimes), increasing the dose further rapidly increases cell killing, because the "extra" dose (above the threshold dose) mostly contributes to "second hits"—the ones that actually cause the cells to die. Given the assumptions described earlier, multiple independent events and the possibility of repair imply that the survival curve will have a *shoulder*, which is what is observed for low-LET radiations, as shown in Fig. 5.9. As LET increases up to the optimum value, the shoulder feature

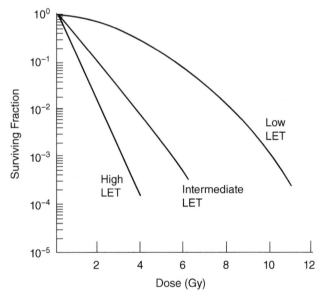

Figure 5.9 Survival curves for three different types of radiation with increasing LET (e.g., 4 MeV alpha particles, 15 MeV neutrons, and 250 kVp X-rays). As the LET approaches the optimal value, the survival curves get steeper, indicating that the killing is greater for a smaller radiation dose.

becomes less prominent, and the survival curve is steeper. For optimal LET radiation (alpha particles, in this case), the survival curve has no detectable shoulder, because cell killing occurs after a single event (one alpha provides multiple hits and no possibility of repair).

Dependence of survival curve shape on RBE/LET:

- Densely ionizing particles have higher RBE/LET (before RBE falloff from overkill).
  - Provides adequate density of ionizations along particle track within a particular cell to hit all required targets for cell death; thus, no threshold dose needed to produce observable effects.
- Sparsely ionizing particles have lower RBE/LET.
  - Inadequate ionization density along particle track to hit all required targets in a particular cell; thus, no effects seen until all required targets hit from more dose.

CHEMICALS

Survival curves are used to study how particular chemicals alter the effect of radiation on cells. Here, we are specifically considering chemicals that are present in the cellular environment at the same time the radiation dose is administered. If the presence of the chemical increases cell survival (compared with the "no chemical" case), then the chemical is said to be a radioprotector. If the presence of the chemical decreases cell survival, then the chemical is referred to as a "radiosensitizer." Although many chemicals have been tested to evaluate their potential as radioprotectors or radiosensitizers, only a few have shown to be consistently important in radiobiology. Furthermore, the fact that some chemicals influence whether cells survive after a radiation dose provides additional evidence that cell repair occurs after exposure to low-LET radiations.

Oxygen: An Important Radiosensitizer

The cell survival curves in Fig. 5.10 display the dramatic effect that oxygen has on the susceptibility of cells to radiation damage. Note that the purpose of the nitrogen in the experiments shown in Fig. 5.10 was to displace oxygen and provide an oxygen-free (anoxic) environment.

The effect of oxygen on the radiation sensitivity of cells is described by the oxygen enhancement ratio (OER). The OER is the ratio of the radiation dose without oxygen to the radiation dose with oxygen that produces the same biological effect. The OER is always greater than or equal to 1:

$$OER = \frac{\text{Dose without oxygen}}{\text{Dose with oxygen}}. \tag{5.11}$$

For example, in an experiment, we find that 100 cGy will kill 50% of cells in air, while in an oxygen-free (anoxic) environment, it takes 300 cGy to kill the same fraction of cells. In this case, the OER for the population would be 3.

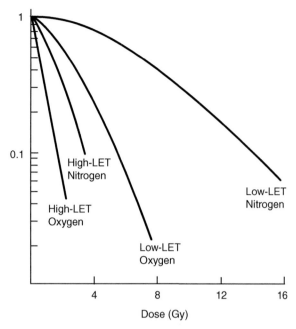

Figure 5.10 Survival curves for HeLa cells irradiated in air and nitrogen with high-LET radiation (e.g., 14 MeV neutrons) and low-LET radiation (e.g., 250 keV X-rays). The presence of oxygen during radiation damage significantly increases cell killing.

The presence of oxygen in the cell medium dramatically influences the effect of radiation, particularly for low-LET radiations. For mammalian cells, the OER is usually between 2 and 3 for low-LET radiations. The OER decreases as LET increases as shown in Fig. 5.11. The OER is approximately one for alpha particles. An explanation for this difference is that high-LET radiations produce a high amount of damage along the particle track. The addition of oxygen does not result in additional cell killing because all the cells along the high-LET path have already been killed. Neutrons typically have an intermediate OER of approximately 1.5.

The mechanism by which oxygen sensitizes cells to radiation is referred to as oxygen "fixing." It appears that oxygen, if present during radiation exposure, makes permanent (i.e., "fixes") otherwise reparable damage from indirect action. In particular, oxygen stabilizes damaging free radicals. Recall that high-LET radiations do not involve free radicals as an intermediate step in producing damage.

For example, as shown in reaction 5.12, the reaction of oxygen with a hydrogen radical can produce the relatively stable superoxide radical, $HO_2\cdot$. Two superoxide radicals may then react to form hydrogen peroxide and an oxygen molecule. Note that the oxygen molecule product in reaction 5.13 is then available as a reactant for another reaction. The products of reaction 5.12 and reaction 5.13, $HO_2\cdot$ and hydrogen peroxide, are both very toxic to biological systems:

$$O_2 + H\cdot \rightarrow HO_2\cdot \tag{5.12}$$

$$2HO_2\cdot \rightarrow H_2O_2 + O_2 \tag{5.13}$$

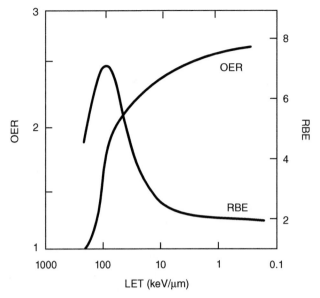

Figure 5.11 A comparison of the dependence of OER and RBE on LET. Oxygen enhancement is most significant for low-LET radiations with low RBE.

In addition to reacting with the products of radiolysis of water, oxygen may also react with organic free radicals:

$$R\cdot + O_2 \rightarrow RO_2\cdot \tag{5.14}$$

The organic radical, $RO_2\cdot$, is more difficult to repair than simply $R\cdot$. Thus, the oxygen essentially "fixes" or makes permanent the damage. This is especially important if $RO_2\cdot$ is a DNA molecule.

The oxygen effect involves a competition between two processes. Damage from radiation-induced free radicals is either made permanent by dissolved oxygen or repaired by hydrogen donors (as discussed later) in the tissue. The competition between these processes will determine the amount of permanent radiation damage. Clinically, the oxygen effect is important in the radiotherapy of tumors. Rapidly growing tumors often outgrow their own blood supply, resulting in areas of the tumor that are poorly oxygenated and therefore more resistant to radiotherapy.

Radioprotectors

Oxygen is a potent *radiosensitizer*, is nontoxic, and has been demonstrated to be very relevant in both the *in vitro* and *in vivo* settings. However, such a potent, non-toxic, and ubiquitous *radioprotector* has not been discovered; although there are naturally occurring and synthetic chemicals that have been shown to have some radioprotective effects. In particular, compounds that readily donate hydrogen, such as the sulfhydryl compounds cysteine and cysteamine, compete with oxygen and can neutralize free radicals, thereby enhancing repair. (Compare reaction 5.15 with reaction 5.14, and note that reaction with the SH group eliminates the free radical.):

$$R\cdot + -SH \rightarrow RH + -S \tag{5.15}$$

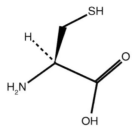

Figure 5.12 The chemical structure of cysteine, a naturally occurring radioprotector. Radioprotectors interfere with indirect action by reacting with free radicals to neutralize their damaging effects. In particular, the hydrogen of the SH group is readily donated in a chemical reaction, enabling the free radical to be neutralized.

As in the case of radiosensitizers, radioprotectors mainly modify indirect action, and they are generally less effective against high-LET radiations.

Sulfhydryl compounds naturally occur at low levels in cells and undoubtedly play a role in normal cellular repair processes. Unfortunately, if the concentration is artificially increased, in order to increase radioprotection, the sulfhydryl compounds are themselves toxic. For example, cysteine (shown in Fig. 5.12) causes nausea and vomiting in humans when administered at levels that would be effective for radioprotection.

The systemic toxicity of sulfhydryl compounds can be reduced if the SH group is "covered" by a phosphate (PO_3) group: for example, PO_3–SH–CH_2–CH–. . . . The so-called thiophosphates are much less systemically toxic, and they act as a "pro-drug," meaning that they are not radioprotective until they are transformed by intracellular enzymes that strip the phosphate group, allowing the SH group to react with free radicals in the cell.

The most successful synthetic radioprotector is amifostine (or WR-2721), which is believed to have been carried by the Apollo astronauts to protect them in case of a large radiation dose due to a "solar event." Amifostine is Food and Drug Administration (FDA) approved for clinical use, where it has been successful in reducing side effects from radiation therapy in head and neck cancer patients. Amifostine is a phosphorothioate compound, and like the thiophosphates, it is a pro-drug that is activated by dephosphorylation *in vivo*. Once activated, amifostine scavenges free radicals generated by ionizing radiation and/or chemotherapy drugs. In the end, amifostine has had only limited clinical success, because it can also confer some protective effect on tumors, and therefore has limited overall therapeutic benefit.

Just as we defined the OER, we can similarly define the dose reduction factor (DRF) for radioprotective compounds. The DRF is the factor by which the radiation dose must be increased, in the presence of the radioprotector, in order to achieve the same biological effect:

$$DRF = (\text{dose of radiation with drug})/(\text{dose of radiation without drug}). \quad (5.16)$$

The best radioprotectors (amifostine and another synthetic compound, WR-638) attain DRF values of 1.6–2.7 for bone marrow or gut in mice exposed to X-rays.

SUMMARY

- In a cell survival experiment, cells are seeded onto petri dishes and exposed to different doses of radiation. The number of cell colonies that subsequently grow is determined. Each colony is assumed to be derived from a single surviving cell.
- A cell survival curve is a plot of the fraction of cells that survive (normalized by the fraction of cells that survive with no radiation exposure) versus the radiation dose; each point on a cell survival curve corresponds to a single dose of radiation. Typically, a semilogarithmic plot is used; that is, the log of the surviving fraction is plotted on the vertical axis versus dose on the horizontal axis.
- Mammalian cell survival curves generally show an exponential response to high doses of radiation with a "shoulder" of varying widths in the low-dose range. An exponential response is a straight line on a semilog plot.
- Densely ionizing radiation produces a "no-threshold" curve (a straight line) while sparsely ionizing radiation results in a curve with a shoulder region (a curve that bends down with increasing dose).
- Cellular repair provides an explanation for the shoulder region of a survival curve.
- Several mathematical models are used to explain the shape of the survival data. These include the single-target model and multiple-target models. The two multiple-target models in common usage are the multitarget (two-component) model and the LQ model.
- In the multitarget model, the exponential slope is described by the parameter D_0, and the shoulder can be described by the extrapolation number, n, or the quasi-threshold dose, D_q.
- The LQ model uses the coefficients α and β to describe the survival curve.
- The multitarget model provides the best fit to data in the high-dose range. The LQ model generally provides the best fit to data in the low-dose range.
- The presence of a radiosensitizer increases the extent of cell death for a given radiation dose. In particular, oxygen "fixes" radiation damage and is a nontoxic and clinically important radiosensitizer.
- The presence of a radioprotector reduces the extent of cell death for a given radiation dose. In particular, hydrogen donor molecules can scavenge free radicals, reducing radiation damage, but they tend to be toxic to normal tissues at useful doses. Thus, there are few clinically useful radioprotectors.

BIBLIOGRAPHY

Broerse JJ, Barendsen GW, van Kersen GR. Survival of cultured human cells after irradiation with fast neutrons of different energies in hypoxic and oxygenated conditions. Int J Radiat Biol Relat Stud Phys Chem Med. 1968;13(6):559–72.

Fajardo LF, Berthrong M, Anderson RE. Radiation pathology. New York: Oxford University Press; 2001.

Hall EJ, Giaccia AJ. Radiobiology for the radiologist. 6th ed. Philadelphia: Lippincott Williams & Wilkins; 2006.

Leaver DT, Washington CM. Principles and practice of radiation therapy. 2nd ed. St. Louis, MO: Mosby; 2004.

Nias AHW. Introduction to radiobiology. 2nd ed. New York: John Wiley & Sons; 1998.

Saha GB. Physics and radiobiology of nuclear medicine. 3rd ed. New York: Springer; 2006.

QUESTIONS

Chapter 5   Questions

1. When referring to cell survival curves, cell death means
   a. loss of reproductive ability.
   b. apoptosis.
   c. necrosis.
   d. loss of function.

2. In a cell survival experiment, the plating efficiency refers to
   a. the fraction of unirradiated cells that survive.
   b. the fraction of irradiated cells that survive.
   c. the number of unirradiated cells that survive.
   d. the number of irradiated cells that survive.

3. The slope of the high-dose exponential region (on a semilog plot) is characterized using which term?
   a. α
   b. β
   c. D_0
   d. D_q

4. The dose at which the linear and quadratic terms contribute equally to cell survival is given by
   a. $\alpha \times \beta$.
   b. $\alpha - \beta$.
   c. α/β.
   d. $\alpha + \beta$.

5. In a traditional *in vitro* cell survival experiment, survival is assessed by
   a. staining cells with a fluorescent dye to determine which are dead and which are alive.
   b. determining whether the cells are still reproducing by viewing the cells through a microscope and counting mitotic cells.
   c. viewing the petri dish with the naked eye and counting the number of cell colonies that have formed after an incubation time of days or weeks.
   d. viewing the petri dish with the naked eye immediately after irradiation to count the dead cells.

6. The shoulder on survival curves for mammalian cells indicates
    a. that the linear–quadratic model is more accurate.
    b. exponential decay of a radioactive source influences cell survival.
    c. the dose region where sublethal damage is being repaired.
    d. that sublethal damage is not being repaired.

7. The lack of a shoulder region on the survival curve for a virus could indicate which of the following?
    a. Viral DNA is much more resistant to radiation damage than mammalian DNA.
    b. Viruses require many "hits" to produce lethal damage.
    c. Viruses do not replicate.
    d. Viruses lack mechanisms to repair radiation damage.

8. Clonogenic cells are
    a. able to proliferate for many generations.
    b. able to undergo at least one mitosis and function properly.
    c. ova and sperm cells.
    d. specialized cells that can generate a new organism without fertilization.

9. What is the main difference between the multicomponent model and the linear–quadratic model? (Assume a semilog plot.)
    a. The linear–quadratic model is linear in the high-dose regime.
    b. The linear–quadratic model curves continuously in the high-dose regime.
    c. The linear–quadratic model cannot be used to fit the shoulder region.
    d. The multitarget model cannot be used to fit the high-dose region.

10. In the figure below, curves A and B have the same
    a. n, extrapolation number.
    b. D_q, quasi-threshold dose.
    c. $1/D_0$, slope.

11. In the figure below, for curve A, the extrapolation number is indicated by which arrow?
    a. 1
    b. 2
    c. 3

12. In the figure below, which cell population is more sensitive to radiation in the low-dose region?
    a. A
    b. B
    c. They are equally sensitive.

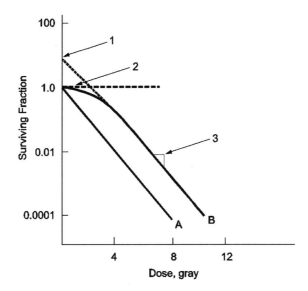

13. If two critical cell targets in the same cell are "hit" by two separate radiation tracks,

   a. the cell will repair itself.

   b. the cell will die.

   c. the cell may repair itself if the time interval between hits is long enough.

   d. the cell will not die.

14. The mechanism by which oxygen increases radiosensitivity is by

   a. making radiation damage more permanent by reacting with free radicals to produce additional chemical species that are more toxic and longer lived.

   b. donating hydrogen atoms to free radicals to increase their potency.

   c. effectively increasing the LET of low-LET radiations by increasing the absorption of energy by the tissue.

   d. neutralizing free radicals that are radioprotective.

15. Cells exposed to radiation and amifostine require 5 Gy to achieve 50% survival. The same cells exposed to radiation alone require 2.5 Gy to achieve 50% survival. Which statement is true?

   a. The dose enhancement factor = 2.

   b. The dose reduction factor = 2.

   c. The dose enhancement factor = 0.5.

   d. The dose reduction factor = 0.5.

16. Radioprotectors and radiosensitizers have little effect on survival curves when high-LET radiations are used, because

    a. radioprotectors and radiosensitizers act directly on DNA.

    b. radioprotectors and radiosensitizers act on the free radicals that mediate indirect action, which is not the primary mechanism of cell killing for high-LET radiations.

    c. radioprotectors and radiosensitizers are destroyed by high-LET radiations.

    d. high-LET radiations cause little cell killing to begin with, so the addition of a radioprotector or radiosensitizer causes little change.

CHAPTER 6

DNA AND GENETICS

KEYWORDS

DNA, DNA structure, DNA breaks, RNA, genes, codons, DNA replication, DNA repair, mutations, genetics, genome stability, epigenetics, telomeres

TOPICS

- A brief history of the discovery of DNA
- The general structure of DNA and RNA and their relationship to each other
- Relationship between genes and codons
- DNA replication and repair and some ramifications of faulty repair
- Differences between genome instability and epigenetics

INTRODUCTION

DNA is the blueprint for life. Blueprints contain all the necessary information needed for the construction of a building. The drawings include lengths of studs, square footage of each room, and location of the stairs. However, blueprints do not contain directions on how to combine which chemicals to grow a tree. There are also no instructions for manufacturing the laminate flooring located on the stairs. This is the main difference between a building blueprint and DNA. DNA contains all the required recipes for each component of the human body. The body cools

Radiation Biology of Medical Imaging, First Edition. Charles A. Kelsey, Philip H. Heintz, Daniel J. Sandoval, Gregory D. Chambers, Natalie L. Adolphi, and Kimberly S. Paffett.
© 2014 John Wiley & Sons, Inc. Published 2014 by John Wiley & Sons, Inc.

itself using sweat glands to produce perspiration. Sweat gland construction utilizes specific genes for manufacturing the proteins used for plasma membranes. These genes, located in the DNA, supply the instructions for the complete construction of the cell and directions for how the cell performs its function. As previously discussed, the cell contains all the processes required for life and is considered the smallest unit of life.

In this chapter, the structure and function of DNA will be addressed in more detail. DNA structure begins with simple molecules and ends with a series of complex bonds. As for function, DNA carries the basic information of life, but transfer of that information undergoes the lengthy processes of transcription and translation.

HISTORY

Although the study of genetics developed during the 20th century, its roots are based on studies from the late 1800s performed by Gregor Mendel. Mendel's research, observation of pea plants in the monastery garden, was performed in relative obscurity. He studied the plants by following physical traits that were carried from one generation to the next. Eventually, Mendel began to interbreed pea plants with differing characteristics to see which would be passed to the next generation. With further observation and interbreeding, Mendel began to propose that each gene, or hereditary trait, was composed of two parts, known now as alleles. Mendel's first breeding of pea plants crossed tall pea plants, growing 2 m in height, with short pea plants, growing only half a meter. The next generation of pea plants was tall, indicating two forms of alleles. The short trait was not seen. As the second generation of pea plants were interbred and grown, the result was a mixture of tall and short plants. Figure 6.1 shows Mendel's pea plant experiment. These results confirmed Mendel's theory of hereditary factors existing in two forms. In 1866, Mendel published his discoveries, but the article was not much noticed and he went on to do other things. Sixteen years after Mendel's death in 1886, his paper was revisited. The study of genetics, as a science, was born and Mendel's research technique was applied to many organisms.

Although Mendel was able to demonstrate inheritance of physical characteristics, his studies did not pursue what was at the root of these traits. In the late 1800s, a German medical student, Johannes Friedrich Miescher, was interested in studying physiological chemistry using lymphocytes. However, he was encouraged by his mentor, Felix Hoppe-Seyler, to study leukocytes instead. Lymphocytes were difficult to obtain in sufficient quantities for study and leukocytes were readily available from puss. Miescher devised a system to isolate leukocytes, from a local hospital's used bandages, without damaging the cells. A series of salt solutions washed the cells from the bandages and isolated the leukocytes. Once the cells were isolated, Miescher lysed the outer membrane and separated the nucleus for further research. When the nuclear membrane was lysed, a gelatinous material precipitated. Miescher called the precipitate nuclein, now known as DNA. As Miescher and his students studied the chemical structure of the nuclein, they were able to determine it contained large amounts of phosphorus and nitrogen but no sulfur. The results, being unlike anything seen before, caused Hoppe-Seyler to repeat all of Miescher's

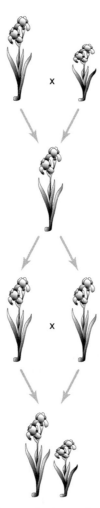

Figure 6.1   A depiction of Mendel's pea plant experiment. Tall and short plants were cross-bred and all progeny were tall. However, crossbreeding the next generation resulted in both tall and short traits. Physical characteristics, such as height, can be easily tracked with minimal effort.

experiments for confirmation. The results were published in Hoppe-Seyler's journal in 1871.

With the discoveries of inheritance and a nuclein made of phosphorus and nitrogen, the big question became "What is a gene?" In 1953, James Watson and Francis Crick tried to answer that question. Watson and Crick had studied DNA and knew nucleotides were connected together. These linkages were the product of chemical bonds between phosphate and sugar molecules located in the nucleotide itself. By linking the nucleotides together, a chain is formed and contains a particular sequence unique to that chain. The sequence differentiates each chain. Having this knowledge in hand, Watson and Crick proposed that DNA molecules consist of two chains of nucleotides, and these chains were held together by weak chemical bonds. In addition to proposing double-stranded DNA, Watson and Crick discovered that the two

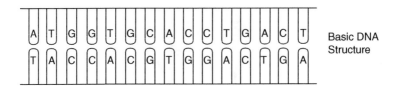

Basic DNA
Structure

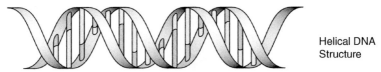

Helical DNA
Structure

Figure 6.2   Basic structure of DNA. The top picture demonstrates the association of nucleotides in a nonhelical fashion. The bottom picture shows the double-helix structure formed by DNA.

strands of DNA were wound around each other in a helical configuration. The structure of DNA, with and without helical arrangement, is shown in Fig. 6.2. Although the structure of DNA was determined, the idea of separate genes that encode traits was still being investigated.

In the early 1900s, geneticists were working at identifying what genes were made of. After Watson and Crick discovered the structure of DNA, geneticists began to work on ways to determine the sequence of bases in DNA molecules. By obtaining the sequence of bases, or sequencing the DNA, all the information necessary to analyze the organism's genes should be present. The collection of DNA molecules that is characteristic to an organism is referred to as its genome. Genome sequencing began with bacteria. Following this success, the Human Genome Project began in 1990 and was a worldwide effort to sequence the approximately 3 billion nucleotide pairs in human DNA. Upon completion of the Human Genome Project in 2003, the human gene number has been placed between 20,000 and 25,000 genes. These genes have been cataloged by location, structure, and potential function. Now, efforts have shifted to the discovery of how genes influence characteristics of the human being.

DNA STRUCTURE

DNA, or deoxyribonucleic acid, is composed of a series of repeating units called nucleotides. Nucleotides consist of carbon, oxygen, hydrogen, nitrogen, and phosphorus. From these molecules, three basic elements are formed and combined to make a single nucleotide. These elements are nucleobase, carbohydrate, and phosphorus units. The nucleobase is made from a combination of nitrogen and carbon atoms that form either five- or six-member rings. Nucleobases are involved in the pairing of DNA polymers, known as complementary base pairing. In the DNA double helix, complementary base pairs occur between nucleobases of opposing DNA strands, which are bound together through hydrogen bonds. Hydrogen bonds are weak and can be broken and rejoined with relative ease. Complementary base

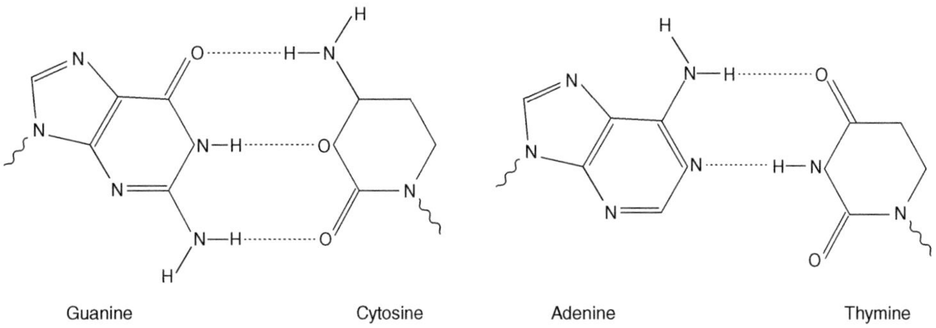

Guanine   Cytosine   Adenine   Thymine

Figure 6.3 Complementary base pairing, indicating hydrogen bonds (dotted lines) between complementary nucleobase pairs. G-C base pairs always contain three hydrogen bonds, while A-T pairs contain two hydrogen bonds. This pairing is invariable throughout all DNA.

pairing only occurs as indicated in Fig. 6.3. Adenine pairs uniquely with thymine (or uracil) and cytosine pairs with guanine. These specific interactions are critical for all functions of DNA. They help maintain the sequence of DNA throughout replication and allow reversible interactions to occur between the bases.

There are five nucleobases, and they are adenine (A), guanine (G), cytosine (C), thymine (T), and uracil (U). Three of the nucleobases are found in both DNA and RNA; however, DNA and RNA each have one unique base. Thymine is found solely in DNA and uracil in RNA. Each nucleobase is bound to a carbohydrate, or sugar, and at least one phosphate group. The carbohydrate is a pentose, or five-carbon, sugar. Deoxyribose is found in DNA while ribose is in RNA. The phosphate is simply a single phosphate atom surrounded by at least four oxygen atoms. With the addition of both a carbohydrate and phosphate, the nucleobase becomes known as a nucleotide. Nucleotides are the basic building blocks of DNA and RNA and will be the focus of further discussion. The basic structure of each nucleotide is shown in Fig. 6.4. Uracil, found only in RNA, contains a ribose sugar while adenine, guanine, cytosine, and thymine are shown with deoxyribose sugar.

Nucleotides are held together through both ester and phosphodiester bonds. These bonds are much stronger than the hydrogen bonds that form between opposing strands of DNA. Ester bonds, which are flexible, bind the carbohydrate to the nucleobase. This bond is flexible and allows DNA strands to move and bend. The phosphate group is then joined to the sugar through phosphodiester bonds. Phosphodiester bonds are strong covalent bonds between one phosphate group and two carbon rings. These bonds act as the linkage between nucleotides to give the polymer defined structure and strength. Phosphodiester bonds are used to form the backbone in both DNA and RNA.

The backbone of DNA is a series of alternating carbohydrate and phosphate groups. Each phosphate of a nucleotide binds to the 5′ carbon of its sugar. The phosphate then binds to the next nucleotide at the 3′ carbon of the sugar. This rope-like structure is called a DNA polymer and, as mentioned earlier, is held together via phosphodiester bonds. Due to the asymmetric bonding nature of the phosphate groups, DNA and RNA molecules are given a direction. The direction is determined by the terminal end of the DNA strand. If a phosphate group is terminal, the phosphate is referred to as the 5′ end. However, if a hydroxyl group from the sugar is

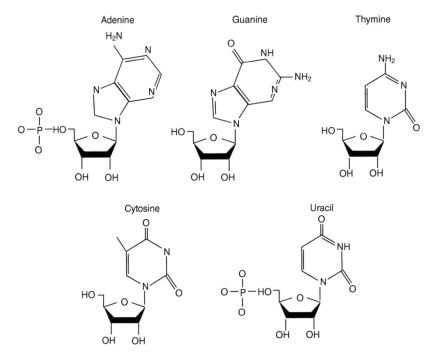

Figure 6.4 Nucleotide structure. All nucleotides shown, except uracil, contain deoxyribose as the carbohydrate. A phosphate group is attached to the carbohydrate in both DNA and RNA polymers. Uracil, found only in RNA, replaces the deoxyribose with a ribose carbohydrate. Nucleotides utilized for RNA contain ribose in place of deoxyribose.

located at the DNA terminus, it is called the 3′ end. Shown in Fig. 6.5 is a picture of a single DNA polymer with labeled 5′ and 3′ ends. The directionality of the DNA polymer is important during transcription and replication, which is discussed later in this chapter.

As complementary DNA strands come together, they form a secondary structure that is similar to a ladder. The sides of the ladder, the DNA backbone, are alternating carbohydrate and phosphate groups. The polymers align, in opposing directions, with each other, and hydrogen bonds are formed between complementary nucleotides. As appropriate hydrogen bonds form, a right-handed double helix is formed. Each base pair, either G-C or A-T, appears as a rung on a ladder.

The DNA double helix includes two strands of DNA and the hydrogen bonds that connect complementary nucleobases. The sugar–phosphate backbone of each DNA polymer is on the outside of the helix, while the bases are on the inside. Each base pair is stacked 0.34 nm from the next and is added in a nearly perpendicular fashion to the long axis of the DNA polymer. As the helix is formed, each complete turn, approximately 10.5 base pairs, fills a 3.4-nm length. The spacing between each nucleotide pair and helical turn are shown in Fig. 6.6. This configuration is the regular structure of DNA found under normal physiological conditions, such as those within the nucleus. Additional DNA structures will not be discussed.

Following organization of the nucleotides into DNA polymers and the double helix, DNA molecules still undergo further packaging. Chromosomal DNA

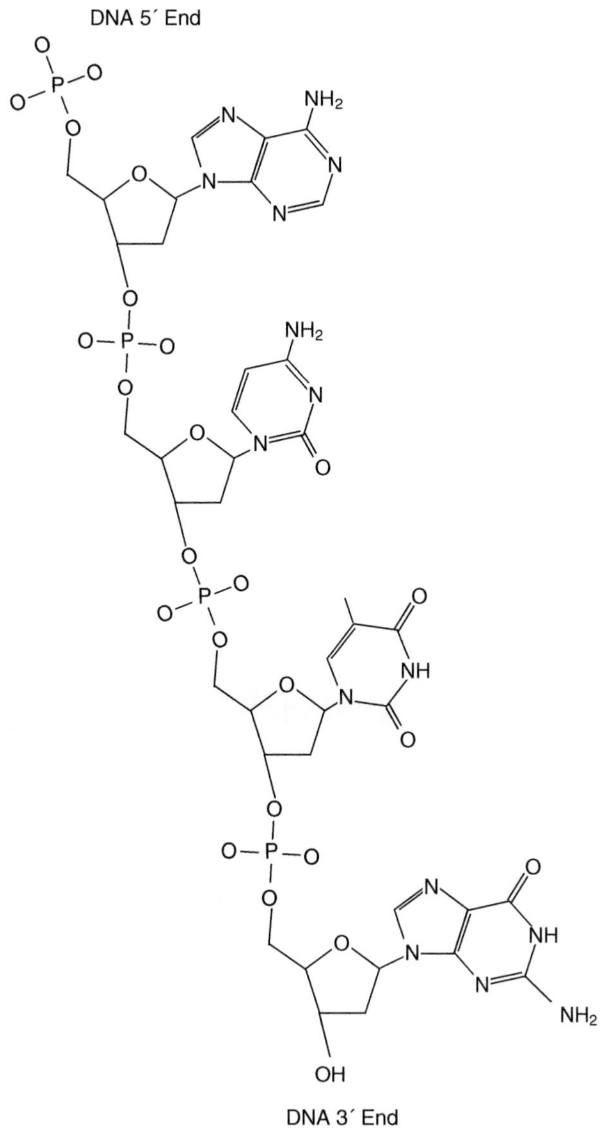

DNA 5′ End

Figure 6.5 Single DNA strand with 5′ and 3′ ends labeled. The 5′ end of DNA terminates with a phosphate group, see top of polymer, and the 3′ end terminates with a sugar group, see bottom of polymer.

molecules are much longer than the diameter of the nucleus itself and must be highly compacted. To begin the process, DNA is coiled around a series of histones. Histones are a set of eight proteins, known as an octomer. DNA winds around the surface of the histone in a helical pathway. The histone complex contains, on average, two complete turns of DNA, which consists of approximately 150 base pairs.

After DNA has successfully wrapped around the histone octamer, the DNA–histone complex is referred to as a nucleosome. Nucleosome structure is often

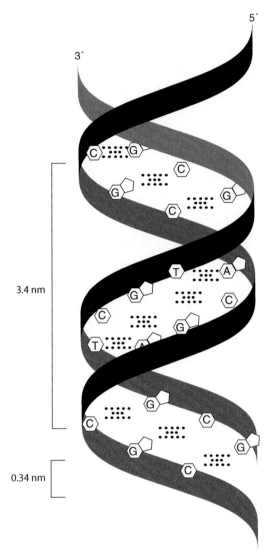

Figure 6.6 Spacing between each nucleotide pair, 0.34 nm, within a DNA helix, and the spacing, 3.4 nm, between complete helical turns are labeled.

compared with a string of beads. The string is free unwound DNA between the nucleosomes and the beads are DNA–histone complexes. A drawing of a nucleosome substructure is shown in Fig. 6.7. As can be seen, formation of nucleosomes reduces the accessibility of DNA to transcription and regulatory proteins. Both strands of DNA must be free for proper DNA binding. Protein factor binding of free DNA has been shown to be 10- to 10^4-fold stronger than histone-bound DNA. This appears to create problems for transcription where long sequences of DNA might be required. However, DNA is unwound from histones when specific sequences are needed. The benefit of nucleosome formation is protection of the DNA strand.

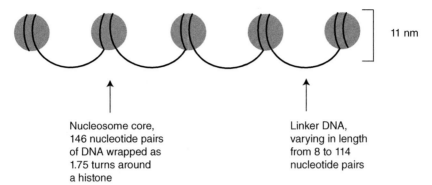

Nucleosome core,
146 nucleotide pairs
of DNA wrapped as
1.75 turns around
a histone

Linker DNA,
varying in length
from 8 to 114
nucleotide pairs

11 nm

Figure 6.7 Illustration of nucleosome substructure, showing approximately two turns of DNA wrapped around each octamer, the linker DNA between each nucleosome and the approximate height of the nucleosome.

The likelihood of a double-strand break (DSB) is greatly diminished without both strands exposed. This could be considered a method of self-preservation.

Although histones are the beginnings of chromosome packaging, further condensation is still required. Chromatin structure beyond the nucleosome is poorly understood due to the fragile nature of DNA. Structural studies are currently under way, and higher levels of chromatin packing, at the moment, can only be theorized.

DNA condensation begins with nucleosome formation and ends with the chromosome. The total length of DNA, in any nucleus, is approximately 2 m. This 2 m must be condensed to fit within a 6-μm-diameter nucleus. Therefore, chromatin must be condensed about 10^4-fold in length. This condensation is similar to trying to fit 100 elephants into the back of a VW Beetle. A summary of DNA organization, beginning with the nucleosome and ending with the chromosome, is shown in Fig. 6.8.

DNA FUNCTIONS

The primary function of DNA is to carry genetic information used during the development and function of an organism. DNA polymers are combinations of gene and nongene sequences. The separation of gene and nongene DNA depends on the sequence at a particular location. Genes contain basic instructions for protein synthesis and organization required by the organism, and there must be a way to move that information out of the nucleus and into the cell for use. This process is transcription. Transcription creates a complementary RNA copy of a specific DNA sequence. Similar to DNA replication, a single DNA strand is used to make an RNA strand. The main difference is only one strand of DNA is copied, and RNA is single stranded. RNA synthesis occurs in a 5′–3′ direction, like DNA, and occurs within five simple steps.

The first step is the unwinding of DNA. Proteins attach to the DNA helix and "unzip" the strands to allow access to the nucleotides. Hydrogen bonds between nucleotides are broken and allow for RNA synthesis. Step two pairs RNA nucleotides with DNA nucleotides. However, thymine is replaced by uracil, as mentioned

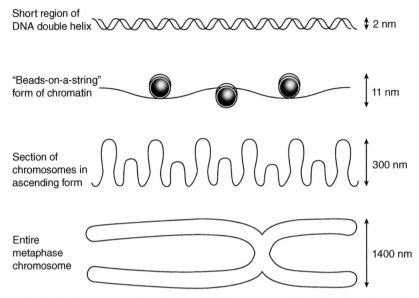

Figure 6.8 Packaging, or condensation, of DNA from a double helix through nucleosome and ending with a chromosome. The double helix, approximately 2 nm in width, is initially wrapped around histones. These nucleosomes undergo further condensation to form chromosomes with a final width of approximately 1400 nm.

previously. RNA polymerase, shown in Fig. 6.9, binds DNA to assist in DNA unwinding and RNA synthesis. As the RNA polymer begins to form, nucleotides are added and form a backbone of alternating carbohydrate and phosphate molecules, completing step three. During step four, hydrogen bonds, formed between DNA and RNA nucleotides, are broken, and the newly synthesized RNA is freed from the template DNA polymer. RNA undergoes further processing to protect the 5′ and 3′ ends and completes step five by exiting the nucleus through a nuclear pore.

As RNA exits the nucleus, it carries information copied from DNA to the ribosomes. Recall from Chapter 2 that ribosomes are sites of protein synthesis. RNA binds to a ribosome and protein synthesis, or translation, begins. Translation is the decoding of RNA sequence by ribosomes to produce specific amino acid chains used for protein synthesis. As in transcription, translation proceeds through distinct steps. They are activation, initiation, elongation, and termination. During activation, amino acids are transferred to the ribosome for attachment to the RNA polymer. RNA binds to a ribosome during initiation and translation begins. Elongation is just what it sounds like. Amino acids are added to a growing chain. At the end of the RNA polymer, termination occurs through a stop codon, and the ribosomal complex disassembles.

The sequence of RNA determines the amino acid sequence for the protein to be produced. Each set of instructions are coded in the DNA by a set of rules, referred to as the genetic code. The genetic code is responsible for defining how DNA sequences are ultimately translated. Rules of the genetic code specify that three nucleotides be read at the same time. This sequence is called a codon. Each codon is specific for a single amino acid utilized during protein synthesis. Codons can be

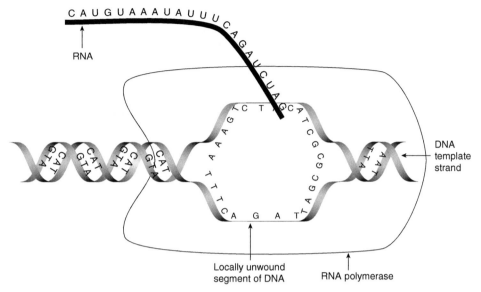

Figure 6.9 RNA polymerase surrounds DNA, unwinds a specific DNA sequence and initiates RNA synthesis. RNA is further processed and then leaves the nucleus for translation.

viewed as a stack of three plates. Each plate is responsible for a single nucleotide within the gene sequence. The start codon, the first three red plates, initiates building the protein. Groups of three plates are then read, at the same time, to continue the construction. At the end of the gene, the stop codon, or final three blue plates, terminates the translation process. The protein is then available for modification and use by the organism.

Although there are numerous proteins throughout the body, there are only 20 amino acids used for each protein. The amino acid sequence dictates what the final protein will be. Due to the limited number of amino acids, degeneracy occurs due to the genetic code. There are 64 possible codes ($4^3 = 64$), four nucleotides read in groups of three. The primary reason behind genomic degeneracy is fault tolerance for point mutations. Point mutations are single-base substitutions that cause one nucleotide to be replaced with another. A point mutation in the third codon position of the amino acid serine, three white plates, would not alter the translation of the DNA sequence. The initial genetic code for serine is TCG, G being a white plate with blue stripes. A point mutation at position three could alter the codon to read TCA, A being a white plate with green polka dots. Serine, three white plates, would still be added to the protein, and this mutation would most likely be silent, not affecting protein synthesis.

DNA REPLICATION AND REPAIR

Several methods of DNA replication have been postulated. They are conservative, dispersive, and semiconservative. Only semiconservative replication will be discussed here since it is the accepted method. The semiconservative method, confirmed by the Meselson–Stahl experiment in 1958, conserves one strand of template

DNA in each replicated helix. That is, as the original helix is broken for replication, the complimentary nucleotides that form the new DNA strand become attached to the template strand via hydrogen bonds. The final two double-strand DNA helices each consist of one original and one newly synthesized strand of DNA.

Now with a basic understanding of semiconservative replication, DNA replication can be described in more detail. DNA replication is the process by which living organisms copy their DNA. It is the basis for inheritance between cell and organism generations. In a similar fashion to RNA and protein synthesis, DNA replication occurs in three steps which are initiation, elongation, and termination.

Initiation of DNA replication occurs at specific sites within the DNA. These sites are called replication origins. Replication origins contain specific DNA sequences that allow replication proteins to attach to the DNA. These initiator proteins recruit additional proteins, such as DNA helicases, to unwind and separate the DNA helix. DNA replication occurs in opposing directions from each origin, which requires two sets of replication proteins. New strands of DNA are synthesized at a rate of about 3000 nucleotides per minute. Even with this speed, multiple origins are needed to allow complete replication within the time allotted for the S phase. If each chromosome contained only one replication origin, approximately 2000 hours would be needed to replicate the entire genome. Clearly, 2000 hours greatly exceeds the time reserved to complete the S phase of the cell cycle. At this point, replication forks have formed and DNA replication moves into the elongation phase. During elongation, DNA synthesis extends the new polymers in a 5′ to 3′ direction. The purpose of directionality is the need to attach nucleotides to the 3′ hydroxyl of the primary strand. DNA polymerases only recognize the hydroxyl end of the polymer, not the phosphate end. DNA polymerases are a family of enzymes that are responsible for DNA replication; however, they do not directly attach to DNA templates. Small strands of RNA, called primers, are attached to the DNA template and used by DNA polymerases for synthesis of new strands of DNA. The new DNA strand is extended in the 3′ direction through the addition of complementary nucleotides.

Elongation of DNA requires a special set of proteins referred to as replication machinery. These proteins include DNA topoisomerases and single-strand binding proteins (SSBPs). DNA topoisomerases are responsible for nicking a single strand of DNA, which allows the polymers to swivel around each other. Strand nicking also removes the buildup of DNA twists during replication. In addition to DNA nicking, topoisomerases cut both backbones, a double-strand cut, which enables one DNA strand to pass through another. The double cut removes knots and entanglements that often form during replication. SSBPs, as their name implies, bind to single-stranded DNA until the second strand is synthesized. By attaching to a single strand of DNA, the SSBP prevents mismatching between strands. When the second strand is complete, the SSBP release the DNA, and hydrogen bonds form to hold the DNA helix together. Once the replication proteins and enzymes have gathered together and attached to DNA, they are called a replication fork. The replication fork forms in the nucleus, only during DNA replication. It is responsible for breaking hydrogen bonds that hold the DNA helix together. As hydrogen bonds are broken, DNA polymerase is able to read each polymer individually. The replication fork moves along the chromosome in a 3′ to 5′ direction along one strand of DNA. Seen in Fig. 6.10 is the basic structure of the replication fork.

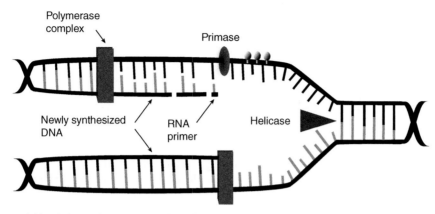

Figure 6.10   Schematic representation of the DNA replication fork. Attachment of the DNA polymerase complex is indicated, as well as an RNA primer and newly synthesized DNA strands.

At the end of each chromosome, a region of DNA is unable to be replicated. This region is known as a telomere. Telomeres are guanine-rich DNA repeats that prevent loss of chromosomal information during replication. The telomeres shorten over time, almost as an indication of when the life of the cell is coming to an end. This shortening has been seen to prevent cellular division and appears to prevent, or greatly reduce, genomic instability. This mechanism is thought to be a natural step toward the prevention of cancer formation.

DNA can be damaged by any number of factors, including normal metabolic activities and environmental radiation. This damage can consist of individual base or structural damage. In any given day, DNA in a single human cell is exposed to anywhere from 1000 to 1,000,000 molecular lesions. These lesions can cause structural damage to DNA, which interferes with genetic transcription. The two types of DNA damage that will be discussed here are single-strand breaks (SSBs) and DSBs. Recall that DNA is a double-stranded helix. In the case of an SSB, one strand of the helix is severed; however, the two DNA strands do not separate from each other. DSBs cleave both DNA strands and results in two free ends of DNA. A DSB is most hazardous to the cell due to an increased possibility of genomic rearrangement. Shown in Fig. 6.11 are examples of both SSB and DSB in the DNA helix.

Repair of DNA damage begins with the identification of damage. As discussed in Chapter 2, two DNA checkpoints monitor for damage at specific points within the cell cycle. These checkpoints halt the cell cycle to allow time for repair of the damage. When an SSB is detected, the repair method uses the same proteins used by the base excision repair (BER) mechanism. BER, briefly, is the repair of a single damaged base. A single base can be damaged by oxidation or hydrolysis, among others. BER removes the damaged base and replaces the missing nucleotide. Once the nucleotide has been replaced, DNA ligase seals the nick in the DNA strand. During repair of an SSB, the BER mechanism skips to the final step of ligation. The broken phosphodiester bonds are reformed, and the break is repaired.

In addition to SSB repair, the cell contains mechanisms to repair DSBs. DSBs are typically more severe than SSBs because the break results in two free ends of

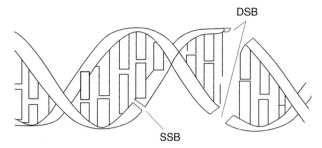

Figure 6.11 Two types of DNA damage. The single-strand break (SSB), severing of a single strand, is shown on the bottom DNA stand, while the double-strand break (DSB) is shown on the right. Both strands of DNA are clearly severed during a DSB. From Missailidis (2007), figure 2.11, p. 42.

DNA. Two DSB repair mechanisms will be briefly discussed here. They are homologous recombination (HR) and nonhomologous end joining (NHEJ). During HR, repair proteins locate homologous DNA, or the sister chromosome. Homologous DNA has the same relative sequence of the damaged DNA. The damaged DNA is resected, and strand invasion occurs. Resection is a process by which DNA surrounding the damage is removed from the 5′ end of the break, while strand invasion takes the 3′ end of the broken DNA and "invades" the homologous DNA. The lost DNA is then synthesized, and the chromosomes separate when repair of the DSB has been completed. NHEJ is called "nonhomologous" because it does not require a homologous template for repair. The broken ends of DNA are simply ligated together. NHEJ repair is mostly accurate but can have some imprecision that leads to the loss of nucleotides. However, this is only seen with DNA overhangs that are not compatible. The first steps of HR are shown in Fig. 6.12.

DNA replication has its own set of inherent errors. Replication slippage is the most common cause of error. During replication, DNA polymerase is responsible for copying DNA. DNA polymerase moves at a speed comparable with the replication fork. However, DNA polymerase can pause briefly during replication. This pause can lead to dissociation between the polymerase and DNA, and dissociation can lead to replication slippage. Replication slippage is a mispairing or displacement of the DNA strand. Replication slippage occurs in regions of DNA that have short, repeated sequences. The dissociated polymerase leads to two types of error. The first is deletion of DNA. A genetic deletion is defined as a mutation in which part of the DNA sequence is missing. The deletion can range from a single base to an entire section of a chromosome. When DNA strands become misaligned, replication can skip over a section of DNA causing deletions. Deletions can lead to frameshift mutations. In the case of p53, a deletion of part of the gene results in the development of Li–Fraumeni syndrome. In addition to deletions, replication slippage can result in insertions. An insertion is the addition of one or more nucleotides into the DNA sequence. One way in which insertions are created is multiple replications of the same DNA sequence. Insertions can also cause frameshift mutations within the DNA sequence, if the number of nucleotides is not divisible by 3. Frameshift mutations alter the normal reading frame of a gene and the amino acids encoded for by the gene.

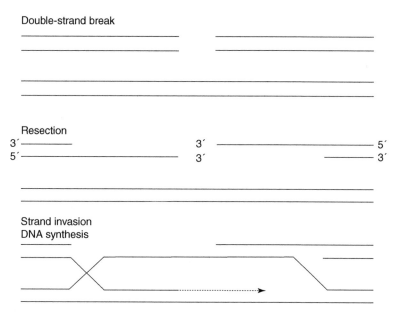

Figure 6.12   Homologous recombination, showing resection, or removal, of damaged DNA followed by strand invasion and synthesis (the dashed line) of new DNA.

GENOME

Maintaining genome integrity is just as important as maintaining genetic accuracy during replication. The genome, on average, is bombarded with up to a million, or 10^6, DNA breaks and lesions per day. Repair, as previously discussed, ensures damage is fixed, and genomic integrity remains intact. In addition to damage repair, a series of checkpoints are in the cell cycle as quality control mechanisms. Mentioned in Chapter 2, two DNA checkpoints in the cell cycle are located in the G1 and G2 phases. The G1 checkpoint locates DNA lesions and, more importantly, breaks. If a single-stranded nick was replicated, the nick could become a full-fledged DSB. Every break in the DNA causes instability within the genome. By pausing the cell cycle, the nick is repaired and replication continues without further damage to the DNA. In the case of the G2 checkpoint, DNA is reviewed for mismatched nucleotides and unreplicated DNA. The cell cycle is, again, paused and repairs are made. Without these vital checkpoints, integrity of the genome is compromised, and mutations are more likely to occur.

Genome instability is commonly caused by chromosomal alterations that can lead to a wide variety of problems. Instability can lead to deletion or insertion of DNA, mentioned earlier, or a change in chromosome number, among other changes. During cell separation, more specifically meiosis, unequal separation of chromosomes can occur. When one daughter cell receives more than one copy of a chromosome, the cell is said to be aneuploid. Aneuploidy is an abnormal number of chromosomes in a cell. The chromosomes themselves have not been altered, but the number is higher, or lower, than expected. A common occurrence of aneuploidy in humans involves chromosome 21. The normal copy number for any chromosome in a human cell is two. When three copies of chromosome 21 appear in a developing fetus, the physical manifestation is Down's syndrome. In addition to aneuploidy, chromosomal structure can be affected by instability.

Instability of chromosomal structure can lead to rearrangements and duplications. Rearrangements most commonly occur between nonhomologous chromosomes. Each of the chromosomes involved receive one part of the nonhomologous partner. In some cases, the chromosomes become fused, a key characteristic of chromosome rearrangement. When fused, the genes on each chromosome are unable to function properly. Genetic fusion is commonly found in DNA of cancer cells. Duplication of DNA is just that, a second unneeded copy. As discussed earlier, DNA duplication, not related to replication, can cause insertions that affect the structure of proteins.

In addition to DNA rearrangements and duplication, DNA expression can be altered in a superficial manner. These changes do not affect the genotype, or genetic sequence, of the individual. Superficial alterations only cause changes in the phenotypic, or physical characteristic, expression of the gene. Epigenetics is the study of gene expression. The Greek prefix *epi-* refers to a feature that is "on top of" or "in addition to" genetics. Figure 6.13 shows several epigenetic factors. One example of an epigenetic manifestation is a scar. The cells of the scar have the same DNA sequence, or genotype, as they did before the injury. During repair of the laceration, the tissue repairs via fibrosis, which alters the phenotypic characteristic of the cell. The skin cell DNA is still intact but genes are being expressed in a different manner. These epigenetic alterations are passed on through each cellular division.

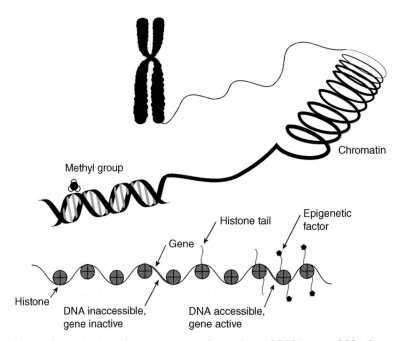

Figure 6.13   Epigenetic alterations appear on the surface of DNA, not within the sequence. For instance, an additional methyl group could lead to activation or suppression of a gene. Most epigenetic mechanisms are influenced by external factors such as pharmaceuticals, aging, and diet. Epigenetic mechanisms have the potential to lead to health end points that include cancer, autoimmune diseases, and diabetes.

SUMMARY

- The role of DNA is to encode proteins and to provide instructions on how to use those proteins.
- DNA was first discovered through studies of physical characteristics, which ultimately lead to the discovery of approximately 20,000 genes in the human genome.
- DNA, and RNA, is based on four specific nucleosomes bound together by a series of hydrogen and ester bonds.
- The double-helix formation of DNA is caused by asymmetric bonds between bases.
- DNA and RNA contain specific orientations based on bonding properties.
- Chromosomal DNA is much larger than the nucleus and requires a high amount of condensation. This begins with winding of DNA around histones.
- The basic function of DNA is to carry genetic information from one generation to the next.
- RNA sequences are read in sets of three nucleotides to form amino acid chains used in protein synthesis.
- RNA is transcribed from DNA for delivery of the message sequence for translation into active proteins.
- DNA is replicated in a semiconservative method.
- Replication of DNA begins at specific points within the strand at a rate of approximately 3000 nucleotides per minute.
- All DNA replication occurs within a replication fork.
- DNA damage can occur during replication, in response to environmental factors and normal metabolic activities.
- Processes are in place to monitor DNA for damage and initiate repair.
- Repair of damage begins with extraction of the damaged base, or series of bases, replacement of those bases, and ligation of the DNA strand.
- Genome stability is critical due to the bombardment of DNA breaks and lesions every day.
- Genomic instability can lead to chromosomal alterations and rearrangements.
- Epigenetics studies the superficial alterations of DNA that do not affect the sequence of DNA.

BIBLIOGRAPHY

Lewin B. Cells. Sudbury, MA: Jones and Bartlett Publishers; 2007.

Missailidis S. The cancer clock. Chichester, UK: John Wiley & Sons; 2007.

Pollard TD, Earnshaw WC. Cell biology. Philadelphia: Saunders; 2002.

Snustad DP, Simmons MJ. Principles of genetics. 5th ed. Hoboken, NJ: John Wiley & Sons; 2009.

QUESTIONS

Chapter 6   Questions

1. Deficiencies in which of the following DNA occurrences could lead to increased genetic instability?
   a. Deletions
   b. Aneuploidy
   c. Insertions
   d. a, b, and c

2. Of the following nucleobases, which are found in *both* DNA and RNA?
   i.   Adenine
   ii. Cytosine
   iii. Uracil
   iv. Thymine
   v.   Guanine
   a. i, ii, iii
   b. i, iii, v
   c. ii, iv, v
   d. i, ii, v

3. The study of genetics began with the publication of whose discoveries?
   a. James Watson
   b. Gregor Mendel
   c. Francis Crick
   d. Rosalind Franklin

4. Which basic elements are common to both DNA and RNA molecules?
   a. Nucleobase, phosphate, carbohydrate
   b. Phosphate, nucleotide, thymisate
   c. Carbohydrate, nucleoside, uracil
   d. Guanine, nucleotide, carbohydrate

5. Of the following base pairs, which are correct?
   a. C-G, A-T
   b. C-T, A-U
   c. A-U, G-C
   d. a and c
   e. a only

6. A codon is a series of _____ nucleotides used to define _____ amino acids for protein synthesis.
   a. three, unique
   b. three, multiple
   c. two, one
   d. four, unique

7. Epigenetics is the study of
   a. alterations in the DNA sequence that lead to changes in phenotypic expression.
   b. alterations not in the DNA sequence caused by environmental factors.
   c. alterations in the DNA sequence caused by environmental factors.
   d. alterations not in the DNA sequence that lead to changes in phenotypic expression.

8. RNA synthesis is similar to DNA replication in that
   a. nucleotides are attached to a sugar–phosphate backbone.
   b. both DNA strands are used as templates.
   c. a single strand of DNA is used to create a single complementary strand.
   d. a and c

9. Protein synthesis occurs by which of the following processes?
   a. Transcription
   b. Elongation
   c. Initiation
   d. Translation

10. Decoding the mRNA sequence occurs during the _____ phase of translation.
   a. transcription
   b. elongation
   c. translation
   d. initiation

11. DNA replication has been postulated to occur in three different ways. Which of the following models has been shown to be the most accurate?
   a. Dispersive
   b. Semiconservative
   c. Conservative
   d. Random

12. Which of the DNA repair mechanisms discussed is used for both single-base repair and single-strand break repair?
   a. NHEJ
   b. BER
   c. HR
   d. None of the above.

13. One trait of genome instability is aneuploidy. Aneuploidy is noted as
 a. change in chromosome length.
 b. abnormal chromosome numbers.
 c. a higher number of chromosomes.
 d. a lower number of chromosomes.

14. One purpose of codon sequences within the DNA is
 a. to signal the start and stop sections of a gene during transcription.
 b. to review the validity of DNA repair mechanisms.
 c. to signal when DNA repairs have been completed.
 d. to differentiate between RNA and DNA.

15. Transcription and translation each follow the basic steps of
 a. initiation, elongation, termination.
 b. initiation, activation, elongation.
 c. initiation, activation, termination.
 d. activation, elongation, termination.

16. The primary function of DNA is
 a. to act as a template for RNA transcription.
 b. to create polymers that allow an organism to survive.
 c. to carry genetic information of an organism.
 d. to attach to proteins.

CHAPTER 7

RADIATION DAMAGE AND REPAIR OF CELLS

KEYWORDS

DNA damage, DNA repair, single-strand break, double-strand break, bystander effect, fractionation, mitotic cycle, radiosensitivity, mutation, genome, chromosome aberration, mutation, potentially lethal damage, sublethal damage

TOPICS

- Types of DNA and chromosome damage and their consequences
- The relationship between radiosensitivity and the mitotic cycle
- The bystander effect
- Classification of radiation damage in terms of the potential for repair
- Evidence of cellular repair from split-dose and dose-rate experiments

INTRODUCTION

This chapter discusses the different types of DNA radiation damage and the evidence for DNA repair. Chapter 5 covered radiation damage at the macroscopic level including macroscopic observations of cell growth in petri dishes; this chapter extends the discussion to the molecular level. Evidence for radiation damage at the molecular level is primarily obtained using modern DNA analysis techniques.

Radiation Biology of Medical Imaging, First Edition. Charles A. Kelsey, Philip H. Heintz, Daniel J. Sandoval, Gregory D. Chambers, Natalie L. Adolphi, and Kimberly S. Paffett.
© 2014 John Wiley & Sons, Inc. Published 2014 by John Wiley & Sons, Inc.

Although radiation can damage the cell membrane, organelles, and other constituents, we will concentrate on damage to nuclear DNA because this damage can
cause reproductive death, as well as mutations and cancer. Each of the over 10 trillion cells in the human body suffers between 10^4 and 10^6 DNA damage events each
day. These events include breaks in the DNA chain and deletions, substitutions, and
inversions in the DNA code. They are due to a variety of agents including ionizing
radiation. Some causes, in addition to ionizing radiation, are environmental chemicals. For example, hydrocarbons in the atmosphere and plant products such as
aflatoxins from moldy peanuts can cause DNA changes. Most of this DNA damage
is repaired correctly with no ill effects. In general, radiation is a significant source
of DNA damage, but it is by no means the only source.

DNA STRAND BREAKS

DNA is a large molecule consisting of a sugar phosphate backbone with nitrogenous
bases. The structure of the bases is shown in Fig. 7.1a. The bases on opposite strands

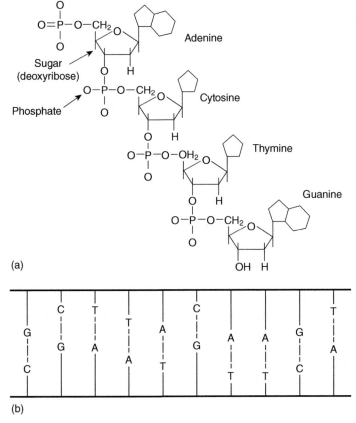

Figure 7.1 (a) The chemical structure of the DNA bases (adenine = A, cytosine = C,
thymine = T, and guanine = G). (b) A 2D representation of DNA, which incorporates the
bases A, C, T, and G in a ladder structure. *Source*: Pasternak (2005), figure 4.1(b).

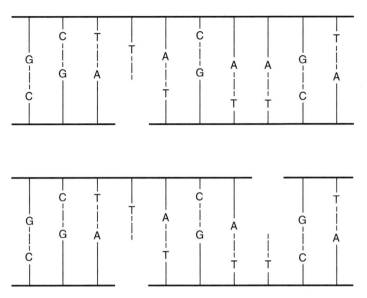

Figure 7.2 A single-strand break (SSB) can be repaired easily, because the opposite strand serves as a template. Two SSBs are also easy to repair if they occur in separate locations, such that the opposite strand is still intact at the location of the damage.

only connect with their complement, that is, adenine–thymine, cytosine–guanine. When the strands are paired, the DNA molecule presents in a double-helix structure. Figure 7.1b shows a 2D view of the DNA double helix if it were untwisted and flattened.

Single-strand breaks (SSBs) involve a break in only one of the DNA strands. Modest doses of low-linear energy transfer (LET) radiations will produce many SSBs. Because the nitrogenous bases are complementary, SSBs are relatively easy to repair, because the intact strand serves as a template. For example, an intact G will attract a C to occupy the break. Figure 7.2 shows schematically how if both strands are broken, but the breaks occur at different locations, the breaks can be readily repaired. This situation could be described as two SSBs on the same molecule.

Double-strand breaks (DSBs) involve breaks in both DNA strands at the same or nearby locations, as shown in Fig. 7.3. Such breaks are more likely to result in faulty repair because the molecule may come apart, and the template for guiding the repair may be lost. DSBs are more likely to occur with high-LET radiations. Most DSBs are lethal because the fragments are stopped at one of the checkpoints in the cell replication cycle.

Base damage includes deletions, substitutions, and additions to one or both of the DNA strands. The alteration of a base in the DNA molecule means that the sequence is disturbed. This changes the storage and transmission of information in the genome. There are many different types of base damage, most of which are detected and repaired before cell replication. However, some forms of base damage escape detection and are passed on to daughter cells. Note that only damage to germ cells, ova or sperm, results in hereditary damage.

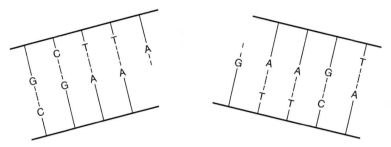

Figure 7.3   A double-strand break (DSB) can sever the DNA molecule, making repair more difficult, because the opposite strand template is lost.

Although SSBs can be damaging to the cell, the DSBs are the source of greatest concern. These are more likely to result in cell killing (DNA too damaged to allow the cell to divide normally), carcinogenesis (DNA damaged enough to damage apoptotic function, leading to cancer), or mutation (DNA incorrectly repaired). However, their occurrence is only 0.04 times that of SSBs after a dose of about 2 Gy.

DNA DAMAGE VERSUS MUTATION

In the past, the terms DNA break, DNA damage, and mutation were used interchangeably. Currently, we understand there is a basic difference between DNA damage and mutation. DNA damage is an aberration in the DNA sequence, for example, SSBs or DSBs and deletions or duplications of the DNA constituents. DNA damage is usually recognized by repair enzymes that constantly monitor the DNA integrity during the replication process. Damage that is recognized is repaired in most cases. Damage that is not recognized or is not repaired correctly will result in cell death or mutation.

Mutation, as opposed to DNA damage, is a change in the DNA base sequence not recognized by the repair enzymes. Thus, the mutation is not repaired and may be replicated. Cells may retain apparently normal reproductive capacity but have altered information in other parts of the genome. For example, a lung cell may still function as a lung cell, but have a defect in one of the genes acting during the cell cycle. The defect is not passed on to the progeny of the host organism, but it is passed on to the descendents of the mutated cell within the host organism. Only mutations that occur in gamete cells (sperm or ova) are passed on to the progeny of the host.

DNA mutations in rapidly proliferating cells may be more likely to lead to cancer simply on the basis of probability, because there are more chances of rapidly replicating cells producing a viable mutation.

CHROMOSOMES AND CELL DIVISION

Radiation may cause chromosomal aberrations, of which there are two types. *Chromosome aberrations* happen early in interphase, before the duplication of the DNA. The break is usually in a single strand of chromatin that will then be duplicated

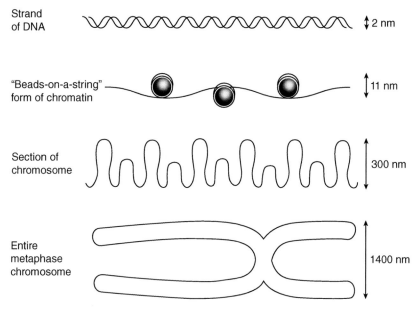

Figure 7.4   Illustration of the relative sizes of portions of the chromosome. Top to bottom: DNA, chromatin, a segment of chromosome, and a full chromosome. The centromere is the point of intersection in the metaphase chromosome and is important in cell replication.

during the S phase. *Chromatid aberrations* happen later in interphase, after the S phase. Usually, one arm of the sister chromatid is broken, but not the other. The relative sizes of chromosome substructures are shown in Fig. 7.4.

Lethal Radiation-Induced Aberrations

Although many types of aberrations can occur, there are generally three lethal types. Two of which, dicentric and ring, are *chromosome* aberrations; the anaphase bridge is a *chromatid* aberration.

Dicentrics form when two separate pre-replication chromosomes suffer breaks and rejoin by illegitimate connections that are subsequently replicated during the S phase. This can produce a pair of sister chromatids with two centromeres (hence the term "dicentric"), as shown in Fig. 7.5 and Fig. 7.6. The problem with the dicentric is that there is more than one centromere for the spindle to grab onto during metaphase, which disrupts the normal process by which the spindles pull the chromatids toward each pole during anaphase.

As shown in Fig. 7.6 and Fig. 7.7, a ring aberration can happen if there are breaks in both arms of a chromosome, such that the chromosome can reconnect to itself. It is replicated in the S phase, but neither the ring nor the acentric fragment has a properly constructed centromere for the spindle to attach to, such that the chromosome cannot be properly divided.

The anaphase bridge occurs late in interphase, after replication. During anaphase, the damaged sister chromatids do not separate properly, but rather stretch to either pole of the cell. The anaphase bridge aberration prevents the separation of the

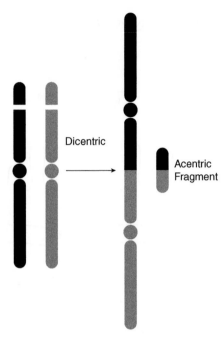

Figure 7.5   Schematic diagram of dicentric and acentric fragment formation demonstrates how broken chromosome ends can rejoin incorrectly.

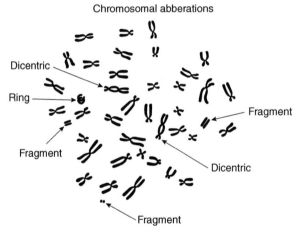

Figure 7.6   Artist's representation of chromosome aberrations observed by electron microscopy, including dicentrics, fragments, and ring.

parent into daughter cells, resulting in reproductive death. An example of an anaphase bridge aberration is shown in Fig. 7.8.

Nonlethal Aberrations

Not all aberrations are lethal to the cell. One of the nonlethal types is *symmetric translocation*, which is a break in two chromosomes that then swap the broken

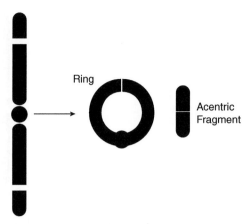

Ring

Acentric
Fragment

Figure 7.7 Schematic diagram of ring and acentric fragment formation, another example of incorrect chromosome structure following a DSB.

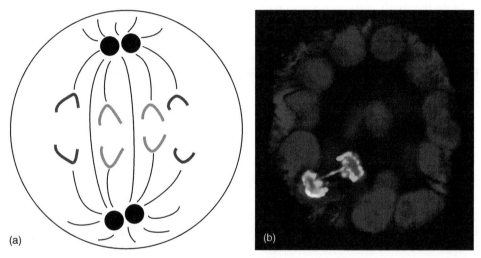

(a)

(b)

Figure 7.8 (a) Diagram of normal anaphase showing the normal separation of all chromosomes. (b) Fluorescent microscope imaging shows an anaphase bridge aberration in a mammary cell. Most of the sister chromatids have separated and are moving toward the opposite poles, but the anaphase bridge (green) cannot separate properly and so prevents mitosis. (Fluorescent micrograph courtesy of Dr. Allison Scaling.)

pieces. The translocation is a fairly stable aberration that can be passed on to progeny; therefore, the translocation can lead to mutation and carcinogenesis. Another nonlethal aberration is the *small interstitial deletion*, in which some genetic information is lost. If the loss of DNA includes the loss of a suppressor gene, the deletion could lead to a malignant change, namely cancer. Figure 7.9 illustrates a translocation, wherein two adjacent pieces of chromosome are broken and exchanged, and an interstitial deletion, wherein a small piece of chromosome is deleted and lost.

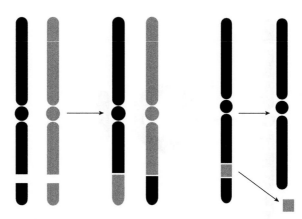

Figure 7.9   Left: Translocation occurs when two adjacent pieces of chromosome are broken and exchanged. Right: Interstitial deletion occurs when a small piece of chromosome is deleted and lost.

Note that both of these nonlethal aberrations are DSBs (both sides of the DNA ladder that makes up each chromatid must break for the chromatid to break). Nevertheless, with these nonlethal aberrations, there remains two sister chromatids with an intact centromere, such that the mechanics of mitosis can proceed normally. The problem with this type of aberration is that the resulting DNA code has some "misspellings" or "missing words," and these errors can be passed on to future generations of cells.

THE BYSTANDER EFFECT

The bystander effect, also called the radiation-induced bystander effect (RIBE), is an effect on cells outside the radiation field. RIBE refers to the observation that cells outside the radiation field can experience damage following radiation exposure to nearby (or even distant) cells in the same organism. The idea that radiation or its free radicals do not have to contact cells to damage the cells goes against traditional radiobiological thinking. Previous radiobiology tenets held that radiation damage was caused only by direct action of the radiation, or by the indirect action of the relatively short-ranged and short-lived radiation products (i.e., free radicals). The bystander mechanisms of action are not well understood, although the effect has been documented both *in vitro* and *in vivo*. Recent developments in DNA analysis have permitted the detection of changes in DNA structure resulting from mutations, which are passed on to future generations of the cell line or offspring of the host. These changes, collectively known as genomic instability, are one of the characteristics of the bystander effect.

Microbeam experiments on cells *in vitro* have allowed experimenters to irradiate very small volumes, for example, just the nucleus of a cell, with one or a few alpha particles. Near and distant cells have shown the genomic instability characteristics of the bystander effect. There is evidence that the irradiated cells exude or secrete some substance(s) that damage unirradiated cells. Experiments show that cells grown in the medium of irradiated cells show genetic instability. Demonstration of the bystander effect is not limited to *in vitro* experiments. Rats whose brains were irradiated with X-rays while their spleens were shielded with lead showed genomic instability in their spleens 7 months after irradiation. These and other experiments show that the bystander effect is present *in vivo*. Some believe that the general fatigue and malaise reported by radiation therapy patients during treatment are a result of the bystander effect. Thus, radiation effects are evident not only in individual exposed cells but also in tissues, organs, and perhaps the entire body.

RADIOSENSITIVITY AND THE MITOTIC CYCLE

The mitotic index is defined as the ratio of cells in mitosis to the total number of cells in the sample. Under a microscope, the condensed chromosomes of cells in mitosis are visible, so that mitotic cells can be distinguished from other cells. A simple equation, shown as follows, defines the mitotic index:

$$\text{Mitotic index} = 100\% \times (P + M + A + T)/N,$$

where $(P + M + A + T)$ is the total number of cells in any phase of mitosis (prophase [P], metaphase [M], anaphase [A], and telophase [T]), and N is the total number of cells in the sample examined.

The mitotic index is an indicator of the reproductive activity of a group of cells. For example, the mitotic index of the cells that line the stomach is high, because the interior of the stomach is a chemically harsh environment, requiring cells to be constantly replaced. By contrast, the mitotic index of skeletal muscle cells is lower, as these cells require only infrequent replacement. Mitotic index can also be used as an indicator of cancer, because most cancer cells replicate rapidly and show a high mitotic index. Radiation sensitivity varies based on mitotic index. It is observed that cell populations with a high mitotic index are generally more sensitive to radiation than those with a lower mitotic index. Table 7.1 shows how normal tissues and cells can be divided roughly into three groups on the basis of their cellular mitotic index.

Some adult tissues remain static with little or no proliferation at all. Neurons are an example of cells with a highly specialized function in which mitosis does not occur and no cell renewal takes place. At the other extreme are epithelial tissues, such as the epidermis and the intestinal mucosa, which rapidly proliferate. The cells of these populations renew themselves throughout adult life.

TABLE 7.1   Classification of Cells on the Basis of Mitotic Index

Mitotic Index Near 0 (Little or No Cell Renewal)	Low Mitotic Index (Slow Cell Renewal)	High Mitotic Index (Rapid Cell Renewal)
Neurons	Thyroid	Epidermis
Some sensory organs	Vascular endothelium	Intestinal epithelium
Cornea	Connective tissue	Bone marrow
Adrenal medulla		Gonads
Red blood cells		

In the middle group are cell populations where rapid renewal is possible on demand, but where cell proliferation normally occurs at a low rate in a healthy individual. Within this middle group of cells are the parenchymal cells of the liver and thyroid, which, together with connective tissue and the vascular endothelial cells, have a low level of cell renewal.

Although DNA was not discovered until the 1950s and the molecular mechanisms of the cell cycle were not elucidated until the 1970s, in 1906, two French scientists, Jean Bergonié, a radiologist, and Louis Tribondeau, a physician, reported on their observations regarding radiation damage to cells. They noticed that some cell types appeared to be more sensitive to radiation than others. The combination of these observations is sometimes referred to as the "law of Bergonié and Tribondeau," although it is not really a physical law (in the same way that "Newton's law" is a law). Bergonié and Tribondeau concluded that cells are most sensitive to radiation when they

- are rapidly dividing
- are undifferentiated (not yet specialized)
- have a long mitotic future.

Subsequently, it was shown by *in vitro* cell survival experiments that cells are most sensitive to radiation during the M and G2 phases and are most resistant during the S phase, as shown in Fig. 7.10. This fact explains why rapidly dividing cells, which spend more time in M phase, appear to be more sensitive to radiation.

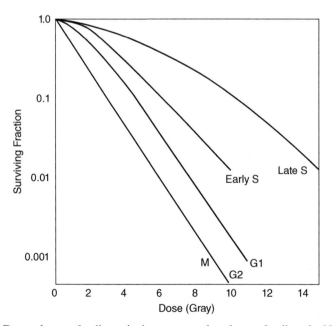

Figure 7.10 Dependence of cell survival curves on the phase of cell cycle. Note that cells are most sensitive in the M phase and least sensitive in the S phase.

(If the mitotic index is high, there are proportionally more cells in the M phase, and these are the cells that die more quickly.) It has also been observed that radiation sensitivity correlates with intracellular levels of sulfhydryl compounds (natural radioprotectors), which rise and fall as a function of phase.

One way to understand the dependence of radiosensitivity on the cell cycle is the following. During the S phase, when DNA is being replicated, is the most suitable time for DNA repair. This is because the biochemical components for replication and repair are similar and are present during the S phase. Thus, radiation damage during the S phase can most likely be quickly repaired. During mitosis (M phase), the chromosomes must have the right configuration to support the various complicated rearrangements occurring during this phase. These rearrangements include condensation, alignment, attachment of spindles, and separation of sister chromatids (but not DNA replication or repair). Failure of any of the critical steps that occur during mitosis means that the cell will fail to divide. Recall that reproductive death (failure to proliferate) is the definition of cell death in experiments designed to determine the effects of radiation on cells. Thus, radiation damage during the M phase has a much greater potential to lead to cell death, compared with radiation damage incurred during other phases of the cell cycle.

CLASSIFICATIONS OF RADIATION DAMAGE AND REPAIR

There are many possible effects following cell irradiation. Figure 7.11 presents some of the possible results. In most cases, the cell either continues to function normally after some delay, or it dies.

Before DNA analysis became available, radiobiological studies were primarily limited to observing the macroscopic effects of radiation damage by observing the response of cells to radiation in cell cultures. Radiation damage is classified on the basis of cell survival. Researchers developed the four classifications of radiation damage based on the survival of irradiated cells shown in Table 7.2.

Lethal damage (LD) is irreversible and fatal. It may result in the cell failing in its function or reproductive capacity. Interphase and mitotic death both result from LD.

Potentially lethal damage (PLD) is reversible depending on the cellular environment. Studies show that the irradiated cells can recover if given time to repair the damage. The results of experiments demonstrating PLD are counterintuitive because cell survival decreases under optimum growth conditions. One explanation of the decreased survival under optimal growth conditions is that cells progress into mitosis before repair is completed. If cells are placed into suboptimal conditions, by cooling the growth medium or adding dilute salt water to the growth medium, the PLD can be repaired. This is because the cells are allowed to "rest and recover" from the radiation damage before resuming their progress through the cell cycle. The result is that cell survival following PLD is greater in suboptimal growth conditions. In suboptimal growth conditions the PLD is not manifested as LD.

Sublethal damage, SLD, may be repaired within hours of the damage if no additional radiation is added during this recovery period. Additional radiation can convert SLD into LD and cell death. Studies of SLD provide a possible explanation of why fractionation in radiation therapy treatments is effective.

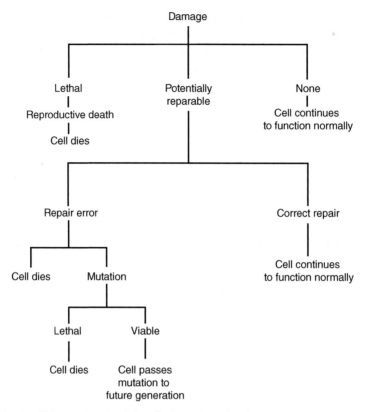

Figure 7.11 Possible results of cell irradiation. Note that in most cases, the cell either continues to function normally after some delay, or it dies.

TABLE 7.2 The Classifications of Cell Damage Based on Cellular Response

Class	Abbreviation	Description
Lethal damage	LD	Leads to death
Potentially lethal damage	PLD	Can be repaired
Sublethal damage	SLD	Can be repaired
Nonlethal damage	NLD	Cell continues to reproduce

Nonlethal damage (NLD) is damage that is assumed to exist but is not observed as a decrease in survival. (Such damage could presumably be observed by DNA analysis.) This concept finds usage in some radiation protection models. These models assume that some molecular damage is likely to have been induced but no damage to the organism is observed.

EVIDENCE OF REPAIR FROM SPLIT DOSES AND FRACTIONATION

The existence of a shoulder region in the cell survival curve implies that some radiation damage can be repaired. It has been estimated that there are more than 100,000

DNA breaks per cell per day in the average human, the vast majority caused by sources other than radiation. Since DNA damage is so common, but mammals exist, mammalian cells must have the ability to repair most damage to DNA, including radiation damage.

Each point on a cell survival curve illustrates the response of a cell population to a *single* dose of radiation. The dose–response curve for multiple doses is different. The response of cells to multiple doses (dose fractionation) depends on a number of factors, including the size of the individual doses (or "fractions"), the time interval between them, and the point in the cell cycle when the cells are exposed. The biological effect of dose fractionation can be predicted from the cell survival curves obtained from *in vitro* cell populations (e.g., breast cancer cell lines) that are relevant to the clinical problem (e.g., breast cancer).

In split-dose experiments, two identical cell groups are irradiated to a given total dose. The first group receives the total dose in a single fraction. The second group receives the same total dose divided into several fractions. This second group is allowed to recover for some time before being irradiated again. The survival of the second group receiving two successive doses is greater than that of the single-dose group. The increase in survival depends on the time interval between the two split doses. This indicates repair of SLD. If the time interval is more than about 6 hours, recovery from the initial SLD caused by the first irradiation is complete. (Cells receiving LD during the first dose do not recover.) In this case, the survival curve produced by the second irradiation will have the same shape as the survival curve produced by the first irradiation. This indicates that the repaired cells show no lasting effects of the previous irradiation. If the interval between doses is short compared with the cell cycle duration, then the recovery is incomplete. In that case, the shape of the second survival curve will not be the same as the initial survival curve. Figure 7.12 compares the survival curve from a single dose and two half doses. The time interval between the two half doses was long enough to permit full repair of SLD.

Further evidence of SLD repair is shown in Fig. 7.13, which shows the surviving fraction as a function of time interval between doses for a split-dose experiment where the cells were held at room temperature between doses. At room temperature (as opposed to body temperature, $37°C$), the cells do not proceed to mitosis. However, repair of SLD does occur, resulting in a significant increase in survival for a delay of 1 hour or more between doses. The delay increases survival, because DNA repair can be completed before the cells are allowed to proceed to the M phase.

As noted earlier, cells are more sensitive to radiation in some phases of the cell cycle compared with others. If an asynchronous cell population is exposed to radiation, cells in the sensitive G2 and M phases will be preferentially killed, and the cells that survive will be more likely to be in the S phase. Thus, a second dose, timed so that the surviving S phase cells have progressed again to G2 and M, will produce significant cell killing, as shown in Fig. 7.14.

A second dose a short time after the first will not have as dramatic an effect, because the cells will have repaired some damage, but will not have entered the sensitive phases yet. Likewise, if the delay between the two doses is very long, the cells will have already gone through the M phase, resulting in repopulation, and they will now be in a less-sensitive phase (G1 or S). This effect has been used to synchronize *in vitro* cell populations for further studies on environmental effects on

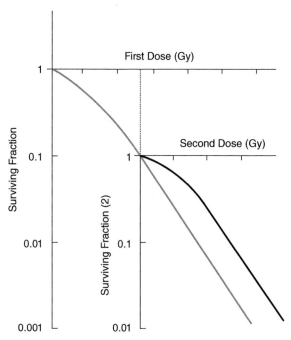

Figure 7.12 Results of a split-dose survival curve. The second half dose curve (black) is similar in shape to the first half dose curve (gray). The gray curve represents the surviving fraction for a single-dose experiment. For the same total dose, the surviving fraction is greater for the split dose, due to complete repair of SLD during the interval between the split doses.

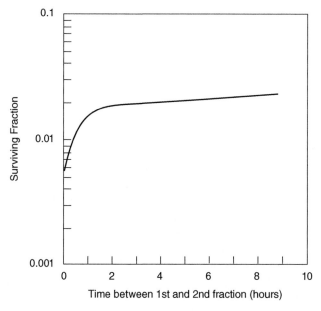

Figure 7.13 *In vitro* cell survival increases if the cells are held at room temperature between doses for >1 hour. At room temperature, the cells are prevented from moving through the cell cycle, which increases the time over which DNA repair can occur.

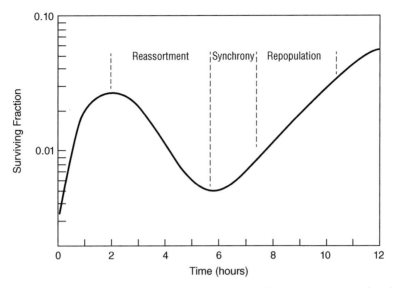

Figure 7.14 Cell survival as a function of time between split doses demonstrating the rapid repair of sublethal damage. Most cells surviving the first dose fraction are in resistant cell phases. A sensitive period for the second dose occurs at approximately 6 hours as cells move into the G2 and M phases.

radiation sensitivity. It has not yet been possible to utilize cell synchronization in human cancer therapy.

Evidence of Repair from the Dose-Rate Effect

One significant modifier of radiation effects is the dose *rate*. Experiments show that dose delivered at high-dose rate produces a different effect than the same dose delivered at a low-dose rate. In particular, it matters if the dose is delivered over many cell cycles as opposed to delivery in a time less than one cell cycle. The dose-rate effect is almost nonexistent for high-LET particles because the high ionization along the particle track is so efficient at cell killing. Figure 7.15 shows how cell survival curves typically change with dose rate for low-LET radiation.

Cells exposed to low-dose rate radiation have time to repair low-LET damage during irradiation. In fact, they may even proliferate during the irradiation. These conditions will result in a wide shoulder in the cell survival curve. A high-dose rate leaves little time for repair. For example, if an SSB occurs on one side of the DNA molecule, a second, nearby SSB may occur nearby before the first is repaired, resulting in a lethal DSB.

SUMMARY

- Single-strand DNA breaks can be readily repaired using opposite strand as template.
- Double-strand DNA breaks are more damaging and may lead to cell death, carcinogenesis, or DNA mutation.

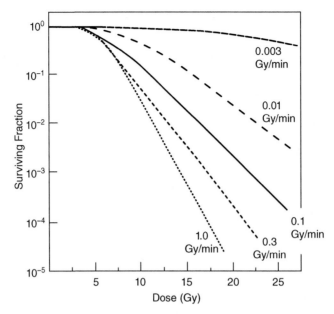

Figure 7.15 Cell survival curves from *in vitro* exposure to different dose rates. At sufficiently low-dose rate, cellular repair and proliferation can occur at a similar rate to cellular damage, resulting in a high survival fraction. As the dose rate is increased, cellular repair cannot occur rapidly enough compared with the rate of damaging events, resulting in reduced survival.

- Lethal chromosomal aberrations include dicentrics, rings, and anaphase bridges.
- Nonlethal aberrations include symmetric translocations and small deletions.
- Radiation damage is classified as nonlethal, sublethal (normally reparable within some hours if no further damage), potentially lethal (can be modified by postradiation conditions), or lethal (not reparable).
- Repair is studied via split-dose experiments with varying time interval.
- The extent of sublethal repair and the survival curve shoulder width are correlated.
- High-LET radiation survival curves exhibit no apparent repair of damage indicating little SLD and a predominance of LD.
- For low-LET radiation, as dose rate is lowered (<30 cGy/h), cell death is reduced due to repair during exposure, resulting in a broad, shallow survival curve.

BIBLIOGRAPHY

Bergonié J, Tribondeau L. Interpretation of a few results of radiotherapy and fixation test of a rational technique. C R Hebd Séanc Acad Sci. 1906 July–December;143:983–5.

Hall EJ, Giaccia AJ. Radiobiology for the radiologist. 6th ed. Philadelphia: Lippincott Williams & Wilkins; 2006.

Lorimore SA, Wright EG. Radiation-induced genomic instability and bystander effects: Related inflammatory-type responses to radiation-induced stress and injury? A review. Int J Radiat Biol. 2003 January;79(1):15–25.

Pasternak JJ. An introduction to human molecular genetics: mechanisms of inherited diseases. 2nd ed. Hoboken, NJ: Wiley-Liss; 2005.

Sinclair WK. Cyclic x-ray responses in mammalian cells *in vitro*. Radiat Res. 1968 March;33(3):620–43.

QUESTIONS

Chapter 7   Questions

1. Single-strand breaks
   a. can be repaired using the opposite strand as a template.
   b. lead to cell death.
   c. will sever the DNA strand completely.
   d. do not happen due to radiation exposure.

2. Symmetric translocation is a chromosomal aberration that
   a. can be passed to future generations.
   b. is always lethal to the cell.
   c. stops anaphase.
   d. involves only a single-strand break.

3. In the cell cycle:
   i.   Cells in the S phase are radioresistant.
   ii.   When the G1 phase has an appreciable length, it has been shown to be resistant in its early part and sensitive in its later part.
   iii. Cells in the G2 phase are the most resistant.
   iv.   The G2 phase is almost as sensitive as the M phase.
   a. i, ii, iii
   b. i, ii, iv
   c. ii, iii, iv
   d. i, ii, iii, iv

4. Mitotic cells under conditions of hypoxia are about as radiosensitive as
   a. mitotic cells that are aerated.
   b. aerated cells in the S phase.
   c. aerated cells in the G2 phase.
   d. Cells are the most radiosensitive in this phase and condition, so there is nothing with which to compare.

5. The variation of radiosensitivity as a function of cell age has been found to be qualitatively similar for X-rays and neutrons but the variation of sensitivity is smaller in the case of neutrons, because

   a. neutrons do not damage DNA and therefore do not affect mitosis.

   b. neutrons have a higher LET and tend to produce lethal damage in all phases of the cell cycle.

   c. neutrons cause little direct damage and therefore cause only single-strand breaks.

   d. neutrons have a lower LET, and the amplitude of variations in radiosensitivity during the cell cycle is a function of LET.

6. The variation of cell radiosensitivity with cell age is understood to be due to cell cycle dependence on

   a. the form of the DNA and the level of naturally occurring sulfhydryl compounds in the cell.

   b. the oxygen enhancement ratio of alpha radiation.

   c. mutations in particular cell phases.

   d. cosmic radiation levels associated with the solar cycle.

7. What is the basic definition of the bystander effect?

   a. Induction of biological effects in unirradiated cells adjacent to irradiated cells

   b. Dose given to medical personnel standing next to treated patients

   c. Mutations in subsequent generations of irradiated cells

   d. Cellular organelle self-shielding

8. In a synchronously dividing culture,

   a. all cells are in the same phase of the cell cycle.

   b. all cells are radiosensitive.

   c. all cells are radioresistant.

   d. cancer cells cannot exist.

9. In which phase are cells the most radiosensitive?

   a. S phase

   b. M phase

   c. G1 phase

   d. G2 phase

10. In which phase are cells the most radioresistant?

   a. S phase

   b. M phase

   c. G1 phase

   d. G2 phase

11. The law of Bergonié and Tribondeau states that cells tend to be most radiosensitive if they have these three properties:

    a. They have a high division rate, a long dividing future, and are of an unspecialized type.

    b. They have a low division rate, a short dividing future, and are highly specialized.

    c. They are cancer cells, are prone to single-strand breaks, and are hypoxic.

    d. They lack natural sulfhydryl compounds, are germ cells, and cannot repair sublethal damage.

12. With normal dose rates, as the dose rate is ____ and the exposure time increased, the biologic effect of a given dose generally is ____.

    a. reduced, reduced

    b. increased, reduced

    c. reduced, increased

    d. None of the above.

13. In a split-dose experiment, the second curve will have the same shape as the first curve if

    a. the time between split doses is long.

    b. the cells repair all SLD before the second dose.

    c. the SLD and PLD values are equal.

    d. a and b

14. Lower-dose rates are generally less effective at cell killing (than higher-dose rates) because

    a. exposure time is longer than cell cycle; repair and proliferation balance cell killing.

    b. there is time for one hit to be repaired before a second, lethal hit occurs.

    c. low-dose rates trigger cells to enter and remain in radioresistant cell cycle phases.

    d. a and b

15. Potentially lethal damage

    a. is repaired under most conditions.

    b. can be repaired, but only under particular conditions (such as suboptimal growth conditions).

    c. is the same as sublethal damage.

    d. a and c

16. Lethal chromosome aberrations involve

    a. DSBs in DNA without gross changes in the structure of the chromosomes.

    b. DSBs in DNA that lead to gross changes in the structure of the chromosomes, such as missing or extra centromeres.

    c. an SSB on each sister chromatid.

    d. mutations that are passed on to future generations.

CHAPTER 8

NORMAL AND MALIGNANT CELLS

KEYWORDS

Normal cell characteristics, cancer cell characteristics, cancer, malignant, mutations, genetic stability, angiogenesis, telomere, apoptosis, aneuploidy

TOPICS

- The difference between normal and cancer cells
- The characteristics of cancer cells
- Four hypotheses of cancer development
- Possible treatments of cancer

INTRODUCTION

This chapter summarizes the current thoughts regarding the origin and development of cancer. The chapter begins with a brief review of normal cells including insight into balance between growth and antigrowth signals controlling normal cell reproduction. This is followed by a discussion of cancer characteristics, the major differences between normal and cancer cells, and the importance of genetic instability in cancer promotion. Then four hypotheses concerning the steps involved in changing a normal cell into a cancer cell are discussed. Finally, the predictions from the different hypotheses regarding prevention and treatment of cancer are presented.

NORMAL CELLS

Before studying the progression toward a full-blown cancer, it is helpful to review the process of normal cell life, error repair, and death.

All cells in the body are closely regulated and must not stray from their form, function, and purpose. As an example, consider cells in the liver. There are many different kinds of cells in the liver, some providing structural support, some producing enzymes and substances to break down digested food, and others to process waste produced during these activities. Regardless of their function, they are all liver cells and are in communication with other liver cells. This communication is either by direct contact or by messenger signals. The balance between growth and antigrowth signals is constantly being altered as circumstances change. If a liver cell is damaged, a signal sends the cell into apoptosis. Growth signals are also sent to a neighboring cell to start the cell cycle for production of a replacement cell. During production of the replacement cell, there are checkpoints to ensure that the replication process is proceeding correctly. At the end of the replacement cycle, antigrowth signals stop the cell cycle, proliferation stops, and the liver continues its function of producing proteins and hormones until another replacement cell is needed. This balance between growth and antigrowth signals maintains homeostasis.

Normal Cells Exhibit Genetic Stability

Genetic stability is the term describing the resistance to change of the genome within the DNA molecule. It represents the absence of errors during cell replication. A high degree of genetic stability means the cell's DNA is passed error free from generation to generation. It is a measure of how well the genome resists change over time.

Genetic stability is important not only to preserve the integrity of the species, but also to maintain the function of the tissues and organs in the body. Genome stability of germ cells protects the species. Genetic stability in the somatic cells maintains the function of all body cells. All cells work for the common good of the whole body. That is, structural stroma cells must continue their function of tissue support, and saliva cells, for example, produce saliva.

Genetic stability is not absolute; some mutations do occur. These mutations increase the diversity of the species and sometimes give a survival advantage. Examples are opposable thumbs and larger brains, which increased survival. Other mutations, including red hair or dimples, are not harmful but have no apparent survival advantage. Most mutations are either repaired or do not survive.

Normal Cell Death

Normal cells die either by apoptosis or necrosis. Apoptosis is also known as programmed cell death and is characterized by bulging of the cell membrane, fracturing of the DNA molecule, formation of apoptotic bodies containing the cell constituents, and finally digestion of the apoptotic bodies by phagocytes. Apoptosis is also known as "cell suicide." Apoptosis is tightly regulated and does not involve inflammation

Cell Progress to Apoptosis

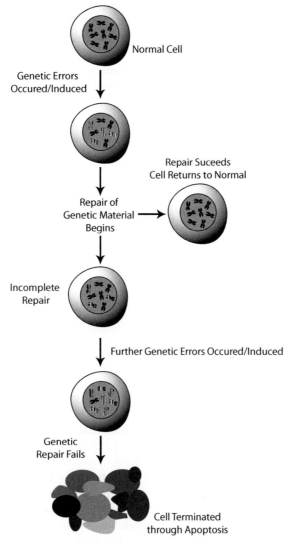

Figure 8.1 Schematic view of a cell's growth, division, mutation, and death. Adapted from the NIH Genetic Home Reference website http://ghr.nlm.nih.gov/.

or swelling of the tissue. Apoptosis is the body's way of recycling the cell's components for reuse (Fig. 8.1).

Necrosis can be considered a "death by trauma" or accidental death caused by injury. Burns, bruises, and cuts are all causes of necrotic death. Necrotic death is characterized by swelling of the cell, membrane rupture, and the uncontrolled release of the cell's contents. This results in inflammation and swelling of neighboring cells and tissues.

Normal Cell Replication Requires an External Growth Signal

Normal cells must wait for an external signal before beginning the reproductive cycle. This is usually either an increase in the strength of an external growth signal or a decrease in an antigrowth signal or some combination of the two. Normal cells do not internally generate growth or antigrowth signals. In all tissues, there is a delicate balance between the growth-promoting genes and the antigrowth-promoting genes. Growth-promoting genes are also called proto-oncogenes. Antigrowth genes are also called tumor suppressor genes.

Normal Cells Obey Antigrowth Signals at Tissue Borders

Cells at the border of an organ receive a different type of antigrowth signal preventing them from extending beyond the boundary surface. As an example, at the surface of the liver, the cells are in contact with nonliver cells. The membranes of the border liver cells send antigrowth signals to their nuclei. Normal cells at the border adjoining a different tissue do not invade across the border because of these border antigrowth signals.

Normal Tissues Have Their Own Blood Supply

The body provides each tissue with its own blood supply to provide food and oxygen for metabolism and to carry away the waste products generated during life.

Normal Cells Are Limited to about 60 Reproductive Cycles

During each reproduction cycle, a cell's DNA loses a small portion of the telomere at the end of the DNA and becomes a bit shorter. This is sometimes called the cell cycle clock.

Telomeres are groups of noncoded ATGC molecules and proteins at the ends of chromosomes. The adenine, thymine, guanine, and cytosine molecules are not in the form of the DNA molecule. They act as counting mechanisms that limit the number of reproductions of a cell, to about 50–70 reproductions. Toward the end of each reproductive cycle, a small section of the telomere is removed. The purpose of the telomere is to mark the end of the DNA molecule. Otherwise, the end of the DNA molecule could stick to another DNA molecule leading to mutations. Alternatively, the DNA repair mechanism could interpret the ends as a double-strand break, which must be repaired or eliminated. Telomeres lose between 50 and 500 base pairs in each replication and eventually are so short the cell's reproduction ceases, leading to senescence or apoptosis. Senescence is a condition where the cell can continue to function, making proteins, hormones, and other products, but does not reproduce. Senescence eventually leads to cell death. The loss of telomeres is part of the natural aging process.

Telomerase counteracts the loss of telomeres during cellular replication. Telomerase is a protein enzyme that adds a DNA sequence to the end of the DNA strand during replication effectively canceling the loss of telomeres. Cells in fetal tissue, very young children, and adult germ cells contain telomerase, so their cells, in effect, do not age. Telomerase is almost undetectable in adult somatic cells, so they undergo aging.

Normal Cells Retain Their Organization

Another trait common to normal cells is the ability to maintain their differentiation. That is, cells always retain their specialty categories whether they are designed for structural support, filtration, protein production, or whatever. This is the way tissues and organs normally function.

CANCER CELLS AND THEIR CHARACTERISTICS

Cancer is a collection of diseases characterized by cells with uncontrolled growth and the ability to spread throughout the body. The name "cancer" comes from ancient physicians who noted that cancers removed from the body had crab-like extensions from the main body of the cancer. Figure 8.2 shows an example of a cancer cell.

Normal cell growth is strictly regulated and controlled. In cancer cells, this control is lost. The cause of cancer is believed to be a series of mutations in cellular DNA. There is strong evidence that each cell in the human body experiences more than 100,000 DNA breaks every day. The vast majority are correctly repaired or sent to apoptosis. Only a tiny fraction of these DNA lesions are repaired incorrectly and survive. Only a small fraction of the surviving lesions are in genes related to cellular repair. Mutations in the cell repair mechanisms are unusually devastating because the repair mechanism is designed to stop mutations.

Damage to the DNA is extremely common and the repair mechanisms are very effective in correcting mistakes in DNA replication. However, given the high frequency of lesions per day in each cell, mistakes in repair are inevitable. Some

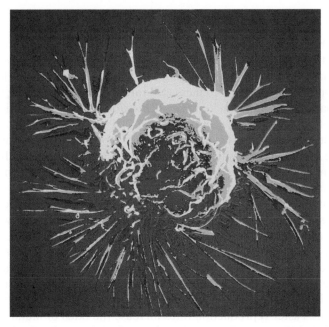

Figure 8.2 Example of extensions from a breast cancer. From a scanning electron microscope image from the National Cancer Institute.

mutated cells may be able to bypass the cell cycle checkpoints and survive. Most survivors die within a few reproductive cycles but Darwin's law comes into play and a few of these survive.

Cancer cells result from a failure of the delicate balance system between growth and antigrowth signals. Almost all cancer cells have at least nine major differences from normal cells. The major difference between benign and cancerous tumors is that cancers spread throughout the body.

THE CHARACTERISTICS OF CANCER CELLS

Cancer cells

- are genetically unstable leading to an increase in replication and mutation rates;
- avoid apoptosis;
- ignore antigrowth signals;
- independently generate internal growth signals. Uncontrolled growth is the first real mark of a cancer;
- ignore boundary signals and become invasive;
- generate signals to develop their own blood supply (angiogenesis);
- live indefinitely, that is, live beyond the normal 50–70 reproductive cycles seen in normal cells;
- spread to distant parts of the body. That is, they metastasize;
- lose differentiation and no longer perform a specific function.

Cancer Cells Exhibit Genetic Instability

Genetic instability is a defining characteristic of cancers. There are two types of genetic instability: *microsatellite instability* (MIN) and *chromosomal instability* (CIN). MIN arises from individual mutations of the DNA chain and leads to elevated mutation rates. CIN refers to increased rates of losing or gaining whole chromosomes or parts of chromosomes during *cell division*. The term "mutation" includes insertion, deletions, duplications, and other "mistakes" in the genome.

Genetic instability has long been hypothesized to be a cardinal feature of cancer. Some of these mutations will add additional "powers" to the offspring. Recent work has strengthened the hypothesis that mutational alterations conferring instability occur early during tumor formation. The genetic instability following a stable mutation drives tumor progression by increasing mutations in proto-oncogenes and tumor suppressor genes. These mutant genes provide cancer cells with survival advantages over normal cells as will be described later in this chapter.

The reason genetic instability is important for cancer growth is that it alters the cell's signals to grow and/or removes some of the cell's growth retardation signals, allowing more errors in DNA replication. In some experimental tumor studies, the mutation rate in cells with genetic instability is five times greater than that of genetically stable cells. Faster reproduction rates increase the odds of mutations, some of which will survive. Thus, genetic instability is thought to increase the chances of cancer developing.

Currently, both chemotherapy and radiation therapy depend on this increased replication rate to differentiate between normal and cancer cells. The success of chemotherapy and radiation therapy depends on the increased replication rate of cancer cells relative to normal cells and the ability of normal cells to more rapidly recover from either chemical or radiation agents.

Genetic instability, a trademark of cancer, allows cancer cells to change their form and function from one generation to the next and to vary greatly from their origin.

The progression from normal cell to cancer cell requires many steps, and the order of these steps is not well established. The basic hypothesis is that there is an initial mutation that escapes the cell's checkpoints and apoptosis. The disagreement is on what comes next. One hypothesis says this first mutation creates a "master gene cell" because it confers the "escape" ability to its offspring who then can undergo additional mutations.

Each of the steps toward a full cancer cell requires a mutation of the DNA molecule at a specific location. The mutation is caused by some internal or external stress. Such stresses include internal waste products from the cell's metabolic activity as well as external factors such as radiation, alcohol, tobacco smoke, and various chemicals. The exact order of these mutations is not clear and may vary considerably. For example, ignoring or bypassing boundary layer antigrowth signals may require a separate mutation. However, the generation of an internal growth signal without an external stress trigger may override the "stop at the border" signal without requiring an additional mutation.

Cancer Cells Evade Apoptosis

Some mutations involve the *p53* gene, one of the genes responsible for initiating apoptosis. With damage to the *p53* gene, or one of the genes responding to the *p53* gene signals, the mutated cell can bypass the repair checkpoints and produces two daughter cells. These daughter cells and their offspring will continue to reproduce whenever an external signal for growth appears. Such a mutation is not, by itself, enough to result in uncontrolled growth because the mutated cells at this stage must still wait for an external growth signal.

Cancer Cells Ignore Antigrowth Signals

Cancer cells ignore antigrowth signals and can keep on replicating once given a growth signal. This mutation triggers uncontrolled growth until limited by the lack of blood supply or the internal cell clock that limits the number of replications allowed.

Cancer Cells Generate Their Own Internal Growth Signals

At some time, the pro- and/or antigrowth genes may be damaged so that once a cell has passed the apoptosis barrier, it can generate its own internal growth signal instead of waiting for an outside stimulus. This means the cell and its descendants can continue to grow until checked by external factors. These factors include a lack of nutrients and oxygen, buildup of waste products, or the presence of a border with another tissue. Of course, if the "stop at the boundary" signal has already been damaged by a previous mutation, growth will continue until lack of oxygen or nutrients or a failure to remove waste products prevents further growth.

Cancer Cells Ignore Antigrowth Signals at Boundaries

At the surface of the liver, the cells are in contact with nonliver cells. The membranes of the border liver cells send antigrowth signals to their nucleus stopping further growth. In cancer cells, the antigrowth signals from the cells at the border are ignored or suppressed, and the cancer cells continue to spread beyond the border.

Cancer Cells Generate Their Own Blood Supply (Angiogenesis)

The ability of cancer cells to generate their own blood supply is a crucial step in their progression. Without the ability to create their own independent blood supply, they would remain just a localized clump of cells smaller than a sesame seed. Tumors depending on an existing blood vessel are limited to about a 100-μm radius, which is the diffusion distance of oxygen, nutrients, and waste products. The development of independent blood vessels is signaled by the release of vascular endothelial growth factor (VEGF), which stimulates the growth of new blood vessels. One of the current areas of cancer research is the use of VEGF suppressors to inhibit the growth of cancer. However, VEGF is needed by the body for wound healing and injury repair, so completely shutting down VEGF is undesirable.

Cancer Cells Reproduce Indefinitely

Cancer cells continue to reproduce because they reset the cellular clock that limits the number of reproductive cycles of a cell. They accomplish this by replacing the telomeres contained on each chromosome. Cancer cells contain telomerase, which replaces lost telomeres in adult cancer cells and so cancer cells can reproduce indefinitely.

Cancer Cells Metastasize

Cancer cells lose some of the components in their membranes that hold them to their neighbors. Cancer cell membranes lose the molecules that keep normal cells in the right place. This means cancer cells can become detached from their neighbors. When the cell membranes are altered, they are then able to leave their origin site and move to other locations through the blood or lymphatic systems. This partially explains how cancer cells spread to other parts of the body. The ability to metastasize is one of the features that make cancers so deadly. Cancers that invade other organs often grow and disrupt vital organ functions, leading to death.

Cancer Cells Lose Their Cell Type or Differentiation

Cancer cells gradually no longer maintain their tissue type. This is partially because they become more and more genetically unstable. With further reproductions, they revert to a more undifferentiated appearance of primitive or stem cells rather than maintaining their highly specialized functions and form. They lose their identity.

TABLE 8.1 Clinical Grades of Cancer and Their Characteristics

Grade	Description
1	Well differentiated
2	Moderately differentiated
3	Poorly differentiated
4	Undifferentiated

These steps from normal cells to a full formed cancer refute to the statement that "one radiation mutation can produce a cancer." Cancer formation requires multiple complex steps.

CANCER GRADE

In clinical cancer treatments, it is common to refer to the "grade" of a cancer. This is a scale used to describe in descriptive terms how far the cancer cell has progressed away from a normal cell when viewed under a microscope. A low-grade cancer looks very much like a normal cell with only minor differences between the cancer and a normal cell from the same tissue. It is referred to as "well differentiated." A higher-grade cancer appears less similar to a normal cell. In general, the more a cancer cell looks like a normal cell, the more likely it will act like a normal cell. Higher-grade cancer cells are more primitive and likely to reproduce faster. Undifferentiated cancer cells have a higher mitotic index. Table 8.1 shows the different cellular pathological grades and their characteristics.

TRADITIONAL HYPOTHESIS OF CANCER DEVELOPMENT

The traditional hypothesis of cancer views cancer development as a linear process with one mutation following another over time. The exact order of the mutations is not clear, but in the traditional hypothesis, some mutations had to occur before others. A mutation's offspring would have to wait until the next mutation in line occurs before the mutated cell could take the next step toward a fully developed cancer.

One problem with this hypothesis is that there does not appear to be enough time for all the necessary mutations to occur during a person's lifetime, where each cell undergoes at most, 50–70 cell divisions. Although a single-cell replication cycle is less than 24 hours, most cells in the body live and function for several months before undergoing a replication.

Thirty years ago, almost all scientists thought that cancer arose following a linear series of gene mutations caused by external factors, including radiation. This is known as the traditional hypothesis. Recently, at least three competing hypotheses on the origin and development of cancer have emerged. They can be termed as the (a) the random multimutation, (b) master gene, and the (c) multichromosome hypotheses. Although similar, the predictions regarding treatment aims and results

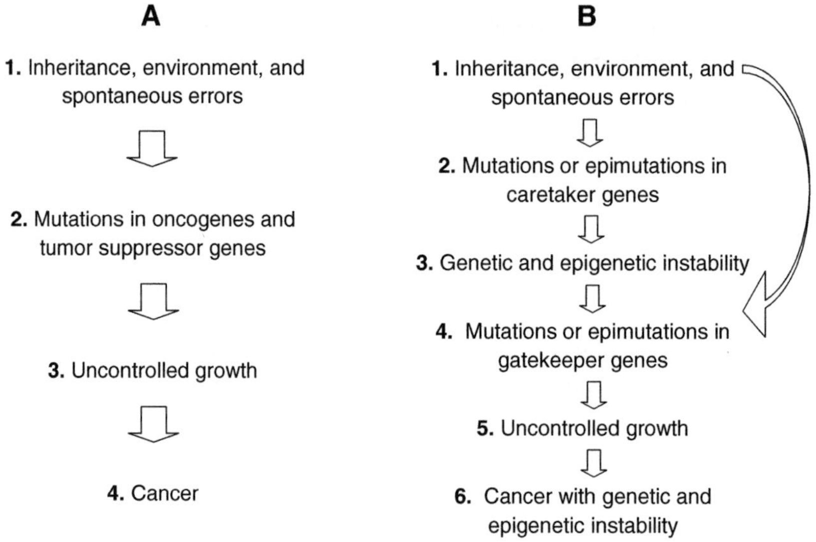

A

1. Inheritance, environment, and spontaneous errors

⇩

2. Mutations in oncogenes and tumor suppressor genes

⇩

3. Uncontrolled growth

⇩

4. Cancer

B

1. Inheritance, environment, and spontaneous errors

⇩

2. Mutations or epimutations in caretaker genes

⇩

3. Genetic and epigenetic instability

⇩

4. Mutations or epimutations in gatekeeper genes

⇩

5. Uncontrolled growth

⇩

6. Cancer with genetic and epigenetic instability

Figure 8.3 Schematic illustration of the traditional and random multimutation models of carcinogenesis. The major difference is that the traditional model suggested the steps from normal to cancer occurred in a 1-2-3... linear series. The random multimutation model postulates that the mutations along the DNA chain can occur in any order and those mutations further down the line are inactive until their turn comes.

are different. Here, we briefly discuss similarities and differences of the three hypotheses and the implications for cancer prevention and treatments (Fig. 8.3).

The Random Multimutation Hypothesis of Cancer Development

The modified hypothesis postulates a series of many random mutations. The random/multimutation hypothesis is similar to the traditional hypothesis except that it does not require a specific order for the mutations to occur. In this hypothesis, a "downstream mutation" could occur first. For example, the mutation permitting metastases or the mutation producing telomerase may be among the first mutations occurring. This hypothesis only requires that a mutation be fixed permanently in the DNA and passed on to future generation of the mutated somatic cells.

The Master Gene Hypothesis of Cancer Development

The master gene hypothesis postulates that few "master genes" control the growth rate of cells, and when one of these is mutated but survives, the regulation of growth rate is lost. Much effort has been expended in searching for a "master gene," but so far none has been found that is present in all tumors.

The Aneuploidy or Multichromosome Hypothesis of Cancer Development

Normal human cells have 46 chromosomes in 23 pairs. They are diploid. Cancer cells however usually have between 60 and 90 chromosomes. This difference in chromosome number causes problems during the cell reproduction cycle. The addition of added chromosomes can be caused by the same stresses (radiation, toxic agents, and free radicals) that cause DNA breaks, deletions, and substitutions in the DNA chain. The mechanisms are still under study, but the result is additional chromosomes in aneuploid cells. Studies show that over 90% of cancers contain aneuploid cells, and some researchers believe all cancers exhibit aneuploidy. The reason aneuploidy is important is that it destroys the genetic stability of the cell. Most aneuploid cells do not survive but a few do, and their descendants can continue to reproduce. It is known that Down's syndrome children have an extra copy of chromosome 21. One extra chromosome is sufficient to cause this syndrome. The aneuploidy hypothesis says that some of the many induced instabilities can eventually lead to all the steps required for a full-blown cancer.

PREDICTIONS REGARDING TREATMENT

Cancer seems to grow in spurts and starts. The mutations may come from a lack of tumor suppressor genes, an excess of oncogenes after a proto-oncogene has been transformed, or some mutations in the genes producing signal proteins. Depending on the particular hypothesis under consideration, the treatment of choice will vary.

Traditional and Random Multimutation Hypotheses

These hypotheses predict that the cancer cells are dependent on the proteins made by the oncogenes, that is, all the signals from the mutated genes that cause uncontrolled growth, generation of independent blood supply, and the production of telomerase for example. Treatments may be directed at breaking this dependence on the products of the oncogenes. If this is not possible, then searching for a way to enhance the effectiveness of the tumor suppressor genes and/or work on ways to delay the growth of tumor cells should be pursued.

Predictions Regarding the Master Gene Hypothesis

If cancer is produced by mutations of a master gene, then after identifying the master gene(s), efforts can be focused on either protecting or repairing the master genes. Screening of high-risk individuals could be followed and their "master genes" studied for characteristic mutations.

Predictions Regarding the Excess Aneuploidy Hypothesis

The excess aneuploidy hypothesis predicts that effective treatments would depend on screening for cells with excess chromosomes and then destroying them. This may not be simple or effective in that there are many naturally occurring aneuploidic cells that do not turn into cancer.

RADIATION AND CANCER

Radiation is one of the first agents shown to cause cancer. Less than 10 years after the discovery of X-rays, Clarence Dally, one of Thomas Edison's assistants, died of cancer caused by exposure to X-rays. Radiation is neither the most prevalent nor the most efficient agent in producing mutations and cancer but is certainly a proven cancer-causing agent at high doses. All studies have shown that small radiation doses do not produce detectable increases in cancer.

SUMMARY AND IMPORTANT POINTS

- Cancer development is a complex process requiring many mutations.
- Cancer cells are genetically unstable leading to an increase in replication and mutation rates.
- Cancer cells avoid apoptosis.
- Cancer cells ignore antigrowth signals.
- Cancer cells independently generate internal growth signals. Uncontrolled growth is the first real mark of a cancer.
- Cancer cells ignore boundary signals and become invasive.
- Cancer cells generate signals to develop their own blood supply (angiogenesis).
- Cancer cells contain telomerase so they can live indefinitely, that is, live beyond the normal 50–70 reproductive cycles seen in normal cells.
- Cancer cells metastasize as they spread to distant parts of the body.
- Cancer cells lose differentiation and no longer perform a specific function.

BIBLIOGRAPHY

Andersen LD, Remington P, Trentham-Dietz A, Reeves M. Assessing a decade of progress in cancer control. Oncologist. 2002;7(3):200–4.

Balmain A, Gray J, Ponder B. The genetics and genomics of cancer. Nat Genet. 2003 Marc; 33(Suppl.):238–44.

Carmeliet P, Jain RK. Angiogenesis in cancer and other diseases. Nature. 2000 September 14;407(6801):249–57.

Couzin J. Medicine. Tracing the steps of metastasis, cancer's menacing ballet. Science. 2003 February 14;299(5609):1002–6.

Fearon ER. Human cancer syndromes: Clues to the origin and nature of cancer. Science. 1997 November 7;278(5340):1043–50.

Gibbs WW. Untangling the roots of cancer. Sci Am. 2003 July;289(1):56–65.

Hanahan D, Weinberg RA. The hallmarks of cancer. Cell. 2000 January 7;100(1):57–70.

Jones PA, Baylin SB. The fundamental role of epigenetic events in cancer. Nat Rev Genet. 2002 June;3(6):415–28.

Kinzler KW, Vogelstein B. Cancer-susceptibility genes. Gatekeepers and caretakers. Nature. 1997 April 24;386(6627):761–3.

Nurse P. The incredible life and times of biological cells. Science. 2000 September 8;289(5485):1711–6.

Trichopoulos D, Li FP, Hunter DJ. What causes cancer? Sci Am. 1996 September; 275(3):80–7.

Vogelstein B, Kinzler KW. Cancer genes and the pathways they control. Nat Med. 2004 September;10(8):789–99.

QUESTIONS

Chapter 8   Questions

1. _____ is a group of coded ATGC molecules and proteins that stops or replaces the telomeres at the end of chromosomes, which are normally snipped off during each reproductive cycle.
   a. Telomeresnip
   b. Oleomerase
   c. Telomerase
   d. Micromase

2. Proto-oncogenes
   a. provide tumor suppressor signals.
   b. provide growth signals.
   c. modify oncogenes in response to stress.
   d. develop into oncogenes with aging.

3. Tumor-promoting genes are known as
   a. tumo-genes.
   b. proto-oncogenes.
   c. promo-genes.
   d. oncogenes.

4. Traditional and modified traditional hypothesis indicate cancer is produced by _____ the cell's DNA.
   a. excess chromosomes on
   b. mutations of
   c. superpowers of
   d. genetic instabilities in

5. Genome stability is required
   a. to initiate mutations.
   b. to maintain species properties.
   c. to prevent mutations.
   d. to prevent emotional instability.

6. Cells die by
   i. leathalocrosis
   ii. necrosis
   iii. fatalist microbism
   iv. apoptosis
   a. i, ii, iii
   b. ii, iv
   c. i, ii, iv
   d. i, ii, iii, iv

7. Cancer cells can reproduce indefinitely because they contain
   a. proto-oncogenes.
   b. telomerase.
   c. cytoplasmic mastics.
   d. aneuploidy bodies.

8. For a cell to metastasize means it
   a. can grow indefinitely.
   b. has made its own blood supply.
   c. has spread outside its tissue borders into the body.
   d. can live indefinitely.

9. Aneuploidy cells have an abnormal number of
   a. chromosomes.
   b. ploidies.
   c. organelles.
   d. nuclei.

10. A fully developed cancer will have a grade of
    a. well differentiated.
    b. unimpacted.
    c. very well developed.
    d. undifferentiated.

11. The current hypotheses of cancer development are the
    i. linear hypothesis of cancer development
    ii. angiogenic hypothesis
    iii. random multimutation hypothesis
    iv. master gene hypothesis
    v. excess aneuploidy hypothesis
    a. i, ii, iii, iv
    b. i, ii, iii, iv, v
    c. i, iii, iv, v
    d. i, ii, iv, v

12. The difference between benign and cancer tumors is that
    a. benign tumors stop growing when they reach a critical size.
    b. cancer tumors develop extraordinarily long blood vessels.
    c. cancer tumors can spread to different parts of the body.
    d. benign tumors quickly show invasive characteristics.

13. When a cell is damaged by radiation,
  a. the damage will probably be repaired.
  b. radiation mitosis results.
  c. there is a high probability of cancer.
  d. there is a more than 50% chance of cell death.

14. Faulty repair of radiation damage usually results in
  a. cancer.
  b. mutations in future generations of offspring.
  c. apoptosis.
  d. giant cell recombination.

15. The most radiosensitive cells are those that divide _____ and are relatively ____ differentiated.
  a. slowly, well
  b. rapidly, well
  c. slowly, poorly
  d. rapidly, poorly

16. The presence of _____ allows cancer cells to reproduce indefinitely.
  a. telomeres
  b. telomerase
  c. micromerase
  d. oncomerase

CHAPTER 9

RADIATION EFFECTS ON TISSUES AND ORGANS

KEYWORDS

Stochastic, deterministic, radiation cataract, thyroid, fetus, latent period, radiation damage, tissue damage

TOPICS

- Radiation latent period
- Stochastic and deterministic effects
- Radiation effects on the blood vessels
- Ionizing radiation effects on the skin
- Radiation cataract formation
- Radiation effects on the thyroid

Following the previous chapters' discussions of microscopic radiation effects on cells, this chapter turns to the larger macroscopic effects on tissues and organs. A tissue is an assembly of cells, which, as an entity, carries out a particular function. An organ is a collection of tissues combined to provide a function or service for the body. Usually, organs are made up of functional tissue, the parenchyma, and the supporting tissues, the stroma. For example, the parenchymal tissue in the heart is the myocardium. It is responsible for pumping blood through the body. The stromal

Radiation Biology of Medical Imaging, First Edition. Charles A. Kelsey, Philip H. Heintz,
Daniel J. Sandoval, Gregory D. Chambers, Natalie L. Adolphi, and Kimberly S. Paffett.
© 2014 John Wiley & Sons, Inc. Published 2014 by John Wiley & Sons, Inc.

tissues of the heart include the connective tissues, blood vessels, and nerves supporting the myocardium. The effects of exposure to the entire body are treated in the next chapter.

Radiation damage is different from most forms of trauma because radiation damage can destroy the cell's ability to reproduce but may not interfere with its function. If a cell cannot complete the cell cycle and does not reproduce, it has undergone reproductive death. This is the most common lethal effect of radiation damage. In reproductive death, the cell may continue its functions, producing hormones, proteins, and so on, but is unable to reproduce. Reproductive death does not lead to cancer.

X-rays were shown to cause biological effects shortly after their discovery by Wilhelm Conrad Roentgen in 1895. In fact, the early researchers often estimated the radiation output of their X-ray tubes by exposing a patch of skin. A dose that produced noticeable skin reddening was known as an erythema dose. In today's units, an erythema dose corresponds to about 7 Gy. Recall that the gray (Gy) is the radiation unit used to measure the radiation energy absorbed by tissue. Less than 10 years after the discovery of X-rays, Clarence Dally, one of Thomas Edison's assistants, died of cancer caused by exposure to X-rays. Dally was working on developing an X-ray fluoroscope. After Dally's death, Edison dropped all research on X-rays.

LATENT PERIOD

Over the years, the "law" of Bergonié and Tribondeau has been modified to more accurately describe the responses seen in humans. We now recognize that the effect of radiation is essentially the same for all tissues and organs, but the time for the damage to be expressed depends on the mitotic index of the cells. That is, cells with higher cell turnover and higher replication rates show radiation damage sooner and hence appear to be more sensitive to radiation. Basically, there is no difference in the radiation damage to cells showing early or late effects. The only difference is the time when the effects appear. Different tissues and organs however will show different responses to radiation depending on the mix of cells in the tissues. The response of an organ and its apparent radiosensitivity varies depending on the mixture of tissues making up the organ.

The latent period is the time between radiation exposure and the appearance of an effect. The latent period is one of the prime indicators of tissue radiosensitivity. This is because early and late effects are easier to observe in a living organism than mitotic indices or cell turnover rates. Tissues with mixed populations can show both early and late effects. In such a case, there may be two latent periods, one for appearance of the early and a second latent period for the late effect. Acute, early effects are those that appear within about a month of exposure. Late effects can appear months or years after exposure. These early and late reactions are important to the clinician because radiation damage may appear bimodal in time with a significant time period between the appearance of early and late effects. Skin is an organ with high turnover dermal cells and lower turnover stromal cells. Skin shows early effects, a period of apparent healing and then in the case of high doses, a late, serious, and difficult-to-heal injury. Figure 9.1 presents a schematic illustration of a bimodal plot

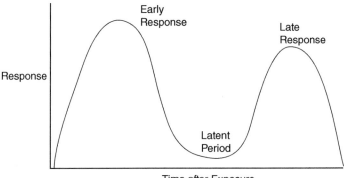

Figure 9.1 A schematic representation of a biphasic response to radiation injury. The intensity of the response and the latent period between the early and late effects is dependent on the radiation dose and the amount of tissue irradiated. The latent periods of the early and late response have been used to provide an estimate of the radiation dose. A shorter time between the exposure and the appearance of radiation effects indicates a larger radiation dose.

showing how the early effect can be separated by a significant time period before the late effects become manifest.

DETERMINISTIC AND STOCHASTIC RADIATION DAMAGE

There are two types of radiation damage: deterministic and stochastic. Deterministic effects are also called tissue reactions because some of the effects are determined before or after the radiation exposure. Tissue reactions or deterministic effects can be modified after the exposure. The damage in a deterministic event or tissue reaction depends on the dose. Radiation burns and cataract induction are examples of deterministic effects; the greater the dose, the more severe the effect. Deterministic effects may have a threshold. A threshold dose is the dose below which no injury is evident. Figure 9.2 shows a schematic illustration of the severity of a deterministic effect as a function of radiation dose with the threshold dose indicated. The latent period is inversely proportional to the dose; that is, a lower dose has a longer period between the radiation exposure and the appearance of the tissue reaction.

STOCHASTIC EFFECTS

In a stochastic effect, increasing the dose increases the probability of damage, but the severity of the effect is independent of the dose. Cancer induction and genetic effects are stochastic effects. Stochastic effects are governed by probability. A particular gene in the DNA is or is not damaged. There is no middle ground. The results of a lottery drawing are similar to a stochastic event. Buying more tickets (higher dose) increases the chances of winning but does not increase the prize.

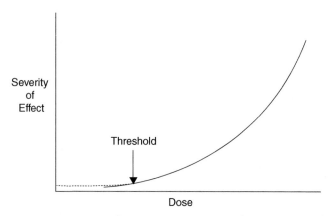

Figure 9.2 Schematic illustration of the relationship between severity of effect and radiation dose for a tissue reaction, formerly called a deterministic effect. The severity of a tissue reaction increases as the dose increases. Note that the existence of a threshold does *not* mean that there is no damage below the threshold, only that it is not evident.

The difference between stochastic and deterministic effects is basically the level of interactions. Stochastic effects arise from interactions at the cellular level, primarily with the DNA molecule. If these interactions result in mutations passed on to future generations, they can lead to cancer or genetic effects. Deterministic effects on the other hand result from damage to groups of cells forming tissues and organs. If damage to cells making up a tissue is large enough to affect the tissue function, the effect will be evident in the loss of tissue function and the threshold dose is exceeded.

RADIATION EFFECTS ON TISSUES

Most information on radiation effects on normal tissues and organs comes from observations during and after radiation therapy treatments. This is because the doses and effects during radiation cancer treatments are carefully monitored. Cancer treatments with radiation began within a few years of Roentgen's discovery. Radiation treatment of cancer is based on the fact that rapidly dividing cells are more sensitive to radiation. Cancer is made up of rapidly dividing cells, so the cancer cells are expected to be more sensitive to radiation than normal tissue. The major challenge in radiation therapy is to eradicate the cancer without unduly damaging surrounding normal tissues. Even today, the amount of radiation delivered to the tumor is limited by the collateral damage to nearby normal tissues. Radiation oncologists have been observing radiation injuries to normal tissues since the birth of the field. Early treatments were limited by the poor penetrating ability of the radiation, so skin reactions limited the dose that could be safely delivered to deeper lying tumors. In the 1950s and 1960s, higher-energy radiation beams became available and data on radiation effects to internal tissues and organs became available.

In radiation oncology, the damage to organs is reported in terms of a tumor dose (TD) that produces complications in normal tissues with 5% probability within 5 years following the end of radiation treatment. This is termed the normal tissue complication probability (NTCP) TD 5/5. Another term used in radiation oncology is NTCP TD 50/5, which is the tumor dose that produces a 50% NTCP in 5 years. These terms are normally not used outside the field of radiation therapy because other medical doses are so much smaller than those used in radiation therapy.

Some important organs, their TD 5/5 and 50/5 values, and the effects of radiation on the tissues are presented here in alphabetical order.

Bladder

The doses for serious complications are 65 Gy TD for NTCP of 5% in 5 years and 80 Gy TD for NTCP of 50% in 5 years. The complications are bladder contraction, volume loss, and difficulty in completely emptying or leaking from the bladder. These are extremely high-radiation doses and will be encountered only in radiation oncology cancer treatments or very serious radiation accidents.

Blood and Blood Vessels

After a significant (>1 Gy) radiation dose from exposure to the whole body, all blood elements are adversely affected. Increases in dose result in an increased effect, and the effects are seen earlier. In the case of a whole body exposure from a radiation accident, the loss of white blood cells means the body's defenses against infection are diminished. Damage to the skin and intestine make the body particularly vulnerable to bacterial infection during the first few weeks following exposures greater than 1 Gy.

A person exposed to 1 Gy has their lymphocyte cell count reduced. He or she will be more susceptible to infection. Early symptoms of such exposures mimic the flu, that is, loss of appetite, nausea, diarrhea, and vomiting. The chapter on whole body radiation treats the effects of decreased white blood cells following radiation exposure more completely.

Most of the long term, late effects on tissues and organs are the result of injury to blood vessels, especially to those making up the microvasculature. Damage to the capillaries bringing oxygen and nutrients to the cells of an organ will inevitably affect its function.

The interior surface of blood and lymphatic vessels is lined with a thin layer of endothelial cells which form a barrier between the circulating blood or lymph inside the vessel and the vessel wall. Damage to the endothelial cells allows white blood cells and fluids to pass through the vessel. Radiation at lower doses can cause damage to the capillary vessels. Such changes can include less flexibility and greater vessel stiffness leading to decreased perfusion. This is especially important in the blood vessels, brain, and skin. Figure 9.3 is a scanning electron microscope image of a blood platelet on interior surface of a damaged blood vessel. The blood platelet illustrated is ready to start the formation of a blood clot.

Bone

The doses for serious complications of bone are 52 Gy TD for NTCP of 5% in 5 years and 65 Gy TD for NTCP of 50% in 5 years. The complications are necrosis and pathologic fractures without any external trauma.

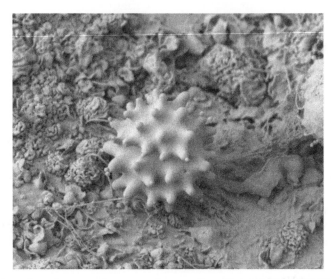

Figure 9.3 Scanning electron microscope image of a platelet on the interior surface of a damaged blood vessel ready to begin clot formation. Image by Mark Turmaine, Department of Cell and Developmental Biology, University College London, reproduced by permission. From Bolsover et al. (2011), chapter 15, figure 15.4, p. 255.

Brain

Because brain cells do not reproduce, they are not significantly damaged unless their blood supply is compromised. The doses for major complications of the brain are 45 Gy TD for NTCP of 5% in 5 years and 60 Gy TD for NTCP of 50% in 5 years. Complications are necrosis and an infarction. An infarction is a group of tissue that dies because of a lack of oxygen caused by an obstruction of the tissue's blood supply. There are reports of decrease in IQ scores of about one IQ point per 4 mSv.

Breast

Radiation treatment for breast cancer is usually spread out over 6 weeks with five 2-Gy treatments per week. This results in a total dose of approximately 60 Gy.

Late side effects from breast irradiation usually appear one or more years after treatment. The two major long-term complications of breast radiation treatments are fibrosis and lymphedema. Fibrosis is a hardening or stiffening of the tissues due to loss of elasticity due to a diffuse scarring. Lymphedema is a swelling due to localized fluid retention caused by damage to the lymphatic system. The complications are the result of blood vessel and connective tissue damage that were in the radiation field. Studies have shown that there is no increase in thyroid cancer following radiation treatment for breast cancer.

Esophagus

The doses for major complications of the esophagus are 55 Gy TD for NTCP of 5% in 5 years and 68 Gy TD for NTCP of 50% in 5 years. These are extremely high-radiation doses and will be encountered only in radiation oncology cancer treatments or very serious radiation accidents.

Major complications include necrosis of the lining of the esophagus. The esophagus, the tube leading from the mouth to the stomach, is located between the lungs in the chest. During radiation to lungs to treat lung cancer, the esophagus is often included in the radiation field. Pain or difficulty with swallowing, heartburn, and a sensation of a lump in the throat are side effects of the radiation. Symptoms usually occur 2–3 weeks into therapy and subside a few weeks after completing treatments.

Eye

Eye doses for complications due to radiation exposure to the eye are 50 Gy TD for NTCP of 5% in 5 years and 65 Gy TD for NTCP of 50% in 5 years. These extremely high doses can lead to blindness.

Cataract Formation   The major complication of radiation to the eye is cataract formation, which is classified as a tissue reaction/deterministic effect with a threshold. Radiation cataracts begin as an opacity near the posterior pole of the eye and progress forward. For many years, the threshold for cataract induction was believed to be about 2 Gy from chronic exposures over many years. Fractionated doses can cause the formation of cataracts after a latent period of 2 years or more depending on the age of the individual and the time period of exposure. Recent studies however have shown that the threshold for cataract formation may be significantly lower. Interventional physicians with exposures spread over many years have shown cataract formation at cumulative doses as low as 0.8 Gy.

The current regulatory limit is set at 150 mGy/year. This limit was established to reduce the risk of radiation-induced cataracts. Recently, in 2011, the International Commission on Radiation Protection (ICRP) has issued a statement that the threshold in absorbed dose for the lens of the eye is now considered to be 0.5 Gy. For occupational exposures, the ICRP now recommends an equivalent dose limit for the lens of the eye of 20 mSv in any 1 year. Although this recommendation does not have the force of law, the recommendation of this international body probably will influence on what is considered good medical practice.

Fetus

Cells most susceptible to radiation damage are those engaged in rapid division and growth. This makes unborn babies particularly sensitive to radiation exposure. There are many possible biological effects of radiation on embryos and fetuses including miscarriage, developmental delays such as smaller head size, mental retardation, and childhood cancer. Fetal doses less than 100 mGy are considered below the level of concern for radiation damage to the fetus. Radiation dose to the fetus is about 25% of the entrance skin dose. Fetal effects from radiation are somatic.

Miscarriage   The effect of a pregnant woman's exposure to radiation depends on the gestational age of the fetus. Radiation exposure during later stages of pregnancy can produce developmental delays and increased incidence of cancer. The newly fertilized conceptus is especially sensitive to radiation damage because each of the cells in the conceptus is vital to the proper development of the fetus. Any significant radiation damage during the first 2 weeks of pregnancy will lead to miscarriage. That is, in utero exposure during the first 2 weeks of pregnancy radiation damage is an "all-or-nothing" effect.

Developmental Delays Radiation damage to the fetus can lead to delayed growth and development of the fetus. The damage may persist as a developmental delay well into childhood. In particular, radiation-exposed fetuses may have smaller than average head, may have brain sizes that are small for their gestational age, and may display cognitive deficits associated with delayed brain development.

One of the most disturbing effects of fetal radiation exposure is either retarded brain growth or mental retardation or both as a result of underdevelopment of brain cells. The fetus is most sensitive to mental retardation due to radiation exposure during the 8–16 weeks of pregnancy. This is when the brain is most rapidly developing. Decrease in mental acuity has been noted only in doses above 100 mGy. During the 8- to 16-week period, the decrease is estimated to be about 30 IQ points per gray.

Childhood Cancer Childhood cancers are more likely in babies who were exposed to radiation in utero or infancy. During this time, their cells are rapidly replicating and are more sensitive to radiation. The rate of cancer deaths from radiation is 5%/Sv for adults and may be as much as twice high for infants and young children.

The consensus of experts has been that abortion due to fear of radiation effects on the fetus should not be considered at radiation doses *to the fetus* of 100 mGy or less. A reasonable estimate of fetal dose from diagnostic plane imaging is one quarter (25%) of the entrance skin dose. The fetal dose from computed tomography (CT) examinations is equal to the computed tomography dose index (CTDI). See Chapter 12 for a discussion of the CTDI.

Genetically Significant Dose (GSD)

The GSD was developed in the 1950s in attempt to provide an estimate of the effect man-made radiation would have on the genetic pool. The GSD (in gray) is an estimated dose, which if given to the gonads of the entire population would produce the same genetic effect as is actually observed. The GSD is *not* an estimate of the genetic effects of radiation. The GSD was developed as a way to compare the importance of various sources of radiation on possible genetic effect. The current estimate of the GSD in the United States is 0.02 mGy (200 µGy). This should be compared with the dose from natural radiation of about 3 mGy.

Heart Damage due to Radiation

The doses for major heart complications are 40 Gy TD for NTCP of 5% in 5 years and 50 Gy TD for NTCP of 50% in 5 years. The ICRP has issued precautionary warnings that damage to the heart, blood vessels, and brain may be seen at doses as low as 0.5 Gy. Such doses can be reached during some complex interventional procedures. Radiation damages the heart by damaging the heart muscle, the valves, or the coronary arteries. A significant complication of heart irradiation is pericarditis. Pericarditis is inflammation of the sac surrounding the heart. The most common symptom of pericarditis is a stabbing, sharp pain in the chest, which becomes stronger when exercising or taking a deep breath.

Damage to the heart muscle, called cardiomyopathy, most often results in a stiff left ventricle, which does not respond to signals to pump more blood. During strenuous physical exercise activity, the stiff left ventricle may not be capable of increased pumping action. When this happens, the blood that is being pumped through the left side of the heart is not pumped out fast enough, and some of the blood backs up in the small blood vessels of the lungs. The oxygen in the lungs is supposed to be transferred to these small blood vessels. When these vessels become engorged with the backlogged blood, the oxygen cannot be transferred to the heart, resulting in congestive heart failure.

Damage to the heart valves is a second problem resulting from radiation exposure. The heart valves lose flexibility and become stiff following radiation exposure. The stiffened valves do not seal properly and leak blood back into the heart chambers, which should be sending blood throughout the body. The amount of blood ejected from the heart during each heartbeat decreases.

Radiation can also cause coronary artery disease. Radiation can damage the small blood vessels, which supply the heart with oxygen and nutrition. The interior lining of healthy blood vessels is smooth. Radiation can roughen the inside of blood vessels. These rough spots provide a site for fatty deposits (plaques) to develop in coronary arteries and other arteries and veins. Calcium deposits can harden the plaques resulting in atherosclerosis (hardening of the arteries). Coronary artery disease occurs when one of the heart vessels is clogged with plaque. If this happens, the heart muscle may begin to weaken and die because it cannot get enough oxygen and nutrition.

If the heart tries to beat faster but is deprived of enough oxygen or nutrition, chest pain (angina) results. The angina may last a few minutes until the oxygen gets through the partially clogged artery. If the heart vessel is completely blocked, that section of the heart muscle may die. If the muscle section is small, then the result is a minor heart attack. Blockage of a larger coronary artery supplying a larger amount of heart muscle is damaged; the heart attack is serious and can be life threatening. The left anterior descending coronary artery is known as the "widow maker" because sudden blockage of it often leads to a fatal heart attack.

Intestine

The major complications of intestinal exposure occur at 40 Gy TD for NTCP of 5% in 5 years and at 55 Gy TD for NTCP of 50% in 5 years. Complications include obstruction and/or perforation leading to massive infection. Radiation damage to the intestinal tract lining will cause nausea, bloody vomiting, and diarrhea. This occurs when the intestine receives an exposure greater than about 2 Gy. The radiation will begin to destroy the rapidly dividing intestinal cells.

The most radiation-sensitive cells in the intestine are the immature stem cells. These immature stem cells are located at the base of the villi (the crypts) in the intestine. They maintain the supply of stem cells for development into mature functioning intestinal cells. The stem cells in the crypts of the intestine develop into intermediate cells, which differentiate into mature cells as they migrate up to the top of the villi. During this migration, they receive signals directing them to develop into specialized cells designed to function as part of an organ. In the mature stage, they actively perform their specialized functions. These functions include absorption of nutrients from the gut and the discharge of waste products into the intestine. This development and migration requires about 14 days. The mature gut cells at the top of the villi are soughed off at the end of their life cycle. Thus, the effects of intestinal radiation become evident about 2 weeks after exposure. The intestine is no longer able to maintain the barrier between the body waste inside the intestine and the bloodstream. This occurs just as the white blood cell population, essential for fighting infection, is dropping. The subsequent infection is often fatal.

Kidneys

Major complication following exposures of the kidney occurs at 23 Gy TD for NTCP of 5% in 5 years and at 28 Gy TD for NTCP of 50% in 5 years. Complications include clinical nephritis and kidney failure. A single dose of 6 Gy to kidneys shows early (within 48 hours) damage. A single dose of 10 Gy results in protein spilling into the urine indicating inadequate filtration by the irradiated kidney. Radiation nephritis usually does not occur until months after the kidneys are exposed.

Liver

The doses for major complications following exposure to the liver are 30 Gy TD for NTCP of 5% in 5 years and 40 Gy TD for NTCP of 50% in 5 years. Major complications include jaundice and liver failure. Jaundice results in a yellow tint of the skin and the whites of the eyes.

Lungs

The doses for major complications of the lungs are 17.5 Gy TD for NTCP of 5% in 5 years and 24.5 Gy TD for NTCP of 50% in 5 years. Complications following radiation treatment for lung cancer include persistent cough and pneumonitis.

Radiation exposure can lower the amount of lung surfactant, a substance that helps the lungs expand. This can result in a dry cough and shortness of breath. Radiation pneumonitis is an inflammatory response of the lungs to radiation, which usually occurs 1–6 months following the completion of radiation therapy. It is often treated with a short course of steroids. Symptoms include a fever, cough, and shortness of breath. Roughly 5–15% of individuals develop this symptom following treatment for lung cancer. In most cases, it resolves over time.

Pulmonary fibrosis refers to the formation of scar tissue in the lungs that can occur for many reasons, including radiation therapy for lung cancer. Symptoms include shortness of breath and a decreased ability to exercise. Pulmonary fibrosis is usually permanent.

Rectum, Bladder, and Prostate

Rectum values are 60 Gy TD for NTCP of 5% in 5 years and 80 Gy TD for NTCP of 50% in 5 years. Exposure to the rectum comes primarily from the treatment of prostate cancer because the rectum and bladder are almost always partially included in external beam therapy of the prostate. Major complications include diarrhea, severe proctitis, necrosis, stenosis, and the formation of a fistula. A rectal fistula is an opening between the rectum and the external skin, which can be very painful and often requires corrective surgery.

Reproductive Organs, Ovaries, and Testicles

Temporary sterility in women occurs above doses of about 1.5 Gy. Doses in excess of 6.0 Gy will permanently sterilize a woman. Prior to the introduction of birth control pills, it was not uncommon for women to request radiation for sterilization as an alternate to surgical sterilization.

Temporary sterility occurs in men at doses above 2.5 Gy and permanent sterility at doses above 5.0 Gy.

Skin

Skin is the most important and largest organ in the body. It usually first shows initial effects of external radiation because the radiation must pass through the skin to reach the internal organs. Radiation doses of about 2 Gy can produce skin reddening. Figure 9.4 shows a representative cross section of the skin and some of the components of the skin.

The thin outer layer of the skin, the epidermis, is about 100 μm thick. It is made up of about 15 layers of epithelial cells, which are continuously regenerating. The epidermis is covered with a layer of protective dead cells, which are continuously sloughed off. The basal or lowest layer of the epidermis contains continually dividing stem cells, which differentiate into skin cells as they migrate up to the skin surface. This migration takes 2–6 weeks depending on the skin thickness. The epidermis layer first shows radiation damage because it is closest to the surface and is made up of rapidly dividing cells.

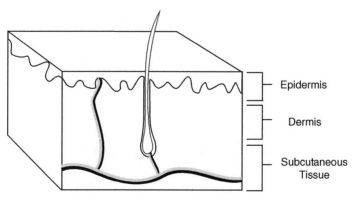

Figure 9.4   The layers of the skin.

The dermis lies below the epidermis and contains muscle fibers, blood and lymph vessels, sweat glands, and hair follicles as well as nerves to respond to touch and pain. The vascular system is limited to the dermis and below.

The epidermis exhibits an early and acute radiation reaction. The underlying dermis shows delayed radiation damage long after the radiation dermatitis of the epidermis has healed. Evidence of dermal injury may not appear until 3 or 4 months later. The amount of damage may not be fully realized for some years. Late skin injuries include chronic skin fibrosis (thickening of the skin by fibrotic tissue), skin contraction, and in rare cases dermal necrosis owing to damage to the dermal capillaries.

The deep redness and the sensitivity caused by radiation fade shortly after the exposure, similar to the effects of sunburn. The skin takes somewhat longer to return completely to its natural color following radiation exposure. In the cases of higher exposure, there may be a second more serious effect that becomes evident many months, or even a few years, after exposure. This is due to the damage to the underlying, slowly dividing cells at the lower skin layers and to the vessels supplying the deeper layers. Such effects that may lead to open sores requiring skin grafts are discussed further in Chapter 12.

Some individuals may continue to have a slightly pinkish or tan hue to their skin for years after exposure. Some individuals may notice a small patch of tiny blood vessels on the skin surface of the radiated area. These vessels—called telangiectasias—look like a tangle of thin red lines. Telangiectasias are *not* a sign of cancer and are usually permanent. Figure 9.5 shows a telangiesia.

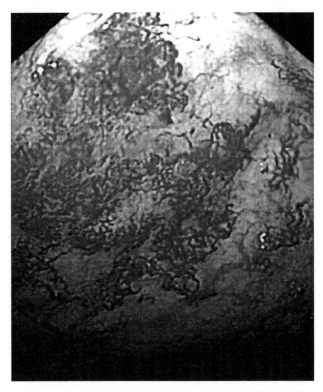

Figure 9.5   Example of telangiectasia, the blotchy vessels appearing on the skin surface following radiation.

Hair loss is another effect following radiation exposure. The loss of hair in clumps occurs with radiation exposures above 2 Gy. Hair regrows within a few months.

Dry desquamation is a condition of itchy dry scaly patches of skin where the patches readily fall off. Dry desquamation is usually the first radiation symptom prompting a patient to seek medical attention, usually from a dermatologist. Few dermatologists consider the possibility of radiation exposure when faced with dry itchy skin. The usual course of treatment for skin not recognized as damaged by radiation consists of trying a few creams and ointments with no improvement. Often the next step is to perform a "punch biopsy" to determine underlying cause. This is consistent with a dermatologist's experience and training. It is also one of the most undesirable things to do because the skin's ability to repair injury has been seriously compromised by the radiation. Patients having repeated or extended interventional procedures should *always* mention this fact to the dermatologist and strongly decline a punch biopsy.

Spinal Cord

The doses for major complications following spinal cord radiation are 47.7 Gy TD for NTCP of 5% in 5 years and 68.3 Gy TD for NTCP of 50% in 5 years. Complications include myelitis, necrosis, and paralysis. The complications increase with the length of cord irradiated. These data are for radiation of 20-cm cord length.

Thyroid

Radiation-induced cancer can come from either external exposure or ingestion of radioactive iodine, which is concentrated by the thyroid. This is especially true of exposure during childhood.

In routine thyroid testing, iodine-131 (written I-131) is given as a capsule swallowed by the patient. The I-131 in the bloodstream can pass through the placental barrier, so exposure to the mother can result in exposure to the fetus. Fetal exposure to I-131 is a hazard only after the 12th week of pregnancy because fetal thyroid is not developed before then.

Potassium iodide, KI, given to the patient before taking the iodine capsule will diminish the uptake by the thyroid. The KI occupies the iodine receptors in the thyroid so the radioactive iodine is not taken up by the gland. Unfortunately, the KI must be given before, or within a few hours of exposure to radioactive iodine, so its protective effects are primarily limited to planned medical exposures. KI does not protect against external radiation.

An individual whose thyroid is exposed to 1 Gy of external radiation is eight times more likely to develop thyroid cancer than an unexposed person. These data come primarily from external medical exposures during the 1930s and 1940s when radiation was used to treat many childhood problems. Medical reasons for exposing children in the 1930s and 1940s included tinea capitis infections (scalp ringworm), enlarged tonsils and thymus glands, and cutaneous hemangiomas. The greatest risk of developing thyroid cancer is between 5 and 29 years after radiation exposure. After this period, the risk decreases.

The dose to the thyroid from a mammographic examination is less than 0.01 mGy per examination. This dose is due to scattered radiation because the thyroid is *never* in the direct beam during a mammographic examination. Thyroid doses from dental examinations are equally low.

SUMMARY

- The latent period is the time between a radiation exposure and the appearance of its effects.
- A stochastic radiation injury is a statistical effect that may or may not occur depending on whether a critical part of the cell's DNA is damaged. The probability of stochastic damage increase with dose but the severity of the effect does not. Cancer induction and genetic damage are stochastic effects. A deterministic effect or tissue reaction describes damage to a group of cells in a tissue, which affects the function of the tissue. Tissue reactions have a threshold dose below which the damage is not evident.
- Radiation damage to blood vessels results in loss of vessel wall flexibility, irritation of the wall linings, and formation of plaques interfering with blood flow. This is especially true in the microvasculature and tiny capillaries. Edema and fibrosis are gross long-term deterministic effects of high exposures.
- Erythema or skin reddening occurs at doses of about 2 Gy. Long-term, hard-to-heal injuries have been seen after repeated multiple interventional procedures. Radiation-induced cataracts due to long-term eye exposures have been implicated in cataracts in interventional physicians. Recent ICRP recommendations suggest limiting eye exposures to less than 20 mSv/year.
- Radiation exposure to the thyroid can occur from either external radiation or exposure via intake of radioactive I-131. External exposure is extremely rare today but was used medically in the 1930s and 1940s providing well-documented data on radiation-induced thyroid cancer. Damage to the thyroid from radioactive iodine can be prevented if nonradioactive iodine in the form of potassium iodine, KI, is administered before the exposure to I-131. The fetal thyroid is not formed before 12 weeks of pregnancy, so inadvertent administration of I-131 to a pregnant woman in the early stages of pregnancy does not endanger her fetus.

BIBLIOGRAPHY

Astakhova LN, Anspaugh LR, Beebe GW, Bouville A, Drozdovitch VV, Garber V, et al. Chernobyl-related thyroid cancer in children of Belarus: A case-control study. Radiat Res. 1998 September;150(3):349–56.

Balter S, Hopewell JW, Miller DL, Wagner LK, Zelefsky MJ. Fluoroscopically guided interventional procedures: A review of radiation effects on patients' skin and hair. Radiology. 2010 February;254(2):326–41.

Boice JD Jr. Radiation and thyroid cancer: What more can be learned? Acta Oncol. 1998;37(4):321–4.

Bolsover SR, Shephard EA, White HA, Hyams JS. Cell biology: A short course. 3rd ed. Chichester, UK: Wiley-Blackwell; 2011.

Cardis E, Kesminiene A, Ivanov V, Malakhova I, Shibata Y, Khrouch V, et al. Risk of thyroid cancer after exposure to 131I in childhood. J Natl Cancer Inst. 2005 May 18;97(10): 724–32.

Conklin HM, Li C, Xiong X, Ogg RJ, Merchant TE. Predicting change in academic abilities after conformal radiation therapy for localized ependymoma. J Clin Oncol. 2008 August 20;26(24):3965–70.

Copeland DR, deMoor C, Moore BD 3rd, Ater JL. Neurocognitive development of children after a cerebellar tumor in infancy: A longitudinal study. J Clin Oncol. 1999 November; 17(11):3476–86.

Davis S, Stepanenko V, Rivkind N, Kopecky KJ, Voilleque P, Shakhtarin V, et al. Risk of thyroid cancer in the Bryansk Oblast of the Russian Federation after the Chernobyl Power Station accident. Radiat Res. 2004 September;162(3):241–8.

Dearnaley DP, Khoo VS, Norman AR, Meyer L, Nahum A, Tait D, et al. Comparison of radiation side-effects of conformal and conventional radiotherapy in prostate cancer: A randomised trial. Lancet. 1999 January 23;353(9149):267–72.

Emami B, Lyman J, Brown A, Coia L, Goitein M, Munzenrider JE, et al. Tolerance of normal tissue to therapeutic irradiation. Int J Radiat Oncol Biol Phys. 1991 May 15;21(1): 109–22.

Fattibene P, Mazzei F, Nuccetelli C, Risica S. Prenatal exposure to ionizing radiation: Sources, effects and regulatory aspects. Acta Paediatr. 1999 July;88(7):693–702.

Frazier TH, Richardson JB, Fabre VC, Callen JP. Fluoroscopy-induced chronic radiation skin injury: A disease perhaps often overlooked. Arch Dermatol. 2007 May;143(5):637–40.

International Commission on Radiological Protection. 1990 recommendations of the International Commission on Radiological Protection: User's edition. 1st ed. Oxford, UK: The International Commission on Radiological Protection by Pergamon Press; 1992.

International Commission on Radiological Protection. Pregnancy and medical radiation. Publication 84. Ann ICRP. 2000;30(1):iii–viii, 1–43.

International Commission on Radiological Protection. Statement on tissue reactions. Publication 118. Ann ICRP Publication 41(1/2)2012.

Jacob P, Kenigsberg Y, Zvonova I, Goulko G, Buglova E, Heidenreich WF, et al. Childhood exposure due to the Chernobyl accident and thyroid cancer risk in contaminated areas of Belarus and Russia. Br J Cancer. 1999 July;80(9):1461–9.

Mao XW. A quantitative study of the effects of ionizing radiation on endothelial cells and capillary-like network formation. Technol Cancer Res Treat. 2006 April;5(2): 127–34.

Merchant TE, Kiehna EN, Li C, Xiong X, Mulhern RK. Radiation dosimetry predicts IQ after conformal radiation therapy in pediatric patients with localized ependymoma. Int J Radiat Oncol Biol Phys. 2005 December 1;63(5):1546–54.

Michalski JM, Gay H, Jackson A, Tucker SL, Deasy JO. Radiation dose-volume effects in radiation-induced rectal injury. Int J Radiat Oncol Biol Phys. 2010 March 1;76(Suppl. 3):S123–9.

Miller RW. Effects of prenatal exposure to ionizing radiation. Health Phys. 1990 July; 59(1):57–61.

Mullenders L, Atkinson M, Paretzke H, Sabatier L, Bouffler S. Assessing cancer risks of low-dose radiation. Nat Rev Cancer. 2009 August;9(8):596–604.

Research Triangle Institute, United States. Agency for Toxic Substances and Disease Registry. Toxicological profile for ionizing radiation. Atlanta, GA: U.S. Department of Health and Human Services, Public Health Service, Agency for Toxic Substances and Disease Registry; 1999.

Ron E, Lubin J, Schneider AB. Thyroid cancer incidence. Nature. 1992 November 12;360(6400):113.

Ron E, Lubin JH, Shore RE, Mabuchi K, Modan B, Pottern LM, et al. Thyroid cancer after exposure to external radiation: A pooled analysis of seven studies. Radiat Res. 1995 March;141(3):259–77.

Sadetzki S, Chetrit A, Lubina A, Stovall M, Novikov I. Risk of thyroid cancer after childhood exposure to ionizing radiation for tinea capitis. J Clin Endocrinol Metab. 2006 December;91(12):4798–804.

Silber JH, Radcliffe J, Peckham V, Perilongo G, Kishnani P, Fridman M, et al. Whole-brain irradiation and decline in intelligence: The influence of dose and age on IQ score. J Clin Oncol. 1992 September;10(9):1390–6.

Streffer C, Shore R, Konermann G, Meadows A, Uma Devi P, Preston Withers J, et al. Biological effects after prenatal irradiation (embryo and fetus). A report of the International Commission on Radiological Protection. Ann ICRP. 2003;33(1–2):5–206.

United Nations. Scientific Committee on the Effects of Atomic Radiation. Sources and effects of ionizing radiation: United Nations Scientific Committee on the Effects of Atomic Radiation: UNSCEAR 2000 report to the General Assembly, with scientific annexes. New York: United Nations; 2000.

Yamashita S, Shibata Y, Sasakawa Kinen Hoken Kyōryoku Zaidan. Chernobyl Sasakawa Health and Medical Cooperation Project. Chernobyl: A decade: Proceedings of the Fifth Chernobyl Sasakawa Medical Cooperation Symposium, Kiev, Ukraine, 14–15 October 1996. Amsterdam; New York: Elsevier; 1997.

QUESTIONS

Chapter 9   Questions

1. An easily observed indication of tissue sensitivity is
   a. cell cycle duration.
   b. latent period between exposure and expression of damage.
   c. mitotic index.
   d. replication rate.

2. The fetus is most sensitive to brain and metal development damage from radiation during the _____ week period of pregnancy.
   a. 0–7
   b. 8–16
   c. 17–24
   d. 25–36

3. During the most sensitive period for radiation damage, the decrease in mental acuity is estimated to be about _____ IQ points per 100 mGy.
   a. 0.3
   b. 3
   c. 30
   d. 300

4. The major complications of radiation exposure result from
   a. damage to the microvasculature.
   b. cell membrane enzyme damage.
   c. contraction of the heart muscle.
   d. plaque formation in the major blood vessels.

5. The chemical ____ can be given to protect the thyroid against absorbing radio-active iodine.
   a. NaI
   b. KI
   c. CrI
   d. H_2I

6. Radiation damage to the conceptus during the first 2 weeks of pregnancy results in
   a. brain damage.
   b. arrested organ development.
   c. an all-or-nothing effect.
   d. late fetal cancer.

7. The probability of a _____ effect, but not the severity, depends on the dose.
   a. stochastic
   b. deterministic/tissue reaction

8. A longer time between the appearance of early and late effects of radiation exposure indicates a relatively _____ radiation dose.
   a. higher
   b. indeterminate
   c. lower
   d. congruent

9. A reasonable estimate of fetal radiation dose from plane diagnostic examination of the abdomen is about
   a. 10% of the X-ray tube output.
   b. 25% of the X-ray tube output.
   c. 10% of the entrance dose.
   d. 25% of the entrance dose.

10. If a fetus is injured by in utero radiation, the injury classified as a _____ injury.
   a. genetic
   b. classical
   c. combination
   d. somatic

11. The thyroid _____ exposed during a mammographic examination.

    a. is

    b. is not

    c. is maximally

12. The two major complications of breast irradiation are

    a. fibrosis and lymphedema.

    b. skin ulcers and fibrosis.

    c. lymphedema and swelling the irradiated tissue.

    d. fibrosis and loss of elasticity due to a diffuse scarring.

13. Current evidence indicates that cataracts can be formed following long-term exposures as low as _____ Gy.

    a. 0.2

    b. 0.8

    c. 2

    d. 8

14. About _____ Gy will produce permanent sterility in women.

    a. 0.2

    b. 2

    c. 0.6

    d. 6

15. Erythema or skin reddening occurs at doses of about

    a. 0.02 Gy.

    b. 0.2 Gy.

    c. 2 Gy.

    d. 25% of the X-ray tube output.

16. Abortion based on fear of fetal radiation exposures should not be considered following fetal doses of less than _____ mGy.

    a. 1

    b. 10

    c. 100

    d. 1000

CHAPTER 10

WHOLE BODY RADIATION EFFECTS

KEYWORDS

Acute radiation syndrome, mean lethal dose, bystander effect, hematopoietic syndrome, manifest illness, gastrointestinal syndrome, neurovascular syndrome, radiation accident

TOPICS

- Conditions for acute radiation syndrome (ARS)
- Symptoms associated with the clinical syndromes of ARS
- Mean lethal dose
- Stages of ARS
- Bystander effect

INTRODUCTION

The effects of radiation are either stochastic or deterministic. Stochastic events are random events. They are thought to be initiated by radiation damage to a single cell, which is then passed on to future generations. The probability, but not the severity, of a stochastic event is a function of dose. The probability of a stochastic event increases with dose, but the precise relation is not known. In this way, stochastic effects are similar to the purchase of lottery tickets. Buying more tickets increases

Radiation Biology of Medical Imaging, First Edition. Charles A. Kelsey, Philip H. Heintz, Daniel J. Sandoval, Gregory D. Chambers, Natalie L. Adolphi, and Kimberly S. Paffett.
© 2014 John Wiley & Sons, Inc. Published 2014 by John Wiley & Sons, Inc.

the chances of winning, but does not increase the amount of the prize. Cancer induction is one of the primary stochastic effects. Greater radiation exposure increases the chances of cancer but does not increase the severity of the cancer.

Children are about twice as sensitive as adults to stochastic effects, probably because they have a more rapid cell turnover during growth. They also have a longer lifetime after exposure to develop stochastic effects. Stochastic effects do not have a threshold because one cell could be damaged even at extremely low doses.

Deterministic effects result from injury to a population of cells leading to loss of tissue and organ function when sufficient cells are damaged. The amount loss is proportional to the radiation dose. Most organs can function with a loss of some functioning cells, and there is often a "threshold dose," below which no loss of organ function is observed.

This chapter focuses on the deterministic effects of high doses of radiation to the whole body over a short period of time.

ACUTE RADIATION SYNDROME (ARS)

In the previous chapter, we discussed how different organs and tissues have different radiosensitivities, and that delivering the dose to a small area in a very short period of time is more damaging (e.g., to the skin) than spreading the dose out over a larger area, or a greater period of time. Radiation sickness, or ARS, is the result of a large dose of radiation delivered to the whole body in a short period (seconds to minutes) of time. The primary cause of ARS is the destruction of immature parenchymal stem cells in the affected tissues.

From the Center for Disease Control website, the required conditions for ARS are as follows:

1. The dose must be large.
2. The dose is usually external.
3. The dose is from penetrating radiation (e.g., X- and gamma rays).
4. The majority of the body receives the dose.
5. The entire dose is received in a short time.

Most of the data and examples we have regarding ARS are taken from the survivors of the Hiroshima and Nagasaki atomic bombings in 1945, as well as the first responders to the Chernobyl Nuclear Power Plant incident in 1986.

ARS is a collection of various deterministic effects that occur in a definite sequence. These effects, as discussed later, result in three distinct syndromes that occur in order, predictably with increasing dose. They are hematopoietic, gastrointestinal, and neurovascular syndromes. As their individual names imply, the syndromes are associated with which organ system is primarily affected by the received dose.

After a significant exposure that will result in ARS, there is a series of events referred to as the "phases of ARS." The phases, discussed in more detail later, are prodromal, latent, manifest illness, and recovery or death.

Though most of the data regarding the stages of ARS come from Japanese atomic bomb survivors, some other clinical examples of ARS are as follows:

1. An explosion at the Chernobyl Nuclear Power Plant in April 1986 resulted in the hospitalization of 237 patients identified as overexposed persons. One hundred thirty-four of them developed ARS. Of these 134 exposed persons, 28 eventually died of ARS-associated injury with extensive radiation burns (Il'in 1995).

2. In September 1987, a shielded radioactive cesium-137 source (50.9 TBq) was removed from the protective housing of an abandoned teletherapy machine in Goiânia, Brazil. Subsequently, the source was ruptured. As a result, many people incurred large doses of radiation by both external and internal contamination. Four of the casualties ultimately died, and 28 people developed local radiation injuries (IAEA 1988).

3. In 1989, a radiological accident occurred at an industrial sterilization facility in San Salvador, El Salvador. The accident occurred when the cobalt-60 source became stuck in the open position. Three workers were exposed to high radiation doses and developed ARS. The immediate acute effects were limited by specialized treatment. Nonetheless, two of the men were so seriously injured that their legs had to be partly or completely amputated. The most highly exposed worker died 6.5 months later, his death attributed to residual lung damage and other injuries (IAEA, Pan American Health Organization 1990).

MEAN LETHAL DOSE (LD$_{50}$)

The mean lethal dose is defined as the amount of dose necessary to cause fatality in 50% of a population within a specified period of time. Because various clinical syndromes run their course in different time periods, the LD$_{50}$ is assessed at different time periods. The time period in which death is assessed is denoted by a subscript denoting the number of days that has elapsed. For example, the LD$_{50/30}$ is the dose necessary to kill 50% of the exposed population within 30 days, whereas the LD$_{100/2}$ would be the dose necessary to kill the entire population within 2 days.

Being a statistical quantity, the LD$_{50}$ varies between species and is not an absolute within the species, as it also depends on body weight and general health of the individual. The LD$_{50}$ is only a guide in assessing the prognosis in any individual or animal. See Table 10.1 for an estimate of mean lethal doses for various species.

TABLE 10.1   Estimates for the Mean Lethal Doses for Various Animals in Gy

Species	LD$_{50/30}$	LD$_{50/8}$	LD$_{50/5}$	LD$_{50/2}$
Mouse	6.4	–	12.6	200
Germ-free mouse	7	20	–	–
Rat	7	–	8.08	200
Monkey	6	15	–	100

It should be noted that the mean lethal dose varies between species and is also dependent on body weight and general health of the individual.

The LD$_{50/30}$ for human whole body irradiation without medical intervention is approximately 5 Gy. However, as with any other clinical reaction, individual patients will respond differently to the same dose based on their overall health.

CLINICAL SYNDROMES OF ARS

As discussed earlier, the effects of radiation depend on the dose received, and this holds for the clinical syndromes associated with ARS.

Hematopoietic Syndrome

When a person is exposed to about 1 Gy, the lymphocyte cell count will be reduced. The body will be more susceptible to infection. Early symptoms of such exposures mimic the flu, that is, loss of appetite, nausea, diarrhea, and vomiting. The chapter on whole body radiation treats the effects of decreased white blood cells following radiation exposure more completely. Figure 10.1 shows the radiation effects on white blood cell counts for ~1–5 Gy.

After a significant radiation dose (usually greater than 1 Gy), all components of the blood were adversely affected. Increases in dose result in an increased effect, and the effects are seen earlier. In the case of a whole body exposure from a radiation accident, the loss of white blood cells occurs just at a time when the body's defenses against infection are most needed. Damage to the skin and intestine make the body particularly vulnerable to bacterial infection during the first 2 weeks following exposure.

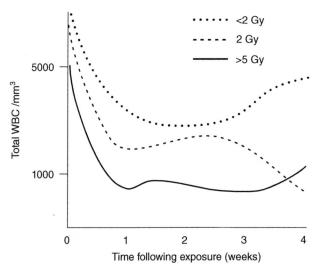

Figure 10.1 White blood count (WBC) as a function of time after exposure. The figure shows plots of white blood cell count over time following exposure to different doses of ionizing radiation. These plots summarize data from the Chernobyl accident.

TABLE 10.2   Summary of the Effects to the Hematopoietic System after Varying Whole Body Radiation Doses

Acute Radiation Effects to the Hematopoietic System	Whole Body Dose (in Gy)
No observable effect	0–0.25
Slight blood changes	0.25–1
Significant reduction in blood platelets and white blood cells (temporary)	1–2
Severe blood damage, nausea, hair loss, hemorrhage, death in many cases	2–5
Death in less than 2 months for >80% ($LD_{80/60}$)	>6

For whole body doses greater than 0.7 Gy, the symptoms of ARS are related to the destruction of the blood producing bone marrow and may manifest as fatigue due to anemia, anorexia, nausea, and vomiting. For doses greater than 2.5 Gy, the supply of mature red blood cells, white blood cells, and platelets is severely damaged and is not adequately resupplied due to the underlying damage done to the hematopoietic stem cells. Death may occur within a few months due to infection, severe anemia, and hemorrhage. The mean lethal dose for death within 2 months due to hematopoietic syndrome is 2.5–5 Gy (Table 10.2).

Following a large-scale radiation accident involving many individuals, the time from exposure to the onset of vomiting can be useful in estimating the magnitude of the radiation exposure. A shorter time between the exposure and the onset of vomiting indicates a higher radiation dose.

Gastrointestinal Syndrome

The stem cells in the crypts of the intestine develop into intermediate cells, which differentiate into mature cells as they migrate up to the top of the villi (Fig. 10.2). During this migration, they receive signals directing them to develop into specialized cells designed to function as part of an organ. In the mature stage, they actively perform their specialized functions. These functions include absorption of nutrients from the gut and the discharge of waste products into the intestine. This migration requires about 14 days. The mature gut cells at the top of the villi are soughed off at the end of their life cycle. Thus, the effects of intestinal radiation exposure become evident about 2 weeks after the exposure. The intestine is no longer able to maintain the barrier between the body waste inside the intestine and the bloodstream. This is just as the white blood cell population, essential for fighting infection, is dropping.

At doses greater than 5–6 Gy, the symptoms associated with ARS are typically severe nausea, vomiting, anorexia, and prolonged diarrhea. These symptoms are brought on due to the injury sustained by the epithelial lining of the gastrointestinal tract. Nausea, vomiting, and anorexia prevent normal food and fluid intake, leading to a severe electrolyte imbalance. Depending on the dose, persistent diarrhea may rapidly progress from loose to watery, to explosive and bloody. Death may occur within weeks due to infection, dehydration, and electrolyte imbalance. The LD_{100} is approximately 10 Gy.

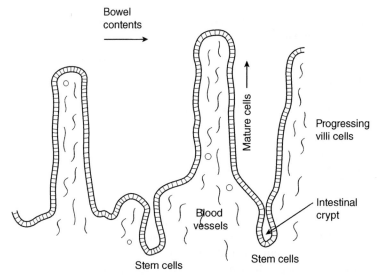

Figure 10.2   Schematic of villi in the intestine. The most radiation-sensitive cells in the intestine are the immature stem cells. These immature stem cells are located at the base of the villi in the intestine. They maintain the supply of stem cells for development into mature functioning cells.

Neurovascular Syndrome (Central Nervous System)

For doses greater than approximately 50 Gy, death occurs usually within 3 days. Although symptoms include nervousness, dizziness, confusion, and other neurological disorders, death most likely occurs due to the destruction of the whole body circulatory system and increased pressure on the brain due to fluid leakage caused by edema, vasculitis, and meningitis.

Keep in mind that these syndromes are not mutually exclusive. A person receiving 50 Gy would most likely experience all three syndromes except for the fact that they may expire before the full onset of each syndrome.

STAGES OF ARS

There are four stages associated with each of the clinical syndromes of ARS: prodromal, latent, manifest illness, and recovery or death. Each of these stages is dose and time dependent, and the severity of each can help in prognosis.

Prodromal Stage

The initial or prodromal stage occurs within minutes or hours after the dose is received. The symptoms of the prodromal syndrome are nausea, vomiting, and diarrhea. The severity of these symptoms, along with time of onset and duration, depends on the size of the dose. A severe prodromal response to a whole body dose will usually indicate a poor clinical prognosis.

Latent Stage

As the early effects begin to subside, there may be a period of time where the subject feels generally healthy for a period of hours to weeks, depending on the dose received. The duration latent period shortens with increasing dose and is a relatively good indicator of clinical prognosis.

Manifest Illness Stage

This stage is dependent on the specific clinical syndrome (hematopoietic, gastrointestinal, central nervous system) and may last for hours up to several months.

Recovery or Death

As shown in Table 10.3, recovery with associated treatment is expected at lower doses (<5 Gy). At doses above 10 Gy, death is expected within weeks.

BYSTANDER EFFECT

The bystander effect has been defined as "the induction of biologic effects in cells that are not directly traversed by a charged particle, but are in close proximity to cells that are" (Hall and Giaccia 2006). Observations of the bystander effect have been noted in experiments with single-particle microbeams targeted to specific cells and resulting in biologic effects being observed in unirradiated close neighbor cells.

Other experiments have shown that if a colony of cells is irradiated, then placed in a colony of unirradiated cells, the result is death of the unirradiated cells. This has also been attributed to the bystander effect.

Although there are many hypotheses to why this bystander effect occurs, there is no one agreed upon theory.

SUMMARY

- Acute radiation syndrome (ARS) is the result of deterministic effects of high doses of radiation to the whole body over a short period of time.
- The required conditions for ARS are the dose must be large, the dose is usually external, the dose is from penetrating radiation (e.g., X- and gamma rays), the majority of the body receives the dose, and the entire dose is received in a short time
- The mean lethal dose is defined as the amount of dose necessary to cause fatality in 50% of a population within a specified period of time. The $LD_{50/30}$ for human whole body irradiation without medical intervention is approximately 5 Gy.
- The hematopoietic syndrome may occur for whole body doses greater than 0.7 Gy.
- The gastrointestinal syndrome may occur for whole body doses greater than 5–6 Gy.

TABLE 10.3   Summary of Acute Radiation Syndromes and Their Associated Symptoms at Various Stages

Syndrome	Equivalent Dose	Prodromal Stage Symptoms	Latent Stage Symptoms	Manifest Illness Stage Symptoms	Recovery or Death
Hematopoietic	>0.7 Gy (some mild symptoms may occur as low as 0.3 Gy)	Anorexia, nausea, and vomiting. Onset occurs 1 hour to 2 days after exposure. Stage lasts for minutes to days.	Stem cells in bone marrow are dying, although patient may appear and feel well. Stage lasts 1–6 weeks.	Anorexia, fever, and malaise. Drop in all blood cell counts occurs for several weeks.	In most cases, bone marrow cells will begin to repopulate the marrow. There should be full recovery for a large percentage of individuals from a few weeks up to 2 years after exposure. Death may occur in some individuals at 1.2 Gy. The $LD_{50/60}$ is about 2.5–5 Gy. Primary cause of death is infection and hemorrhage. Most deaths occur within a few months after exposure.
Gastrointestinal (GI)	>10 Gy (some symptoms may occur as low as 6 Gy)	Anorexia, severe nausea, vomiting, cramps, and diarrhea. Onset occurs within a few hours after exposure. Stage lasts about 2 days.	Stem cells in bone marrow and cells lining the GI tract are dying, although patient may appear and feel well. Stage lasts less than 1 week.	Anorexia, severe diarrhea, fever, dehydration, and electrolyte imbalance.	Death is due to infection, dehydration, and electrolyte imbalance. Death occurs within 2 weeks of exposure. The LD_{100} is about 10 Gy.
Neurovascular syndrome (central nervous system)	>50 Gy (some symptoms may occur as low as 20 Gy)	Extreme nervousness and confusion; severe nausea, vomiting, and watery diarrhea; loss of consciousness; and burning sensations of the skin. Onset occurs within minutes of exposure. Stage lasts for minutes to hours.	Patient may return to partial functionality. Stage may last for hours but often is less.	Return of watery diarrhea, convulsions, and coma. Onset occurs 5–6 hours after exposure.	No recovery is expected. Death occurs within 3 days of exposure.

Adapted from CDC (2005).

- The neurovascular syndrome may occur for whole body doses greater than 50 Gy.
- There are four stages associated with each of the clinical syndromes of ARS: prodromal, latent, manifest illness, and recovery or death. Each of these stages is dose and time dependent, and the severity of each can help in prognosis.

BIBLIOGRAPHY

Bushberg JT. The essential physics of medical imaging. 2nd ed. Philadelphia: Lippincott Williams & Wilkins; 2002.

CDC. Acute radiation syndrome: A fact sheet for physicians. Atlanta, GA: Centers for Disease Control and Prevention; 2005 [updated March 18, 2005; cited March 28, 2013]. Available from: http://www.bt.cdc.gov/radiation/arsphysicianfactsheet.asp.

Hall EJ, Giaccia AJ. Radiobiology for the radiologist. 6th ed. Philadelphia: Lippincott Williams & Wilkins; 2006.

Il'in LA. Chernobyl: Myth and reality. Moscow: Megapolis; 1995.

International Atomic Energy Agency (IAEA). The radiological accident in Goiânia. Vienna Lanham, MD: International Atomic Energy Agency; UNIPUB, distributor; 1988.

International Atomic Energy Agency (IAEA), Pan American Health Organization. The radiological accident in San Salvador: A report. Vienna Lanham, MD: International Atomic Energy Agency; UNIPUB distributor; 1990.

International Atomic Energy Agency, World Health Organization. Diagnosis and treatment of radiation injuries. Vienna Lanham, MD: International Atomic Energy Agency; 1998.

Nias AHW. An introduction to radiobiology. 2nd ed. Chichester: Wiley; 1998.

QUESTIONS

Chaper 10   Questions

1. The time to death from the _____ syndrome is _____.
   a. hematopoietic, 1–2 months
   b. cerebrovascular, 2–4 weeks
   c. gastrointestinal, 2–4 months
   d. prodromal, 1–2 hours

2. The main cause of death from the hematopoietic syndrome is
   a. hypotension arising from microvascular destruction.
   b. hemolytic anemia.
   c. infection and hemorrhage resulting from loss of white cells and platelets.
   d. loss of erythrocytes resulting in organ ischemia.

3. An individual who received a single whole body dose of 50 mGy would be expected to exhibit the following symptoms:

    i. nausea

    ii. vomiting

    iii. death within 1 week

    iv. depressed white blood count

  a. i, ii

  b. i, ii, iv

  c. i, ii, iii, iv

  d. None of the above.

4. Regarding the human $LD_{50/30}$:

  a. The $LD_{50/30}$ associated with an acute whole body irradiation is approximately 4–5 Gy for individuals without medical care following irradiation.

  b. Even with optimal medical care, the $LD_{50/30}$ cannot be increased.

  c. The most common cause of death in people who receive a dose close to the $LD_{50/30}$ is severe anemia.

  d. The $LD_{50/30}$ is the dose that leads to death within 50 days of 30% of the population.

5. A reactor accident exposes workers to different whole body radiation doses. The group exposed to doses greater than 50 Gy will be expected to exhibit _____ within the first week.

    i. nausea and vomiting

    ii. depressed white blood count

    iii. prolonged diarrhea

    iv. convulsions

  a. i, ii

  b. i, ii, iii

  c. ii, iii, iv

  d. i, ii, iii, iv

6. The death of an individual 21–28 days after a whole body irradiation dose of 5 Gy would likely be due to damage to the _____ organ system.

  a. gastrointestinal

  b. central nervous system

  c. cardiovascular

  d. hematopoietic

7. In humans exposed to a total body dose of 10 Gy, which of the following symptoms would be expected during the first 48 hours after the exposure?

   i. Nausea

   ii. Fatigue

   iii. Depressed or enhanced motor activity

   iv. Apathy

   v. Vomiting

   a. i, ii, iii

   b. i, iii, iv, v

   c. i, ii, iv, v

   d. i, ii, iii, iv, v

8. The mean lethal dose for humans is about _____ Gy.

   a. 0.5

   b. 5

   c. 50

   d. 500

9. Which one of the following is not a listed phase of acute radiation syndrome?

   i. Latent

   ii. Euphoric

   iii. Recovery

   iv. Prodromal

   a. i, ii, iii

   b. i, ii, iv

   c. ii, iii, iv

   d. i, ii, iii, iv

10. Following a large radiological accident, the _____ could be used to estimate the radiation dose to victims.

   a. results of blood samples sent to the lab for assay

   b. lack of vomiting within 12 hours after the exposure

   c. degree of erythema

   d. presence of anxiety and confusion

11. Most of our current understanding of whole body irradiation effects come from

   a. experiments conducted on rats and mice.

   b. the accident at Three Mile Island.

   c. atomic bomb survivors.

   d. Monte Carlo simulations.

12. At doses close to the dose that would be lethal to 50% of the human population, the principal components of the prodromal syndrome are
    a. extreme nervousness and confusion.
    b. explosive bloody diarrhea and moist desquamation.
    c. anorexia, nausea, and vomiting.
    d. burning sensations of the skin and loss of consciousness.

13. The bystander effect describes the effect of radiation on
    a. future generation of irradiated cells.
    b. cells and tissues outside the irradiated site.
    c. cells nearby that are protected by oxygen.
    d. tissues with a partially depleted oxygen supply.

14. Death is expected within 2 weeks following at whole body doses of ___ Gy or greater.
    a. 0.1
    b. 1
    c. 10
    d. 100

15. During the ___ period between the ARS stages, the individual appears to recover and may show no ill effects.
    a. latent
    b. prodromal
    c. manifest illness
    d. confusion

16. The usual increasing order of stages of the ARS is
    i. prodromal
    ii. latent
    iii. manifest illness
    iv. recovery/death
    a. iv, iii, ii, i
    b. i, ii, iv, iii
    c. ii, iii, iv, i
    d. i, ii, iii, iv

CHAPTER 11

RADIATION TREATMENT OF CANCER

KEYWORDS

Radiation therapy, radiation oncology, linear accelerator, radiation therapy radiation biology, HDR, brachytherapy

TOPICS

- Describe the biological principles of radiation cancer treatments
- Differentiate between external beam and internal radiation therapy
- Describe the techniques and equipment used to perform radiation oncology treatments
- Describe some of the side effects of radiation therapy

This chapter on radiation treatment of cancer is included in a book on the biological effects of medical imaging because inevitably, the reader will be considered an expert or at least knowledgeable in all things concerning radiation. Half of all cancer patients receive radiation therapy at some point in their course of the disease. It is likely that the reader or their friends and family will ask about someone who has, is, or will be receiving radiation therapy treatments. This chapter covers the basics of the biology, equipment, and complications of radiation therapy so the reader can answer some basic questions regarding radiation treatment of cancer.

Radiation therapy, also called radiation oncology, surgery, and chemotherapy are the three primary methods to eradicate cancer. Both surgery and radiation therapy

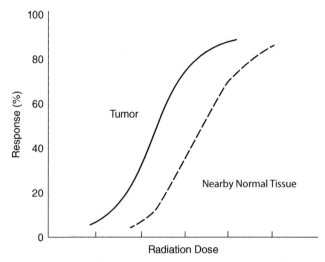

Figure 11.1 Tumor and normal tissue dose–response curves showing that normal tissue response occurs at higher doses than tumor response but that high tumor response inevitably involves some normal tissue response.

are local control procedures. They treat cancer either by cutting it completely out or killing "all" the cells in the treatment volume. Chemotherapy is a systemic treatment that aims to kill all the cancer cells distributed throughout the body. All three modes of treatment attempt to kill the cancer cells without too much damage to normal cells.

Within a year of Wilhelm Roentgen's discovery of X-rays, reports were published on the use of X-rays to treat skin cancer. For over 100 years, physicians have been studying the effects of radiation on normal and cancerous tissues. Radiation damages all cell components, but damage to the tumor cell's DNA can prevent reproduction and halt cancer growth. Radiation therapy treatments are designed to maximize damage to tumor cells while restricting damage to the surrounding normal tissues to a tolerable level. Figure 11.1 presents a comparison of the dose–response of tumor cells and nearby normal tissues. Notice that the response of normal tissue rises above a few percent before the tumor response reaches 50%. This means that some normal tissue damage is inevitable in all radiation therapy treatment. In most cases, the normal tissue damage is tolerable and illustrates the difficulty in balancing tumor killing against normal tissue damage.

Early studies quickly established that rapidly dividing tissues are more sensitive to radiation than tissues with cells that divide more slowly. They also showed that a series of fractionated doses killed more cancer cells than the same dose delivered in a single exposure. The explanation was that several fractions of the total dose over time allowed normal cells to recover whereas the tumor cells did not recover from the radiation as quickly.

Figure 11.2 shows a schematic representation of a fractionated versus single-dose cell survival curve experiment. Notice the higher survival of cells exposed to a series of fractionated doses compared with those receiving a single dose. This allows normal tissue cells to survive or recover from the radiation dose.

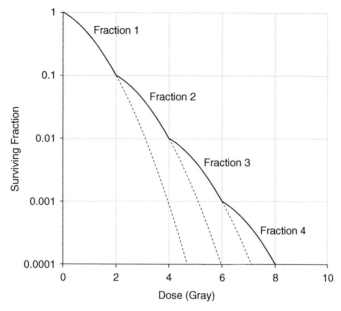

Figure 11.2 Representative cell survival curves showing the effect of fractionation. Cells exposed to the same total dose divided into two reactions show a greater survival than the cells receiving a single dose.

Observations of *in vivo* tumors showed that many solid tumors have a necrotic central portion surrounded by a ring of hypoxic cells that are not proliferating but are still viable if reoxygenated. Figure 11.3 shows an idealized sketch of such a tumor with a necrotic center, a ring of hypoxic cells surrounded by oxygenated viable tumor cells. Actual tumors are not all perfectly spherical, but Fig. 11.3 is drawn to emphasize the important points of the anoxic (without oxygen) necrotic center and the hypoxic (lower than normal) rim around the necrotic center. The oxygen diffusion distance is about 200 μ. Although most solid tumors have developed their own blood supply through angiogenesis, they still "piggyback" on the existing blood vessels to obtain oxygen and nutrients.

THE FOUR Rs OF RADIATION ONCOLOGY

To explain the observations following fractionation experiments and treatments, radiation biologists developed the four Rs of radiation therapy or radiation biology. Table 11.1 lists these four observations.

Repair is the process of rejoining DNA strands. Most repairs occur within 15 minutes to 1 hour. Split-dose experiments show that repair is completed within about 6 hours.

Redistribution refers to the change in the fraction of cells in each phase of the cell cycle. Cells in different parts of the reproductive cycle have different sensitivities. M is the most sensitive, and late S is the least sensitive. Radiation exposure kills more of the cells in the M phase, and more cells in the S phase survive. This effect has not been shown to be advantageous in radiation therapy.

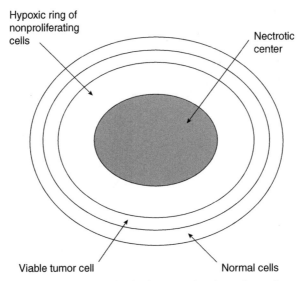

Figure 11.3 A schematic view of a spherical tumor showing a hypoxic necrotic center surrounded by a ring of hypoxic, radioresistant tumor cells and an outer ring of oxygenated tumor cells.

TABLE 11.1   The Four Rs of Radiation Therapy
Repair
Repopulation
Redistribution
Reoxygenation

Reoxygenation occurs as the sensitive, well-oxygenated tumor cells are killed and the tumor shrinks. The outer layers die, and anoxic cells are reintroduced to oxygen. Reoxygenation does not affect treatments with high linear energy transfer (LET) radiation because the higher-density radiation tracks kill hypoxic tumor cells as well as well-oxygenated tumor cells.

Repopulation of the clonogenic cells occurs during the course of fractionated radiation therapy. Each radiation fraction reduces the total tumor population while repopulation rebuilds it. The desired effect is a reduction in the total tumor population. Repopulation of the tumor may occur because the vascularity of the tumor increases as the tumor shrinks. Reoxygenation may counteract the effect of repopulation.

CELL SURVIVAL CURVES AND FRACTIONATION

Models have been developed to reproduce the curved portion of the cell survival curve. One of the more popular models is the linear–quadratic or LQ model. In the LQ model, the survival S after a dose of D is given in Equation 11.1:

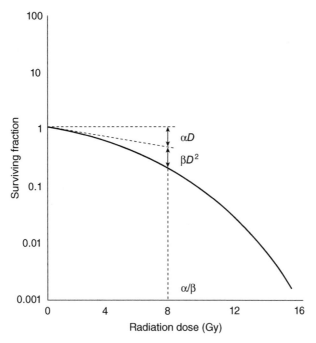

Figure 11.4 Example showing how the parameters α and β can be used to fit the curved portion of the cell survival curve.

$$(S) = \exp(-\alpha D - \beta D^2), \tag{11.1}$$

where α represents the linear portion of the survival curve and β represents the quadratic portion of the survival curve. Tissues with higher mitotic indices are classified as "early responders" or more radiosensitive and tend to have higher α/β ratios.

The LQ or α/β model shown in Equation 11.1 fits the curved portion of the survival curve up to doses of 5–6 Gy, which includes the doses used in radiation therapy.

Figure 11.4 shows how the LQ model fits the lower-dose curved portion of the cell survival curve, which is the dose range used in radiation therapy treatments.

The α/β ratio can be used to describe the shape of the survival curve. A low α/β (0.5–6 Gy) ratio is usually characteristic of late-responding normal tissues with lower mitotic indices. The higher α/β ratio is usually characteristic of tissues with higher mitotic indices including early-responding normal tissues and rapidly proliferating tumors.

FRACTIONATION

External beam radiation therapy employs daily fractionated doses with fraction sizes varying from 1.8 to 2.0 Gy per treatment. Fractionation allows more of the normal cells surrounding the tumor to recover from the radiation damage than the tumor cells.

The LQ model can be successfully used for dose estimation in routine radiation therapy treatments. This model can be used to calculate the dose using different fractionation schemes. This is important when the fractionation schedule must be changed such as when the patient requires a break in the treatments. The LQ model can be used to adjust the subsequent treatment doses to attain the same ultimate tumor dose. The LQ model has also been used for correcting errors in treatments when one or a few treatment fractions were incorrect.

HYPERFRACTIONATION

Hyperfractionation refers to the treatment of a patient with more than one treatment fraction per day. Hyperfractionation usually employs two treatments per day with at least a 6-hour interval between treatments. This interval is designed to allow normal tissues to recover but is aimed at reducing tumor reoxygenation and repopulation. As with conventional fractionation, the treatments are limited by adverse normal tissue reactions.

HYPOFRACTIONATION OR CONTINUOUS RADIATION

Hypofractionation refers to a treatment scheme that uses a slightly reduced dose per fraction with fewer fractions in a shorter time. As an example, an experiment to compare standard and hypofraction results of postmastectomy radiation therapy used 50-Gy fractions for 25 treatments over 35 days against 42-Gy fractions in 16 treatments over 22 days. At 10-year follow-up, there was no difference in recurrences or cosmetic results between the standard and hypofractioned treatments.

COMPLICATIONS FROM RADIATION THERAPY

The goal of radiation therapy is to kill as many tumor cells as possible while minimizing the acceptable amount of normal tissue damage. Through experience, the radiation therapy community has developed measures of the doses that can be delivered to the tumor while producing specified complications. The measure developed is termed the normal tissue complication probability (NTCP) and is expressed as the tumor dose which when delivered to a tumor type will produce either a probability of either 5% or 50% complications. For example, delivering a tumor dose of 60 Gy is expected to produce complications in 5% of the patients in 5 years. This would be expressed as the 5% NTCP for the rectum is a dose delivered to the tumor of 60 Gy. The 50% NTCP for the rectum is 80 Gy means that a tumor dose of 80 Gy is expected to produce complications in 50% of the patients.

Normal tissue complications depend on the volume of tissue irradiated, the fractionation of the normal tissue irradiated, the dose delivered, and the fractionation scheme.

TECHNIQUES USED TO TREAT CANCER

There are two types of treatment techniques used to deliver radiation therapy: external beam and implant therapy or brachytherapy.

The external beam technique uses fractionated treatments. The dose delivered depends on the intent of treatment. If the intent of the treatment is cure, then a high dose of 60–70 Gy is used. If the treatment is palliation, then a lower dose of 30–50 Gy is often used. These are usually administered in daily fractions during the work week, commonly 5 days per week. The treatment extends from 3 to 7 weeks. The radiation biology of these two intents is different in that palliative treatment is often given in higher doses per fraction ignoring the late effects on normal tissue.

An alternate treatment schedule called hyperfractionation treats the patient twice a day with at least a 6-hour interval between treatments. The interval between treatments is designed to allow the normal tissues to recover. The advantage of hyperfractionation is that the patient treatments are completed in about half the time.

EXTERNAL BEAM TREATMENT

The primary method of delivering external beam radiation treatment to the patient is from a linear accelerator. Figure 11.5 shows a photo of a modern external beam radiation therapy accelerator.

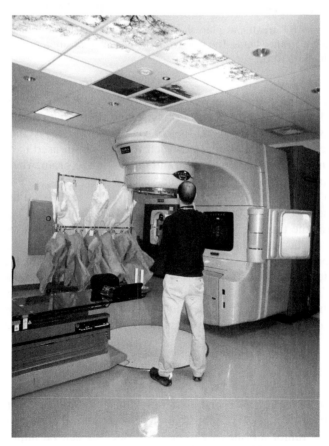

Figure 11.5   Photograph of a modern linear accelerator used in external beam radiation therapy.

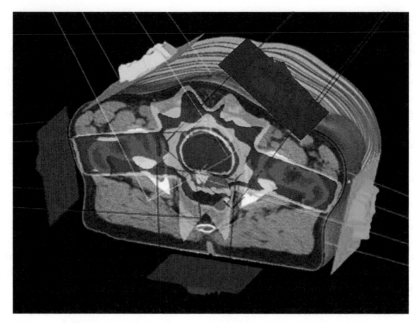

Figure 11.6   An IMRT treatment plan showing the radiation distribution at the prostate resulting from five entrance fields. The field from the posterior position has a reduced intensity to reduce the dose to the rectum.

The newest and most widely used method of external beam therapy is intensity modulated radiation therapy (IMRT), which shapes the radiation field and modulates the intensity of the X-ray beam to achieve a uniform dose to the tumor while minimizing the dose to critical normal structures. It is often used to treat prostate cancer, lung tumors near the spinal cord, and tumors in the brain, where tumors are near critical structures such as the optic nerve.

Figure 11.6 presents an example IMRT plan used to treat prostate cancer. The plan shown uses five 6-MV X-ray beams. Many IMRT treatments employ continuous radiation as the therapy machine rotates around the patient. A multileaf collimator is used to shape the radiation fields to avoid the radiosensitive rectum and bladder. The beam intensity is decreased while passing through the rectum.

Particle external beam therapy using proton beams has been introduced in the last few years. The primary advantage of this technology is that it can provide better geometric distribution of dose to the cancer while minimizing the dose to normal tissue. The relative biological effectiveness (RBE) is similar to that of X-ray beams.

BRACHYTHERAPY OR IMPLANT THERAPY

Brachytherapy is a treatment technique using radioactive sources directly implanted into the tumor. The sources are placed in or near the tumor so the radiation dose is limited to the tumor and nearby tissues. The sources can be implanted permanently or for a limited amount of time. There are two forms of brachytherapy: permanent and temporary.

Permanent brachytherapy involves implanting small radioactive seeds or pellets into the tumor. It is primarily used in the treatment of prostate cancer. In the operating room, the seeds are inserted into the tumor through carefully positioned needles. The patient is discharged from the hospital after a few days of recovery. The seeds are left in place permanently. The radioactivity inside the patient decays away within a few weeks, continuously delivering radiation dose until the seeds are fully decayed.

Temporary brachytherapy uses small radioactive sources about the size of a grain of wheat sealed in a plastic wire or a short metal container the diameter of telephone wire. The sources are placed in either catheters or containers called after-loaders to hold the radioactive sources in the proper position in or near the tumor while the radiation dose is delivered. The catheters or after-loaders containing nonradioactive sources are placed in the patient, the positioning is checked with X-rays, and then the radioactive sources are placed in the catheters or after-loaders to actually deliver the radiation dose.

Temporary brachytherapy is divided into two categories: low- or high-dose brachytherapy.

High-dose brachytherapy uses two different dose rates known as high-dose rate, known as HDR, and low-dose rate, known as LDR. Each HDR treatment requires less than an hour and may be repeated weekly for 3 or 4 weeks. The catheter or after-loader is removed after each treatment, and the patient is not radioactive after the treatment.

During LDR treatments, the radioactive sources remain in the catheter or after-loader for 2–4 days while the patient remains in the hospital. After the treatment is completed, the holder and sources are removed. The patient does not contain any radioactivity after the treatment.

SUMMARY

- The objective is to deliver a very high dose to the tumor while minimizing the dose to normal tissue.
- There are two types of treatments: external beam and brachytherapy.
- External beam treatments are given with a fractionated schedule.
- The four Rs of radiation treatment are recovery, repopulation, redistribution, and reoxygenation.
- The predominant external beam therapy modality uses a linear accelerator generating an IMRT treatment plan.
- Brachytherapy involves implanting radioactive sources in and near the tumor.
- Complications of radiation therapy depend on the part of the body irradiated, total dose delivered, the fractionation schedule and the volume of tissue irradiated, and previous and subsequent therapy.

BIBLIOGRAPHY

Joiner M, van der Kogel A. Basic clinical radiobiology. 4th ed. London: Hodder Arnold; 2009.

Perez CA, Breaux S, Bedwinek JM, Madoc-Jones H, Camel HM, Purdy JA, et al. Radiation therapy alone in the treatment of carcinoma of the uterine cervix. II. Analysis of complications. Cancer. 1984 July 15;54(2):235–46.

Whelan TJ, Pignol JP, Levine MN, Julian JA, MacKenzie R, Parpia S, et al. Long-term results of hypofractionated radiation therapy for breast cancer. N Engl J Med. 2010 February 11;362(6):513–20.

Withers HR, Taylor JM, Maciejewski B. Treatment volume and tissue tolerance. Int J Radiat Oncol Biol Phys. 1988 April;14(4):751–9.

QUESTIONS

Chapter 11   Questions

1. Which one of the following cell inactivation parameters best correlates with killing of tumor cell population by fractionated radiation?

   a. β component

   b. α component

   c. D_0

   d. D_q

   e. None of the above.

2. The alpha/beta ratio is

   a. the same as the flexure dose.

   b. large for actively dividing cells compared with nondividing cells.

   c. large for cells exposed to X-ray compared with cells exposed to alpha particles.

   d. larger for cells of the lung than for bone marrow cells.

3. D_0 is the dose of radiation that

   a. if fully used (no wasted radiation) would be sufficient to kill 100% of the exposed cells.

   b. is necessary to kill 37% of the original cells.

   c. is necessary to exceed the quasi-threshold dose.

   d. reduces survival to 10% of the original number.

4. D_q is the threshold dose

   a. that is given to cancer therapy patients.

   b. that theoretically must be reached before cell inactivation occurs.

   c. at which double-strand breaks begin.

   d. that is responsible for Poisson statistics.

5. How many cells will remain if 10^6 cells are irradiated to 6 Gy of X-rays that reduce survival to 0.1?

   a. 5×10^5 cells

   b. 10^5 cells

   c. 5×10^4 cells

   d. Not enough information is given to calculate.

6. The shape of a tumor control probability curve for a series of identical tumors, as a function of total dose above a particular threshold would best be described as

   a. parabolic.

   b. sigmoidal.

   c. linear.

   d. linear–quadratic.

7. The ratio of the number of cells in a 6-mm-diameter solid tumor compared with a 2-mm-diameter tumor will be closest to

   a. 3.

   b. 6.

   c. 9.

   d. 27.

8. As the dose rate for X-rays increases from 1 to 100 cGy/min,

   a. survival increases.

   b. repair is saturated for rates above 10 cGy/min.

   c. cell killing increases.

   d. survival depends on the extrapolation number.

9. Reoxygenation

   a. occurs in normal tissue near tumors.

   b. makes some tumor tissues more resistant to neutrons.

   c. occurs as the result of fractionation of the radiation dose.

   d. makes cells more sensitive to alpha particles.

10. Oxygen must be present

   a. during or very shortly after radiation to be effective.

   b. at a minimum of 120 mmHg to elicit maximum effect.

   c. for maximal killing of alpha particles.

   d. in order for tirapazamine to effectively kill cells.

11. One of the main reasons for continued interest in high-LET radiation therapy is

   a. the relatively low energies required to produce excellent depth dose curves.

   b. independence of cell killing on oxygen concentration.

   c. lower cost than conventional low-LET radiotherapy.

   d. better control rates for rapidly growing tumors.

12. IMRT is a form of
    a. brachytherapy.
    b. external beam therapy.
    c. heavy ion therapy.
    d. chemotherapy.

13. All of the modalities listed are used to treat cancer patients. The most common form of external beam therapy is
    a. protons from a cyclotron.
    b. photons from a linear accelerator.
    c. alpha particles from a cyclotron.
    d. carbon nuclei from a cyclotron.

14. HDR is a form of
    a. brachytherapy.
    b. external beam therapy.
    c. heavy ion therapy.
    d. chemotherapy.

15. What modality is used to treat the skin or superficial lesion?
    a. Electrons
    b. Photons
    c. Alpha particles
    d. HDR
    e. IMRT

16. What isotope is used for prostate seed implants?
    a. Ir-192
    b. I-131
    c. Pd-103
    d. Cs-137
    e. Co-60

CHAPTER 12

RADIATION BIOLOGY OF DIAGNOSTIC IMAGING

KEYWORDS

Diagnostic radiology, biology of diagnostic radiology, fluoroscopy, planar imaging, mammography, CT

TOPICS

- Biological effects of planar X-ray imaging
- Biological effects of fluoroscopic imaging
- Biological effects of mammographic imaging
- Biological effects of computed tomographic imaging
- Equipment and techniques to acquire diagnostic X-ray images

DIAGNOSTIC PROCEDURES

Almost all medical imaging procedures come from one of the six major diagnostic procedures: planar, fluoroscopic, computed tomographic, mammographic, magnetic resonance, or ultrasound imaging. The first four modalities use X-rays, magnetic resonance imaging uses radio frequency radiation, and ultrasound imaging uses high-frequency sound waves. Only procedures using X-rays are covered in this chapter.

Radiation Biology of Medical Imaging, First Edition. Charles A. Kelsey, Philip H. Heintz,
Daniel J. Sandoval, Gregory D. Chambers, Natalie L. Adolphi, and Kimberly S. Paffett.
© 2014 John Wiley & Sons, Inc. Published 2014 by John Wiley & Sons, Inc.

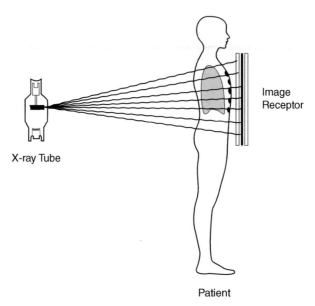

Figure 12.1   Schematic diagram of the geometry used to generate a planar radiographic image.

Medical diagnostic procedures expose more people to radiation than any other source of man-made radiation. In the United States, almost half (48%) of the population exposure is from diagnostic X-ray procedures. The frequency and amount of radiation the population gets from medical exposure increases with patient age.

The geometry of the four X-ray modalities is similar. A radiation source outside the patient sends X-rays through the patient to an image receptor on the other side of the patient's body. The transmitted radiation is detected, converted into a digital image, and presented on a video monitor. Less than 2% of the incident radiation reaches the detector on the exit side of the patient. The majority of the remaining 98% is absorbed in the patient where it may produce biological effects.

Figure 12.1 presents a schematic view of the planar image geometry where the X-rays pass through the patient and are detected in an image receptor on the exit side of the patient.

The dose to a particular patient depends on many factors including type of procedure, patient thickness, size of the X-ray beam, distance to the patient's skin, and technique factors used to make the exposure. Although determining the dose received by a specific patient requires detailed and complex calculations, it is possible to provide general values for various procedures for average-sized patients. Table 12.1 shows typical patient doses for several common radiographic procedures. The patient dose can vary by as much as a factor of 2 or 3 from these values. The table has two dose columns. The first column gives the typical entrance dose in mGy, and the second column gives the effective whole body dose in mSv. Recall that the effective dose is the whole body dose that would produce the same biological effect as the actual dose from the examination. The entrance dose is a close approximation to the maximum dose at the skin. Organ doses below the skin will be less. For diagnostic energies, the dose at the patient's midline is only about 10% of the maximum.

TABLE 12.1 List of Selected Diagnostic X-ray Examinations Showing Typical Entrance Skin Doses and Whole Body Effective Doses

Examination	Entrance Dose mGy	Effective Dose mSv
Abdomen	3	1
Chest	0.4	0.1
Head	1	0.1
Pelvis	3	2
Mammography	2	0.1
Spine	2	1
Dental	3	0.005

FLUOROSCOPY

Fluoroscopy is used to observe and record moving anatomy with the X-ray tube located on one side of the patient and the detector on the opposite side. Fluoroscopy is often used in cardiology and radiology to place catheters or stents in the patient. Sometimes, these procedures are difficult and require a great deal of time. In these cases, the patient may receive a large dose of radiation. Recall the patient receives the highest dose on the entrance side of the beam and that is often the posterior side of the patient.

Figure 12.2 shows a schematic diagram of a fluoroscopy system and a picture of fluoroscopic unit. The X-ray tube is located beneath the patient and the imaging device is above the patient. When using fluoroscopy units, which can be oriented horizontally, the operator should stand on the side opposite the X-ray tube. This is because the X-ray beam scatters both forward and backward. Standing opposite the X-ray tube allows the forward scattered X-rays to be attenuated in the patient before striking the operator.

The patient receives the primary dose, and greater than 98% of the radiation is absorbed or scattered in the patient. This scattered radiation is the greatest source of radiation dose that the operator receives during the fluoroscopy procedure. During fluoroscopy procedures, all individuals in the room must be wearing protective shielding. Protection reduces the operator dose to less than 10% of the scatter dose. During fluoroscopy, the X-ray beam is strictly collimated to pass through the patient and strike the image receptor.

The greatest source of radiation to the operator and staff during fluoroscopy is scattered from the patient. Stepping back from the patient reduces the scatter dose significantly. One step backward (from 1 to 2 m from the patient) reduces the scattered dose by about a factor of 4. A rule of thumb is that 1/1000 (0.001) of the patient entrance dose is received by the operator at 1 m from the patient. Physicians specializing in interventional procedures are recommended to wear protective glasses.

Table 12.2 presents some typical entrance and effective doses from representative fluoroscopic examinations.

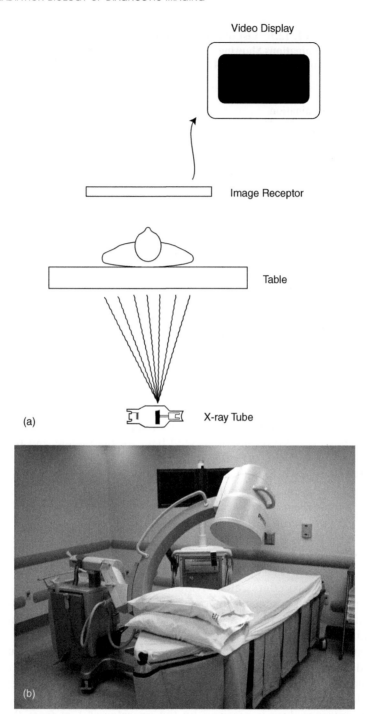

Figure 12.2   (a) The image on the left shows a schematic diagram of fluoroscopy equipment showing the patient on the table. (b) The figure shows a C-arm fluoroscopy room used for interventional radiology or cardiology procedures.

**TABLE 12.2   Typical Fluoroscopy X-ray Exams
Showing Typical Entrance Skin Doses and Whole Body
Effective Doses**

Examination	Entrance Dose mGy	Effective Dose mSv
Upper GI		6
Barium enema	60	8
IVP	4	2
Cardiac CTA		16
Interventional head		5

GI, gastrointestinal; IVP, intravenous pyelogram; CTA, CT angiogram.

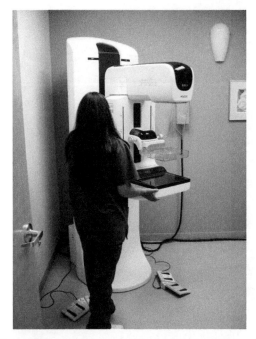

Figure 12.3   Picture of a digital mammography unit.

MAMMOGRAPHY

The breast is thinner than most other parts of the body and is relatively uniform and composed primarily of soft tissue. Mammographic examinations must detect small, submillimeter, higher-density calcium deposits and also larger cysts and cancers having almost the same density as normal breast tissue. To accomplish this difficult task, a specially designed unit is used to optimize the image with minimum dose. Figure 12.3 shows a picture of a mammography unit.

The mammography unit produces high-quality images that can show the difference between normal and cancerous tissues. Figure 12.4 illustrates a mammogram of a normal breast and one with a breast cancer.

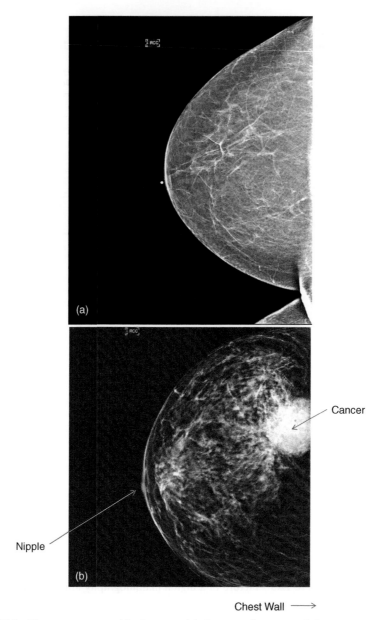

Figure 12.4 Two mammographic images. (a) Image of a normal breast mammogram; (b) image of a patient with a breast cancer.

During the mammographic examination, the breast is compressed to create a thinner, more uniform object. Lower-energy radiation is used because less penetration is needed. The mammography unit is designed to image the entire breast up to the chest wall. Mammographic doses are regulated by the U.S. Food and Drug Authority (FDA). Every mammographic facility must be accredited by the FDA before it can legally take mammograms. FDA regulations set maximum dose for a single image at 3 mGy. This is considerably higher than the 1–1.5 mGy used in most digital mammographic units. In a typical mammography screening exam, each breast is imaged twice. One image is in the cranial–caudal (CC) direction and the other is in the medial–lateral oblique (MLO) direction. In a screening mammographic examination, each breast should receive less than 2–3 mGy.

There has been some concern in the popular media that mammographic examinations might cause thyroid cancer because of the scattered radiation from the breast reaching the thyroid, which is known to be sensitive to radiation. Measurements have shown that the scattered radiation reaching the thyroid from a two-view mammographic examination is <0.04 mGy.

Background radiation is higher at higher altitude and that the annual background radiation in Denver or Salt Lake City is about 1 mGy/year, higher than at sea level. So the dose to the thyroid from a mammogram is about the same as a 2-week vacation in Denver or Salt Lake City. Most people would not be concerned about the extra radiation exposure during a 2-week vacation in the Rocky Mountains.

COMPUTERIZED TOMOGRAPHY (CT)

CT scanning uses a tightly collimated X-ray beam directed through the patient to a digital detector. The detector and the X-ray tube rotate about the patient as the patient moves continuously through the scanner. Figure 12.5 shows a schematic view of the CT geometry together with a photo of a clinical unit with a technician standing beside the unit. The transmission data collected during the rotation around the patient are processed in the CT computer and presented as a series of slice images.

CT examinations are the largest contributor of medical dose to the general public, and CT examinations of the head are the most common CT examination. CT doses are measured using the computed tomography dose index (CTDI). The CTDI takes into account the contributions from all the entrance beams as the source rotates around the patient. Typical CTDI is shown in Table 12.3. The CTDI is a

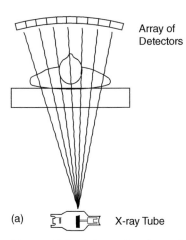
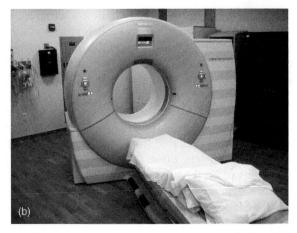

Figure 12.5 Schematic view of the CT geometry (a) and a photo of a clinical CT scanner (b).

TABLE 12.3   List of Selected CT Examinations Showing Typical CTDI (Organ) Doses and Whole Body Effective Doses

Examination	CTDI mGy	Effective Dose mSv
Abdomen	20	6
Chest	15	7
Head	50	2
Pelvis	20	7

representative dose to the tissue being irradiated. For example, it may represent the fetal dose for an abdominal scan of a pregnant patient. The table also shows the effective dose for each scan. This is representative of the effective whole body dose.

Figure 12.6 compares a conventional planar chest image and a CT image of the chest. The two images of the same anatomy are different in part because they are views perpendicular to each other.

RADIOBIOLOGY OF RADIOGRAPHIC IMAGING

The doses from most individual radiographic imaging procedures are actually quite low. However, multiple CT or specialized interventional or cardiology procedures can possibly deliver doses that result in noticeable damage. The organs at risk from diagnostic radiology and cardiology procedures are the skin, reproductive organs, eye, thyroid, and the female breast.

Skin

Skin damage from medical radiation is different from skin damage from the sun because medical radiations are much more penetrating. It is interesting that radiation exposures from interventional and diagnostic exposures are more damaging to the skin than radiation therapy exposures. This is because radiation therapy X-ray energies are so much more penetrating; they do less damage to the sensitive layers of the skin.

The highest dose from diagnostic procedures is at the skin surface where the X-rays enter. Most effects on the skin such as reddening, hair loss, and desquamation are tissue reaction or deterministic effects. Induction of skin cancer is a less frequent, long-term stochastic effect. The threshold for deterministic skin effects such as skin reddening or erythema is about 2 Gy. However, the actual skin reaction in a particular case depends on many factors including location of the skin, size of the area irradiated, dose fractionation, patient sensitivity, previous exposure, and any drugs the patient is taking.

Figure 12.7 shows radiation injury to the back of a patient who underwent three separate fluoroscopic procedures to improve his heart efficiency. The X-ray beam

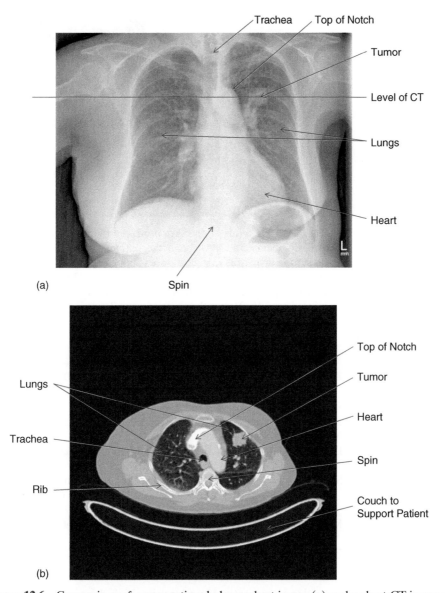

Figure 12.6 Comparison of a conventional planar chest image (a) and a chest CT image of the chest (b). The two images of the same anatomy are different in part because they are views perpendicular to each other. The CT image is conceptually displayed as a view from the patient's feet.

entered through his back, and the three entrance ports overlapped resulting in an area of excess dose.

One of the problems with excess skin exposure is that serious long-term effects are often not evident for months after the exposure. In the case shown in Fig. 12.7, there was some superficial redness apparent within a week after the last exposure. This early redness subsided within a week. The itching and open sore did not develop until several months after the last procedure.

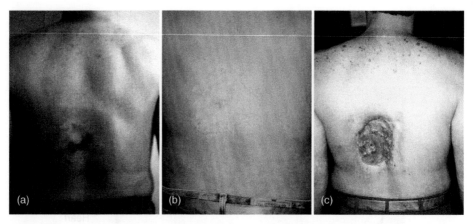

Figure 12.7 An example of a radiation injury to the skin produced by three separate interventional procedures. The X-ray beam entered through the patient's back, and the three entrance ports overlapped resulting in an area of excess dose (Shope). (a) The patient's back 6–8 weeks after exposure. The outline of the radiation field is evident. (b) The patient's back 16–21 weeks after exposure. The exposed area appears to be healed with only a small ulcerated area visible. (c) The injured area 18–21 months postexposure. The injury required skin grafts.

TABLE 12.4 Advice Physicians Can Give to Patients Undergoing High-Dose Procedures

Skin Dose (Gy)	Advice to Patient
0–2	No advice because no effects are expected.
2–5	Erythema may occur but should fade within a few weeks. If itching lasts beyond a few weeks, call the physician.
5–15	Some reaction may be expected. Be sure to observe the irradiated entrance area. If skin erythema and itching occur, patient should call the radiologist's office.
>15	Medical follow-up is essential, nature and frequency of which depending on estimated radiation dose.

Physicians should consider giving patients undergoing high-dose or difficult procedures advice about the possible side effects, especially if they previously had similar procedures that may have exposed the same skin area.

Perfusion head CT scans study the amount of blood reaching various parts of the brain by following a radio-opaque dye as it is transported into, through, and out of the brain. Perfusion studies require multiple CT scans in a short time resulting in a higher dose than used in a conventional CT head scan. The skin dose from a perfusion study is in the range of 300 mGy as compared with a dose of about 2 mGy from a conventional head scan. Multiple procedures may result in a significantly higher dose.

Table 12.4 provides general advice physicians should provide to patient undergoing high-dose X-ray procedures.

Reproductive Organs

The gonads, in general, are very radiosensitive. For male gonads, temporary sterility occurs at acute doses of at least 500 mGy, and permanent sterility can occur after acute doses of 6 Gy. To create permanent sterility in females, a dose of 6 Gy is required.

For many years, there was concern that pregnant women or potentially pregnant women should not undergo X-ray procedures that irradiate the embryo. Today, each female patient of childbearing age is asked if she is pregnant or could be pregnant. The current thinking is that if a female patient is pregnant or could be pregnant, then a physician will discuss the risks and benefits of the procedure before making a decision to postpone the procedure. Most diagnostic procedures pose little risk to the unborn child and if medically necessary should not be delayed.

Eye

Current regulations are based on older studies on the radiation sensitivity of the eye, which indicated that 2 Gy for acute and 5 Gy for chronic exposure are required to produce a cataract. Recent data show that doses as low as 0.5 Gy may produce a cataract. The current regulatory dose limit to the eye is 150 mSv/year. New data and International Commission on Radiological Protection (ICRP) recommendations may soon reduce this limit to 20 mSv/year. Based on these new findings, it may be prudent for physicians working in the high-dose areas to consider using eye shield protection. Only patients receiving many head scans would be at risk of eye damage and cataract formation.

Thyroid

The dose to the thyroid from any of the diagnostic X-ray procedures other than CT scans, which include the neck, is very small. Therefore, there is no real biological danger of thyroid cancer formation from non-CT procedures. CT examinations that do not include the neck only irradiated the thyroid with scattered radiation. The radiation dose from scattered radiation is very small, usually less than a few percent of the entrance dose, so is not of concern. If the neck is being examined during the CT scan, a thyroid protective shield is *not* recommended because a shield usually degrades scan image quality. The dose to the thyroid from mammography or dental exams is exceedingly small and is not a matter of concern.

Female Breast

Cancer can be induced by X-rays from a normal chest X-ray, chest CT, or mammogram. Fortunately, the normal chest X-ray is performed in the posterior–anterior (PA) projection. This means the breast receives the exit dose that is about 1% of the entrance dose and is quite low. Chest CT procedures produce a fairly uniform irradiation though the chest. In fact, the breast may receive the highest dose because it is near the surface. The breast dose from a typical chest CT is 10–12 mGy. The breast dose from a single planar PA chest image is about 5 µGy. Although the CT

TABLE 12.5 Tips on What to Tell Patients Concerned about Radiation

Patient Questions	Tip
What are you going to do?	Give the name of the procedure and its purpose
Why am I getting this procedure?	To find out what's wrong or to fix your problem
How much radiation will I get?	Give the dose in general terms, not specifically from Table 12.1, Table 12.2, or Table 12.3.
What does that mean? Or What is the risk?	Explain in terms of natural background. For example, it is about the same as living in Denver for 2 years instead of at sea level.
Will it hurt?	No, just lie still; there may be some noise.

dose is 4 orders of magnitude larger than the PA chest dose, both of these doses are relatively small and of little cause for concern regarding cancer induction.

PATIENT CONCERNS AND QUESTIONS

The medical community has recommended that any procedure involving X-rays that has a dose less than 100 mGy is not a risk. This is because a 100-mGy level is only four to five times larger than the natural background radiation dose in the United States.

Chapter 14 compares doses from medical radiation to doses from natural radiation sources.

The issue of answering patient's concerns and questions is always troublesome. Table 12.5 gives some tips and points designed to aid when these situations arise.

SUMMARY OF DIAGNOSTIC X-RAY RADIATION EFFECTS

- Diagnostic procedures, when done properly, do not pose a significant risk.
- Radiation-induced skin injuries may not become fully manifest until months after the radiation dose was administered.
- The diagnosis of a radiation-induced skin injury is often delayed.
- The lens of the eye is one of the most radiation-sensitive tissues.
- Diagnostic imaging adds some additional risk to the patient; however, the risk of dying from undiagnosed disease is much worse.
- CT scans produce the largest dose to the patient.

BIBLIOGRAPHY

Balter S, Hopewell JW, Miller DL, Wagner LK, Zelefsky MJ. Fluoroscopy guided intervention procedures: A review of radiation effects on patients' skin and hair. Radiology. 2010 February;254(2):326–41.

Bushberg JT, Seibert JA, Leidholdt EM, Boone JM. The essential physics of medical imaging. 3rd ed. Lippincott Williams & Wilkins; 2002.

Cousins C, et al. TG: 62 patient and staff radiation protection in cardiology. ICRP Report 2010.

Koenig TR, Mettler FA, Wagner LK. Skin injuries from fluoroscopically guided procedures: Part 2, review of 73 cases and recommendation for minimizing dose delivered to patient. Am J Roentgenol. 2001;117:13–20.

Mettler FA, Huda W, Yoshimumi TT, Mahesh M. Effective doses in radiology and diagnostic nuclear medicine: A catalog. Radiology. 2008 July;248(1):254–63.

Radiology Info.org. Available from: http://www.radiologyinfo.org/en/safety/.

Shope T. FDA report "Radiation-induced skin injuries from flouroscopy. FDA web site "Radiation_Emitting Products." 1995. http://www.fda.gov/radiation-emittingproducts/radiationemittingproductsandprocedures/medicalimaging/medicalx-rays/ucm116682.htm.

Wagner LK, Eifel PJ, Geise RA. Potential biological effects following high x-ray dose interventional procedures. J Vasc Interv Radiol. 1994;5:71–84.

Whelan C, McLean D, Poulos A. Investigation of thyroid dose due to mammography. Australas Radiol. 1999;43:307–10.

QUESTIONS

Chapter 12   Questions

1. Radiation-induced cataracts can arise at doses as low as _____ Gy.
   a. 0.2
   b. 0.5
   c. 2
   d. 5

2. A thyroid protective shield is _____ during a CT examination of the neck.
   a. always recommended
   b. never recommended
   c. recommended only for children
   d. necessary only for obese patients

3. The fetal exposure from a planar abdominal X-ray of a pregnant woman would be expected to be about _____ Gy.
   a. 0.3
   b. 0.8
   c. 1.5
   d. 3

4. The usual views of each breast during routine mammography examination are the _____ views.
   a. cranial–caudal (CC) and the anterior–posterior (AP)
   b. anterior–posterior (AP) and medial–lateral oblique (MLO)
   c. cranial–caudal (CC) and the medial–lateral oblique (MLO)
   d. cranial–caudal (CC), medial–lateral oblique (MLO), anterior–posterior (AP), and the left lateral (LL)

5. The entrance skin exposure for a PA chest X-ray will typically be about _____ mGy.
 a. 0.004
 b. 0.04
 c. 0.4
 d. 4.0
 e. 40.0

6. The effective dose for a PA chest X-ray will typically be about _____ mSv.
 a. 0.001
 b. 0.01
 c. 0.1
 d. 1.0
 e. 10

7. The typical dose per breast from a two-view screening mammography (CC and MLO) using a digital mammography system is
 a. 0.2 mGy.
 b. 0.5 mGy.
 c. 1.0 mGy.
 d. 2.0 mGy.
 e. 0.3 Gy.

8. A patient undergoing fluoroscopy receives an entrance skin dose of 850 mGy. The radiologist who performed the study was standing about 1 m away. The exposure to the radiologist, outside her lead apron, would be about _____ mGy.
 a. 85
 b. 8.5
 c. 0.85
 d. 0.085
 e. 0.0085

9. The threshold dose causing prompt erythema of the skin is approximately ____ Gy.
 a. 0.02
 b. 0.20
 c. 2
 d. 20
 e. 200

10. The computed tomography dose index (CTDI) or organ dose measured in the center of a *body* CT scan is about _____ mGy.
 a. 0.3
 b. 1.0
 c. 15
 d. 30
 e. 60

11. The computed tomography dose index (CTDI) or organ dose measured in the center of a *head* CT scan is about _____ mGy.

   a. 1.0

   b. 15

   c. 30

   d. 50

12. The imaging procedure that accounts for most of the medical dose to the general public is

   a. CT.

   b. mammography.

   c. chest.

   d. barium enema.

13. The most common CT procedure is

   a. head.

   b. chest.

   c. abdomen.

   d. dental.

14. Temporary sterility in male patients can be produced at doses as low as _____ Gy.

   a. 0.1

   b. 0.5

   c. 1

   d. 2

   e. 6

15. Changes in the eye have been seen at doses as low as _____ mGy.

   a. 100

   b. 200

   c. 500

   d. 1000

   e. 2000

16. The biological risk for a woman who has a screening mammogram annually is

   a. high.

   b. minimal.

   c. low.

CHAPTER 13

NUCLEAR MEDICINE
RADIATION BIOLOGY

KEYWORDS

Radiopharmaceutical, isotope, nuclide, SPECT, PET, MIRD, I-131, half-life, cumulated activity, internal dosimetry, dosimetry, radioisotope imaging, nuclear medicine imaging, nuclear medicine therapy, radionuclides, exposure rate, fetal dose, thyroid dose

TOPICS

- The underlying principles of nuclear medicine imaging and therapy
- The biological aspects of nuclear medicine
- External dosimetry issues specific to nuclear medicine
- Internal dosimetry in nuclear medicine
- The medical internal radiation dosimetry (MIRD) method

INTRODUCTION

Nuclear medicine is a branch of radiology that uses radioactive pharmaccuticals in the diagnosis and treatment of patients. Radioactive pharmaceuticals or "radiopharmaceuticals" are usually compounds that have been labeled with a radioactive nuclide. The pharmaceutical properties of a radiopharmaceutical determine where the material will localize within the patient. The photons or electrons emitted by

Radiation Biology of Medical Imaging, First Edition. Charles A. Kelsey, Philip H. Heintz, Daniel J. Sandoval, Gregory D. Chambers, Natalie L. Adolphi, and Kimberly S. Paffett.
© 2014 John Wiley & Sons, Inc. Published 2014 by John Wiley & Sons, Inc.

the radiopharmaceutical during radioactive decay are used to either provide information regarding the patient's physiology or to deliver a therapeutic radiation dose to tissue. The risk of detrimental effects due to nuclear medicine exams is comparable with those from other modalities such as computed tomography (CT) and intervention radiology.

The route of administration of the radiopharmaceutical depends on the particular procedure. In most nuclear medicine procedures, the radiopharmaceutical is administered by intravenous injection. Some procedures require the radiopharmaceutical to be inhaled, ingested with food or liquid, or injected into regions of the body other than a vein.

The majority of nuclear medicine procedures are for diagnostic rather than therapeutic purposes. In diagnostic nuclear medicine, the biological distribution of the radiopharmaceutical within the patient is used for diagnosis. This "biodistribution" of the radiopharmaceutical depends on the physiologic processes occurring within the patient. The biodistribution of a radiopharmaceutical should be different between a normal patient and a patient with a disease. The different biodistribution between normal and diseased states should register as a difference on nuclear medicine images.

Nuclear medicine imaging can be done in a variety of ways. These include planar studies that are analogous to radiographs. Tomographic nuclear medicine studies are performed with single-photon emission computed tomography (SPECT) and positron emission tomography (PET). Regardless of the specific method used to obtain the images, the basic work flow remains the same. The radiopharmaceutical is administered to the patient. Images are acquired of the radiopharmaceutical within the patient. The images of the biodistribution of the radiopharmaceutical within the patient are then used for diagnosis.

Nuclear medicine therapy involves the use of radiopharmaceuticals that are selectively taken up in diseased tissue and emit high-energy electrons during beta-minus decay. These high-energy electrons have an average range in tissue of less than a centimeter. Thus, the radiopharmaceutical can deliver a large amount of energy to the diseased tissue.

ISOTOPES AND RADIOPHARMACEUTICALS

The nucleus of an atom contains protons and neutrons. These particles are collectively known as nucleons. In standard nomenclature, the symbol for a generic element is $_Z^A X$. In this notation, the atomic number, Z, is the number of protons in the nucleus. The atomic mass, A, is the total number of nucleons in the nucleus. For example, $_6^{13}C$ signifies that the carbon nucleus has a total of 13 nucleons. Six of these nucleons are protons. By subtracting Z from A, we find there are seven neutrons in the $_6^{13}C$ nucleus. Often, the number of protons is not written since the chemical symbol implies the number of protons. For instance, $_6^{13}C$ is usually written as ^{13}C. All carbon nuclei have six protons. Another widely used nomenclature is the element followed by a hyphen and the atomic mass. For instance, ^{13}C can also be written as C-13.

Isotopes of an element have the same number of protons, Z, but different numbers of neutrons. The number of protons in the nucleus determines the number of electrons in the outer shells. The electron structure of an atom determines its chemical properties. Thus, all isotopes of an element have the same chemical properties. The difference between isotopes is in the number of neutrons within the nucleus. Among isotopes of a given element, the nuclear properties can be significantly different. For example, isotopes of carbon include ^{11}C, ^{12}C, ^{13}C, and ^{14}C. All of these isotopes of carbon have six protons and six electrons and have the same chemical properties. The nuclear properties of these isotopes are very different. The isotopes ^{12}C and ^{13}C are stable while ^{11}C and ^{14}C are radioactive.

The nucleus of a radioactive element has too much energy and is unstable. The nucleus can change to a more stable state by undergoing radioactive decay and emitting particles and energy. Radioactive decay products include alpha particles, electrons, positrons, and gamma photons. Radionuclides used in nuclear medicine decay by gamma emission, beta-minus, electron capture, or positron decay. Radionuclides that emit alpha or neutrons are not used in nuclear medicine.

In nuclear medicine, radioactive nuclei are used to radiolabel molecules. For example, if one were to take glucose and replace some of the stable carbon atoms with a radioactive version such as ^{11}C, then one would have a radioactive version of glucose that would have the same chemical behavior as normal glucose. The radioactive glucose could potentially be used as a tracer to study glucose uptake and metabolism in a patient. There is a wide variety of methods that can be used to add a radioactive atom to a molecule. As a result, there is a large arsenal of imaging agents that have been developed over the decades since the introduction of nuclear medicine imaging.

Gamma rays are high-energy, electromagnetic radiation. A particle or "quantum" of electromagnetic radiation is the photon. Gamma photons have zero charge and zero mass. The difference between X-ray photons and gamma photons is the point of origin. X-rays are produced from electron reactions, and gamma photons originate in nuclear reactions. The interaction of high-energy photons with matter is the same for both X-rays and gamma rays. In other words, X-rays and gamma rays undergo photoelectric absorption and Compton scattering.

The radionuclides used in nuclear medicine imaging emit gamma photons with specific, characteristic energies. For example, the most widely used radionuclide in nuclear medicine imaging is technetium-99m, Tc-99m or ^{99m}Tc. The "m" means that the nuclide is "metastable." A Tc-99m nucleus will undergo radioactive decay to Tc-99 by emitting a gamma photon. After the emission of the gamma photon, the nucleus is left in the "ground" or lowest energy state. The energy of the photon emitted by the transition of Tc-99m to Tc-99 is 140 keV (Table 13.1). Scattering of the emitted photons within the patient leads to a spread in the energies emitted from the patient. Photons with energies corresponding to the primary emitted energy are used to form the images. Scattered photons contribute to image noise.

Some radionuclides used in nuclear medicine decay by beta-minus decay. In this type of decay, the emitted particles are an electron and an antineutrino. The antineutrino will likely not interact with tissue and will leave the patient. However, the electron will interact with the tissue. An electron has a relatively low mass and is negatively charged. Electrons emitted by radionuclides used in nuclear medicine will typically slow and stop in less than a centimeter of tissue. The energy transferred to the surrounding tissue by the slowing electron can be relatively large. In therapy, the goal is to use this energy to destroy diseased cells.

TABLE 13.1   Listed Are Several Radionuclides Commonly Used in Nuclear Medicine

Radionuclide	Energy of Gamma Emission (keV)
Tc-99m	140
F-18	511
Xe-133	81
In-111	172, 247
I-131	364 (also emits β-)
I-123	159

Radionuclides that undergo radioactive decay by gamma emission produce gamma rays with characteristic energies.

When a radionuclide undergoes beta-minus decay, a neutron is effectively converted into a proton. As a result, beta-minus decay does not change the atomic mass, A, of the decaying nucleus. Beta-minus decay increases the atomic number, Z, by 1. In the following reaction notation, X signifies the original, parent nucleus and Y is the resulting daughter nucleus. In beta-minus decay, the increase in the number of protons in the nucleus results in an element that is different from the parent element.

Beta-minus decay:

$$_Z^A X \rightarrow {}_{Z+1}^A Y$$

Beta-plus decay is also known as positron decay. In this decay, the emitted particles are an energetic positron and a neutrino. A positron is a positive electron and is the antiparticle of the electron. Sometimes the positron is written as β^+. Beta-plus or positron decay effectively converts a proton into a neutron. As a result the atomic mass, A, remains unchanged and the atomic number, Z, decreases by 1.

Beta-plus decay:

$$_Z^A X \rightarrow {}_{Z-1}^A Y$$

When a positron and electron interact, they undergo annihilation and emit two photons. The photons move away from each other in opposite directions, and each of these annihilation photons has 511 keV in energy. The energy of the reaction is carried away from the point of annihilation by the two photons. This characteristic feature of positron-electron annihilation is the basis for PET imaging (Fig. 13.1).

An alternative reaction to beta-plus decay is electron capture. In this type of decay, the nucleus captures a K-shell electron and emits a neutrino. In this reaction, a proton is effectively converted to a neutron. The capture of the K-shell electron by the nucleus leaves a vacancy in the K-shell. Subsequent filling of this vacancy by outer shell electrons produces characteristic X-rays and Auger electrons. After electron capture, the nucleus may be left in an excited state. The nucleus may then de-excite by gamma emission. Some medical radionuclides such as I-123 and Tl-201 decay by electron capture.

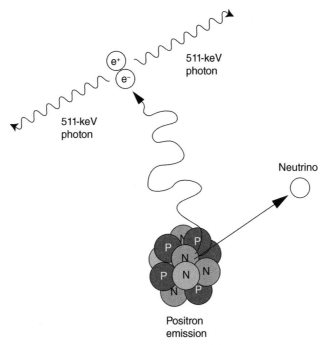

Figure 13.1 When a positron slows in matter, it will eventually interact with an electron. The result is a positron-electron annihilation event. The two particles are converted into two photons. Each photon has an energy of 511 keV. The photons move in opposite directions. This reaction is the basis for positron emission tomography (PET).

RADIOACTIVE DECAY

Radioactive decay is a random process. It is impossible to predict exactly when a specific radioactive nucleus will undergo radioactive decay. However, statistical methods can be used to describe the behavior of large groups of radioactive nuclei. For a collection of radioactive nuclei, the "activity" is a quantity that describes the number of radioactive decays occurring at a certain point in time. The activity can be defined as

$$A(t) = \lambda \cdot N(t),$$

where $A(t)$ is the activity at time t. The factor $N(t)$ is the number of radioactive nuclei present at time t. The activity of a radioactive material exponentially decreases with time. The rate at which the exponential decay occurs is governed by the decay constant, λ. The decay constant, λ, is a unique value for each nuclide. The rate of decay is not affected by temperature, pressure, and electrical or magnetic fields. The Système International (SI) unit for activity is the becquerel (Bq), which is equal to 1 disintegration per second. In the United States, the common unit of activity is the curie. One curie is equivalent to 3.7×10^{10} disintegrations per second.

TABLE 13.2 Half-Lives for Several Radionuclides Commonly Used in Nuclear Medicine

Radionuclide	Half-Life
Tc-99m	6.02 hours
F-18	109 minutes
Xe-133	5.3 days
In-111	67 hours
I-131	8.06 days
I-123	13.2 hours

Every radionuclide has a unique, characteristic half-life.

Units of activity:

Becquerel: 1 Bq = 1 disintegration per second = 1 dps

Curie: 1 Ci = 3.7×10^{10} disintegrations per second = 3.7×10^{10} Bq

The following exponential equation is known as the decay equation and describes how the activity changes with time:

$$A(t) = A_0 \cdot e^{-[\lambda \cdot t]}.$$

Here, A_0 is the initial activity of the sample at an arbitrary time, $t = 0$. This time is often referred to as the calibration time. The term $A(t)$ is the activity at a time, t, subsequent to the calibration time.

It is common to refer to the half-life of a radionuclide. The half-life is the time for half of the radioactive nuclei present at time $t = 0$ to undergo radioactive decay. Each radioactive nuclide has a characteristic half-life. Table 13.2 shows the characteristic half-life of some of the most common radioactive nuclides used in nuclear medicine.

The half-life, $T_{1/2}$, is equal to the natural logarithm of 2, ln(2), divided by the decay constant, λ:

$$T_{1/2} = \ln(2)/\lambda$$

or

$$\lambda = \ln(2)/T_{1/2}.$$

The decay equation is commonly written in terms of the half-life instead of the decay constant:

$$A(t) = A_0 \cdot e^{-[(\ln(2)/T_{1/2}) \cdot t]}.$$

Figure 13.2 shows the activity of any radionuclide as a function time. In this case, the time is expressed as the number of half-lives that have passed since the initial time, $t = 0$. For example, if we have 20 mCi of Tc-99m in a vial at noon, what activity

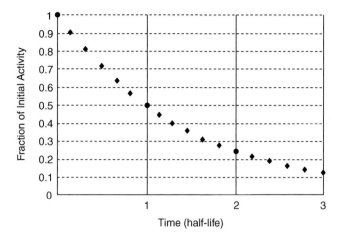

Figure 13.2 The activity of a radioactive material plotted as a function of time. After one half-life, the activity will be 50% of the activity at time, $t = 0$. After two half-lives, the activity will be 25% of the initial activity.

can we expect to have at midnight? The half-life of Tc-99m is 6 hours. After 12 hours, or two half-lives, only 25% of the initial radioactive nuclei will remain. Thus, at midnight, only 5 mCi of Tc-99m will remain in the vial.

The activity administered to a patient depends on the procedure. The amount of activity given to a patient may be modified by the physician to take into account the patient age, weight, metabolic status, and other factors that may affect the uptake and elimination of the radiopharmaceutical. Activities commonly administered in nuclear medicine range from a few microcuries, μCi, to a few hundred millicuries, mCi. Most imaging doses are in the neighborhood of 1–30 mCi. Some therapy doses can be up to several hundred millicuries. There is no upper limit to the amount of activity a nuclear medicine physician may prescribe for a patient. Like all medical procedures, the nuclear medicine physician must weigh the risk to the patient and the potential benefit to the patient from doing the procedure.

EXTERNAL DOSIMETRY

External dosimetry in nuclear medicine is limited to exposures from gamma rays or beta particles. Most instances of exposure are from gamma rays. Like X-rays, these are energetic photons. In matter, gamma ray photons are absorbed and scattered by the same mechanisms that act on X-rays, yet there are significant differences between X-ray-emitting sources and gamma-emitting sources that may impact external dosimetry.

The average energy of a gamma ray spectrum is usually much higher than the spectrum from a typical medical X-ray source. For instance, as a rule of thumb, the average energy of an X-ray beam used in radiographic imaging is 1/3 to 1/2 the peak X-ray energy. In some CT scans, the peak X-ray energy may be set to 140 kVp. In this case, the average energy of the X-ray beam is likely in the neighborhood of 70 keV. When imaging with gamma emitters such as Tc-99m, all of the photons emitted by the source will be at the characteristic energy. Tc-99m is monoenergetic and only emits a 140-keV gamma photon. Compton scattering in the patient will produce lower-energy photons, but for the most part, the average energy will remain much higher than the average energy of a comparable diagnostic X-ray beam.

In nuclear medicine, the source of gamma photons is always "on." In X-ray modalities, the X-ray tube only produces X-rays when the appropriate voltage and current are applied. Cutting the power supplied to the tube terminates the exposure, and X-rays are no longer produced in the X-ray tube. In nuclear medicine, the radiopharmaceutical always emits radiation. During transport and storage, the radiopharmaceuticals are kept in shielded containers. After administration, the patient becomes a source of radiation. If the administered radiopharmaceutical is a gamma emitter, the exposure rate at a distance from the patient may be significant. If the administered radiopharmaceutical is a beta-minus emitter, the likelihood of high-energy electrons escaping the body and traveling a significant distance is low. However, in this case, the body fluids of the patient may contain beta-minus-emitting radionuclides and can pose a potential radiation hazard.

Significant exposure to energetic electrons from beta-minus emitters rarely occurs. When it does occur, it is usually after an adverse event such as spill. Although the range of beta in tissue is fairly small, in air the range is approximately 800 times that in tissue. The range of the beta from Y-90 is several meters in air. The range is long enough that beta particles emitted by Y-90 on the floor could enter the lens of the eye. Another hazard of working with beta emitters is the possibility of intake via ingestion or inhalation.

If the amount of activity of a radionuclide is known, it is possible to calculate the exposure rate at a distance, d, from source using the following equation:

$$\dot{X} = \frac{A \cdot \Gamma}{d^2}.$$

In this equation, $\dot{X}$ is the exposure rate in roentgen per second. The term A is the activity in either mCi or Bq. The distance from the source to the point of interest is d, and Γ is the exposure rate constant. In this equation, the assumption is made that the source is a point source of activity and that the exposure rate decreases as $1/d^2$. The exposure rate constant, Γ, is a unique value for each nuclide. Values have been experimentally determined and these values may be found in the literature (Table 13.3).

TABLE 13.3 Exposure Rate Constants for Several Radionuclides Commonly Used in Nuclear Medicine

Radionuclide	Exposure Rate Constant Γ (R-cm^2/mCi-h)
Tc-99m	0.795
F-18	5.68
Xe-133	0.568
In-111	3.46
I-131	2.2
I-123	1.78

Adapted from Smith and Stabin (2012).

Example:
A syringe contains 20 mCi of a Tc-99m radiopharmaceutical. Calculate the exposure rate at a distance of 1 m. The value of Γ for Tc-99m is 0.795 R cm^2/mCi·h.

Solution:
At a distance of 1 m, the source can be treated as a point source:

$$\dot{X} = \frac{A \cdot \Gamma}{d^2} = 20 \text{ mCi } (0.795 \text{ R-cm}^2/\text{mCi-h})/(100 \text{ cm})^2 = 0.00159 \text{ R/h} = 1.59 \text{ mR/h}.$$

It is common in radiography and other X-ray modalities for technologists, nurses, and physicians to wear protective "lead" vests. A typical lead vest like those used in radiography and interventional medicine weighs approximately 10 lb and stops 90% of the scattered X-rays. Wearing one of these vests often becomes uncomfortable after a few hours. In PET imaging, the radiopharmaceuticals emit 511-keV gamma photons. To effectively reduce the dose to the technologists, the vest would have to be very thick. The weight of the vest then becomes so great that the vest would be impossible to use on a regular basis.

Rather than wearing personal shielding all day long, most nuclear medicine technologists employ other methods to reduce their exposure to radiation. Nuclear medicine technologists are trained to minimize their time around the patients once the radiopharmaceutical has been administered. They also regularly use equipment designed to help minimize the external exposure to radiation. Specially designed containers called "pigs" are used to store radiopharmaceuticals until use. The pigs are usually lined with lead or tungsten to attenuate the gamma photons. When the technologist is preparing to inject the patient, the radiopharmaceutical is measured and prepared behind a shield called an L-block. The L-block shields the body but still allows for manipulation of the syringe. A syringe containing a radiopharmaceutical is then placed in a syringe shield, which provides some amount of protection during injection. Stainless steel syringe shields are commonly used for gamma-emitting radiopharmaceuticals. For beta-emitting radiopharmaceuticals, low-Z materials such as plastic are used to shield against the high-energy electrons emitted by the source. High-Z materials such as steel should not be used to shield against high-energy electrons. There is a potential that the shield would become a source of bremsstrahlung X-rays produced by the electrons.

Checking for contamination and prompt cleanup of radioactive spills is another measure that helps minimize the radiation dose to occupational workers and the public. Surveys for contamination are made daily in a nuclear medicine department and all technologists receive training on how to clean up and decontaminate after spilling radioactive material. Frequent surveys and wipe testing in the nuclear medicine department help ensure that radioactive contamination is not being spread into nonrestricted areas. This helps minimize the risk of inadvertent and unnecessary external and internal exposures to the public, workers, and patients.

Nuclear medicine technologists and others who work with radiopharmaceuticals on a regular basis are aware of the hazards of radiation. Every nuclear medicine technologist has training in radiation safety. Throughout the nuclear medicine department, the philosophy of ALARA is used. ALARA stands for as low as reasonably achievable. Those working with radionuclides should be familiar with the phrase "time, distance, shielding." That is, minimize the time spent around a radioactive source. Maximize the distance between oneself and the source, and use shielding when it is reasonable to do so.

INTERNAL DOSIMETRY

The techniques of internal dosimetry are used for the determination of the radiation dose produced by a radioactive source within the body. Occupational internal exposures are infrequent but may occur. Occupational workers are trained to minimize the risk of intake of radiopharmaceuticals. To avoid ingestion or inhalation of radioactive materials, workers in nuclear medicine adhere to several simple rules. These include no eating, drinking, smoking, or application of cosmetics where radiopharmaceuticals are being handled. All radioactive materials should be labeled and stored properly. Spills of radioactive materials should be reported and cleaned immediately.

A bioassay is a test to measure the amount of radioactive material that has been ingested or inhaled. A bioassay may be necessary when there has been a possible unintentional intake of radioactive materials. This may occur during administration of volatile radiotherapy agents or after an accident or spill. In most cases where a bioassay is warranted, the radionuclide of concern is I-131. In this case, the bioassay consists of using a thyroid probe to measure the amount of radioactive iodine in the thyroid gland.

HALF-LIFE AND CUMULATED ACTIVITY

An important parameter in internal dosimetry is the cumulated activity. This is the total number of nuclei that have undergone radioactive disintegration within an organ that has absorbed a radioactive material. For those familiar with calculus, the total number of disintegrations that will occur with a sample of activity, A_0, can be calculated by integration of the decay equation from time = 0 to time = ∞. Another, perhaps more intuitive approach, is to realize that in an infinite amount of time, every radioactive nuclei present at time = 0 will eventually undergo radioactive decay. Thus, the total number of disintegrations is equal to N_0, which is the total number of radioactive nuclei present at time = 0. The total number of radioactive nuclei in a sample, N, is usually unknown. However, it is possible to measure the activity of a sample, and the half-life for a radionuclide is available in the literature. The relationship, $A = \lambda N$, can be rearranged and rewritten in terms of the half-life:

$$N = A/\lambda = A \cdot (T_{1/2}/\ln(2)) = A \cdot 1.44 \cdot T_{1/2}.$$

The value of N_0 is found to be

$$N_0 = A_0 \cdot 1.44 \cdot T_{1/2}.$$

Graphically, this is shown in Fig. 13.3. The number of radioactive disintegrations is the area under each curve.

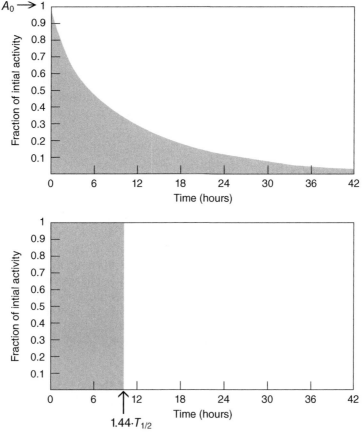

Figure 13.3 The total number of disintegrations is equal to the area under each curve (shaded area). In this figure, the areas under the two curves are the same.

THE BIOLOGICAL HALF-LIFE AND EFFECTIVE HALF-LIFE

After administration, the amount of radioactivity within a patient decreases through two processes. One process is radioactive decay. The other process is biological excretion. Many radiopharmaceuticals are eliminated via the urinary or digestive systems. The biological half-life, T_b, is the time that it takes a person to eliminate one-half of the administered radiopharmaceutical via biological processes. The biological half-life can have a wide range of values depending on the radiopharmaceutical and route of administration. For instance, the radioactive gas Xe-133 is used to image the ventilation properties of the lungs. In this study, the patient inhales the gas and then exhales. Here, the patient eliminates half of the administered activity in a relatively short amount of time. The biological half-life for ventilation studies is approximately 30 seconds. There are radiopharmaceuticals with biological half-lives that are effectively infinite. For instance, the radiopharmaceutical Tc-99m sulfur colloid is used to image the liver. After administration, the radiolabeled sulfur colloid enters cells in the liver, and the sulfur may remain in the liver for years.

The combined effect of biological elimination and radioactive decay is described by the effective half-life, T_e. The effective half-life may be calculated as follows:

$$1/T_e = 1/T_b + 1/T_p.$$

In this equation, T_p is the physical half-life. It is the same as the half-life from previous discussions, $T_{1/2}$. Note that $1/T_e$ is the rate of elimination, which is simply the sum of the biological rate of elimination, $1/T_b$, and the rate of elimination due to radioactive decay, $1/T_p$.

MEDICAL INTERNAL RADIATION DOSIMETRY (MIRD)

Perhaps the most widely used method for calculating internal dose to a patient is with the MIRD method formulated by the Society of Nuclear Medicine (SNM). The MIRD methodology is conceptually simple. In it, we want to calculate the amount of energy deposited in a "target" organ by the radiation emitted by one or more "source" organs. To perform such calculations, we need to make a number of assumptions regarding the biodistribution of the radiopharmaceutical within the patient, the size of the organs, and the distance between organs (Fig. 13.4).

The general MIRD equation for dose to a target organ, r_k, is shown as follows:

$$Dr_k = \sum_h \tilde{A}_h S(r_k \leftarrow r_h).$$

The dose to the target organ, Dr_k, is the sum of the contributions from each source organ, r_h. The term $\tilde{A}_h$ is the cumulated activity. It is the total number of

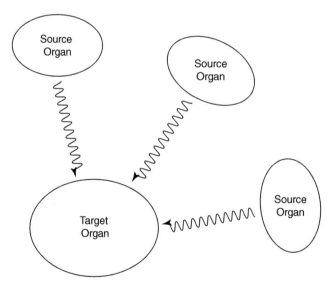

Figure 13.4 An illustration of the idea underlying the MIRD method. The dose to the target organ is the sum of all the contributions of radiation from source organs. The contribution from each source organ depends on a variety of factors including the amount of radiopharmaceutical uptake and distance to the target organ.

disintegrations that occur in a source organ, r_h. The units of $\tilde{A}_h$ are mCi·h. The cumulated activity, $\tilde{A}_h$, can be rewritten as

$$\tilde{A}_h = f_h \cdot A_0 \cdot 1.44 \cdot T_e.$$

Here, A_0 is the initial activity administered to the patient and f_h is the fraction of the initial activity that accumulates in the source organ. The term T_e is the effective half-life. Note that $A_0 \cdot 1.44 \cdot T_e$ is simply the total number of disintegrations between time $t = 0$ and $t = \infty$, where the rate of decay is governed by the effective half-life.

In the MIRD nomenclature, the term "$S(r_k \leftarrow r_h)$" is the "S-value" for source organ, r_h, and irradiating target organ, r_k. The S-value is the mean absorbed dose in the target organ per cumulated activity in the source organ. The absorbed dose in a target organ is calculated by multiplying the cumulated activity in each source organ by the corresponding S-value and summing the contributions from each source organ. S-values have the units rad/μCi-h or mGy/MBq·s. The S-values are calculated with the use of computer models known as Monte Carlo simulations. The computer simulations track the number of radioactive emissions that leave the source organ and deposit energy within the target organ. The tally of the simulated energy deposition in the target organ is the absorbed dose. The organ size, mass, and positions used in the MIRD simulations are for an idealized person. No person will exactly match the values used in the simulations. In addition, the radiopharmaceutical is assumed to be uniformly distributed in the source organ, which may not be a valid assumption in some cases. S-values and other data are published in MIRD pamphlets and are available at the SNM website. Perhaps an example will better illustrate the factors used in the MIRD method.

Example:
A hypothetical radiopharmaceutical is radiolabeled with Tc-99m. A patient is injected with 10 mCi of this radiopharmaceutical. When this radiopharmaceutical is injected into a patient, 60% instantaneously localizes in the thyroid gland and the remaining activity is rapidly removed from the blood by the kidneys and accumulates in the bladder. Once the radiopharmaceutical has localized in the thyroid gland, it remains there for a very long time. Thus, the biological half-life is effectively infinite and the effective half-life is equivalent to the physical half-life. Calculate the absorbed dose in the lungs from the gamma emissions from the thyroid (Table 13.4).

The S-value is found from MIRD pamphlet No. 11. For the case where the thyroid is the source organ and the lungs are the target organs, the S-value is 9.4×10^{-7} rad/μCi-h.

Solution:

$$A_0 = 10 \text{ mCi}$$

$$T_e = 6 \text{ hours}$$

$$f_h = 0.60$$

$$\tilde{A}_h = f_h \cdot A_0 \cdot 1.44 \cdot T_e = 0.60 \times 10 \text{ mCi} \times 1.44 \times 6 \text{ hours} = 51.8 \text{ mCi-h} = 51,800 \text{ μCi-h}$$

$$\text{Dose}_{(\text{lungs}\leftarrow\text{thyroid})} = (51,800 \text{ μCi-h}) \times (9.4 \times 10^{-7} \text{ rad/μCi-h}) = 0.049 \text{ rad} = 49 \text{ mrad}$$

TABLE 13.4 S-Values for Some Source and Target Organs

S, Absorbed Dose Per Unit Cumulated Activity (rad/μCi·h)

For Technetium-99m

Target Organs	Source Organs						
	Ovaries	Pancreas	Skin	Spleen	Testes	Thyroid	Bladder Contents
Kidneys	9.2E − 07	6.6E − 06	5.7E − 07	9.1E − 06	4.0E − 08	3.4E − 08	2.6E − 07
Liver	5.4E − 07	4.4E − 06	5.3E − 07	9.8E − 07	3.1E − 08	9.3E − 08	1.7E − 07
Lungs	6.0E − 08	2.5E − 06	5.8E − 07	2.3E − 06	6.6E − 09	9.4E − 07	2.4E − 08
Ovaries	4.2E − 03	4.1E − 07	3.8E − 07	4.0E − 07	0.0E + 00	4.9E − 09	7.3E − 06
Pancreas	5.0E − 07	5.8E − 04	4.4E − 07	1.9E − 05	5.5E − 08	7.2E − 08	2.3E − 07
Skin	4.1E − 07	4.0E − 07	1.6E − 05	4.7E − 07	1.4E − 06	7.3E − 07	5.5E − 07
Spleen	4.9E − 07	1.9E − 05	5.4E − 07	3.3E − 04	1.7E − 08	1.1E − 07	6.6E − 07
Testes	0.0E + 00	5.5E − 08	9.1E − 07	4.8E − 08	1.4E − 03	5.0E − 10	4.7E − 06
Thyroid	4.9E − 09	1.2E − 07	6.9E − 07	8.7E − 08	5.0E − 10	2.3E − 03	2.1E − 09
Uterus (nongravid)	2.1E − 05	5.3E − 07	4.0E − 07	4.0E − 07	0.0E + 00	4.6E − 09	1.6E − 05

Table adapted from MIRD pamphlet No. 11, Society of Nuclear Medicine.

Assume that the only other contribution to the absorbed dose in the lungs is from the remaining activity that has accumulated in the bladder. To simplify calculations, assume that the activity arrived in the bladder instantaneously and the activity remains in the bladder indefinitely. The S-value for the case where the bladder is the source organ and the lungs are the target organ is 2.4×10^{-8} rad/μCi-h:

$$A_0 = 10 \text{ mCi}$$

$$T_e = 6 \text{ hours}$$

$$f_h = 0.40$$

$$\tilde{A}_h = f_h \cdot A_0 \cdot 1.44 \cdot T_e = 0.40 \times 10 \text{ mCi} \times 1.44 \times 6 \text{ hours} = 34.6 \text{ mCi-h} = 34{,}600 \text{ μCi-h}$$

$$\text{Dose}_{(\text{lungs}\leftarrow\text{bladder})} = (34{,}600 \text{ μCi-h}) \times (2.4 \times 10^{-8} \text{ rad/μCi-h}) = 0.0008 \text{ rad} = 0.8 \text{ mrad}$$

Thus, the total absorbed dose to the lungs from this radiopharmaceutical is the sum of the thyroid contribution and the contribution from the contents of the bladder:

$$\text{Absorbed dose in lungs} = 49 \text{ mrad} + 0.8 \text{ mrad} = 49.8 \text{ mrad}.$$

An organ can be both a source organ and a target organ at the same time. For instance, in the previous example, we can calculate the absorbed dose to the thyroid from the radiopharmaceutical that localized in the thyroid. In this case, the thyroid is both the source organ and target organ. The S-value for the case where the thyroid is both the source and target organ is 2.3×10^{-3} rad/μCi-h. For radionuclides that undergo beta-minus decay, it can be assumed that all energy deposition is in the region where the radiopharmaceutical localizes.

Some limitations of the MIRD method include assumptions regarding kinetics of the radiopharmaceutical. This includes uptake and effective half-life of the radio-pharmaceutical. In some cases, the biokinetics of a radiopharmaceutical are based on methods such as animal studies, which may or may not translate well to humans. Also, the S-values and biokinetics are based on models of a healthy person. Disease within the patient may alter the biodistribution and biokinetics of the radiopharmaceutical.

FETAL DOSE

Due to the relative radiation sensitivity of the fetus, caution must be applied in situations where the fetus may be exposed to radiation or radiopharmaceuticals. The MIRD method may also be used to calculate the dose to the fetus from either maternal organs or from uptake in fetal organs.

In the case where the radiopharmaceutical does not cross the placenta, the radiation dose to the fetus will only be from radiation emitted by the maternal organs. Many radiopharmaceuticals are removed from the body by the urinary system and accumulate in the urinary bladder. The mother's bladder is in close proximity to the uterus and fetus. The dose to the uterus by radiopharmaceuticals in a variety of source organs can be calculated using tabulated S-values and the MIRD method.

In the case where the radiopharmaceutical does cross the placenta, the radiation dose to the fetus is the sum of the contributions from radiation emitted by the mother and the radiation emitted by the radiopharmaceutical absorbed by the fetal organs. The radiopharmaceutical of primary concern is radioiodine. Dietary iodine is necessary for proper functioning of the normal thyroid gland. The thyroid extracts iodine from the blood and incorporates the element into several very important hormones. Diseases of the thyroid gland may afflict women of childbearing age. Radioactive iodine distributes within the body in the same manner as stable, dietary iodine. The radioactive iodine is often used to diagnose and treat diseases of the thyroid. There are two widely used versions of radioiodine: I-123 and I-131. Iodine-123 emits a 159-keV gamma photon and has a half-life of 13.2 hours. The photon energy is very good for imaging and the relatively short half-life contributes to rapid elimination of the radioactivity from the patient. For these reasons, I-123 is widely used for diagnostic purposes. Iodine-131 emits gamma photons of several different energies. The most frequently emitted of these has an energy of 364 keV. Not only does I-131 emit gamma rays, but it also emits an energetic electron in 90% of radio-active decays. Most of the electrons emitted only travel a few millimeters while depositing energy within the tissue. For this reason, I-131 is widely used in therapy where the thyroid tissue function needs to be reduced or where the thyroid tissue needs to be destroyed.

Data are available for the absorbed dose to the fetus from radiopharmaceuticals administered to the mother as shown in Table 13.5. These values take into account the S-values for the mother's contribution to the fetal dose, the biodistribution within the mother, and in some cases placental crossover and the resulting biodistribution within the fetus. Results from these types of studies greatly simplify the calculation of the fetal dose.

The fetal thyroid begins to absorb iodine at the 10th to 12th week of gestation. The percent uptake by the fetal thyroid can exceed that of the mother. Uptake in the fetal thyroid can easily result in doses that can damage or destroy the gland. Notice the difference in magnitude of the values for I-123 and I-131 in Table 13.6. It only takes a small amount of I-131 activity to produce a significant absorbed dose

TABLE 13.5 Absorbed Dose Estimates to the Embryo/Fetus per Unit Activity of Radiopharmaceutical Administered to the Mother

Radiopharmaceutical	Early mGy/MBq	3 Months mGy/MBq	6 Months mGy/MBq	9 Months mGy/MBq
I-123 sodium iodide	2.0E – 02	1.4E – 02	1.1E – 02	9.8E – 03
I-131 sodium iodide	7.2E – 02	6.8E – 02	2.3E – 01	2.7E – 01
F-18 FDG	2.2E – 02	2.2E – 02	1.7E – 02	1.7E – 02
T-99m pertechnetate	1.1E – 02	2.2E – 02	1.4E – 02	9.3E – 03
Tc-99m MDP	6.1E – 03	5.4E – 03	2.7E – 03	2.4E – 03
Tc-99m MAA	2.8E – 03	4.0E – 03	5.0E – 03	4.0E – 03
Xe-133, 5-minute rebreathing, 7.5-L spirometer volume	2.2E – 04	2.6E – 05	1.9E – 05	1.5E – 05

Adapted from Russell et al. (1997).

TABLE 13.6   Fetal Thyroid Dose for Two Different Isotopes of Iodine

Absorbed Dose in Fetal Thyroid from Radionuclides Administered to the Pregnant Woman		
(mGy/MBq Administered to the Woman)		
Gestational Age (Months)	I-123	I-131
3	2.7	230
4	2.6	260
5	6.4	580
6	6.4	550
7	4.1	390
8	4.0	350
9	2.9	270

I-131 undergoes beta-minus decay and emits a high-energy electron. This is responsible for the relatively large dose to the thyroid tissue. Adapted from Watson (1992).

in the fetal thyroid. This is of special concern since the hormones produced by the thyroid are important for neurological development. If damage to the fetal thyroid occurs, there is a chance that the child will develop hypothyroidism and possibly cretinism.

In general, the radiation dose to the fetus due to uptake of radioiodine is dependent on the age of the fetus and the status of the mother. In the literature, more tabulated data like those shown are available. Data for special cases such as hyperthyroidism in the mother are also available.

Example:
A mother receives a thyroid uptake and imaging study to evaluate the possibility of Grave's disease. Several months after the study, the mother discovers that she is pregnant. After determination of the age of the fetus, it is estimated that the fetus was 11 weeks old at the time of the nuclear medicine study. During the procedure, 10 μCi of I-131 and 12 mCi of Tc-99m pertechnetate were administered to the mother. Calculate the radiation dose to the fetus and the absorbed dose to the fetal thyroid.

Solution:

$$10 \, \mu Ci = 370,000 \, Bq = 0.37 \, MBq$$

$$12 \, mCi = 444 \, MBq$$

Whole body dose:

Using the 3-month value for I-131,
$$D = (6.8 \times 10^{-2} \, mGy/MBq)(0.37 \, MBq) = 0.025 \, mGy.$$

Using the 3-month value for Tc-99m pertechnetate,

$$D = (2.2 \times 10^{-2} \text{ mGy/MBq})(444 \text{ MBq}) = 9.8 \text{ mGy}.$$

The total whole body absorbed dose is 9.8 mGy.
For the fetal thyroid:
The 3-month value for I-131 is 230 mGy/MBq.

$$\text{Dose} = (230 \text{ mGy/MBq})(0.37 \text{ MBq}) = 85 \text{ mGy}.$$

The exposure of a fetus to ionizing radiation has been known to produce lethal effects in the preimplantation stage, induction of malformations, and detrimental effects to intelligence. The International Commission on Radiological Protection (ICRP) has taken the position that there is little practical risk to the embryo and fetus for deterministic effects for radiation doses under 100 mGy (ICRP Publication 103). The lifetime cancer risk for *in utero* irradiation is about three times the risk as for the entire population. This is similar to the value obtained for exposure in early childhood. In the previous example, an absorbed dose of 9.8 mGy is substantially less than the threshold dose of 100 mGy; thus, no deterministic effects should occur. However, stochastic effects cannot be ruled out.

For breastfeeding, the primary radionuclide of concern is I-131. It accumulates in breast milk and can be passed to the nursing infant. Other radiopharmaceuticals either do not accumulate in breast milk or are in such quantities that cessation of breast-feeding is usually not necessary. In cases where the mother may be significantly radioactive after a nuclear medicine study, the mother is often advised to avoid breast-feeding due to the close contact with the child. In this case, the breast milk may be pumped, and the child may be fed by another individual. In many cases, the mother is given instructions so as to keep the exposure to the infant as low as reasonably achievable.

CONCLUSION

External dosimetry in nuclear medicine is unique in that the patient is often the primary source of radiation. The nuclear medicine department is also the only place in the radiology department where personnel will likely encounter unsealed sources of radioactive materials. Internal dosimetry in nuclear medicine can be a complex issue that involves the biokinetics of the radiopharmaceutical within the patient. A common method for internal dosimetry calculations is the MIRD model. The MIRD model has been used in conjunction with other data to calculate the dose to the fetus due to activity being administered to the mother. A topic of special concert is the unintentional administration of I-131 to the pregnant female due to the high uptake in the fetal thyroid and high potential for damage to the gland.

For further readings and references on these topics, the RADAR website and the SNM website are both excellent places to begin further investigation.

BIBLIOGRAPHY

Russell JR, Stabin MG, Sparks RB, Watson E. Radiation absorbed dose to the embryo/fetus from radiopharmaceuticals. Health Phys. 1997 November;73(5):756–69.

Smith DS, Stabin MG. Exposure rate constants and lead shielding values for over 1,100 radionuclides. Health Phys. 2012 March;102(3):271–91.

SNM. Society of Nuclear Medicine. Reston: SNM; 2012 [cited March 29, 2013]. Available from: http://www.snm.org/.

Snyder WS. "S," absorbed dose per unit cumulated activity for selected radionuclides and organs. New York: Society of Nuclear Medicine; 1975.

Stabin MG, Siegel JA, Hunt J, Sparks R, Lipsztein J, Eckerman KF. Radar: The radiation dose assessment resource. An online source of dose information for nuclear medicine and occupational radiation safety. J Nucl Med. 2001 May;42(5):243.

Watson E. Radiation absorbed dose to the human fetal thyroid. Fifth International Radiopharmaceutical Dosimetry Symposium. Oak Ridge, TN: Oak Ridge Associated Universities; 1992, pp. 179–87.

QUESTIONS

Chapter 13   Questions

1. A sample of a Tc-99m-labeled radiopharmaceutical is measured at 8:00 a.m. and is found to have an activity of 1 mCi. What will be the activity of the sample 12 hours later at 8:00 p.m.? The half-life of Tc-99m is 6 hours.

   a. 0 mCi

   b. 1 mCi

   c. 0.5 mCi

   d. 0.25 mCi

2. How many radioactive nuclei, N, are in a 1 GBq sample of F-18? The decay constant of F-18 is 1.05×10^{-4} per second.

   a. 9.5×10^{12} F-18 nuclei

   b. 1.6×10^{11} F-18 nuclei

   c. 500 F-18 nuclei

   d. 2.6×10^{9} F-18 nuclei

3. Which of the following would be the most chemically similar to the stable nuclide C-12?

   a. Carbon-14

   b. Nitrogen-12

   c. Fluorine-12

   d. Oxygen-18

4. The MIRD method is used to calculate

   a. the activity of a radiopharmaceutical.

   b. the time required for a procedure.

   c. the organ doses from internal radiopharmaceuticals.

   d. the effective half-life.

5. What is the cumulated activity, $\tilde{A}_h = 1.44 \times A_0 \times T_e$, for 100 Bq of activity in an organ and an effective half-life of 10 minutes? Assume a fractional uptake, f_h, of 1.0.

   a. 86,400 disintegrations

   b. 1440 disintegrations

   c. 14.4 disintegrations

   d. 5.3×10^{11} disintegrations

6. What is the cumulated activity, $\tilde{A}_h = 1.44 \times A_0 \times T_e$, for 5 μCi of activity in an organ and an effective half-life of 2 hours? Assume a fractional uptake, f_h, of 1.0.

   a. 0.069 μCi-h

   b. 14.4 μCi-h

   c. 2.67 μCi-h

   d. 86,400 μCi-h

7. What is the effective half-life of a radiopharmaceutical that has a physical half-life of 6 hours and a biological half-life of 1 hour?

   a. 7 hours

   b. 0.14 hours

   c. 1.17 hours

   d. 0.86 hours

8. What is the effective half-life of a radiopharmaceutical that has a physical half-life of 6 hours and a biological half-life of 1 year?

   a. 6 hours

   b. 0.17 hours

   c. 6 years

   d. 0.17 years

9. The exposure rate constant, Γ, for Tc-99m is 0.795 R·cm^2/mCi·h. What is the exposure rate 10 cm from a 1-mCi point source?

   a. 0.00795 R/h

   b. 0.00795 mR/s

   c. 161 R/h

   d. 161 mR/s

10. The exposure rate constant, Γ, for F-18 is 5.68 R·cm^2/mCi·h. What is the exposure rate 100 cm from a 15-mCi point source?

    a. 0.0085 R/s

    b. 8.5 mR/h

    c. 117 R/h

    d. 117 mR/s

11. The fetal thyroid has avid uptake of iodine after what period of time?

    a. Immediately after conception

    b. The 2nd to 3rd week of gestation

    c. The 10th to 13th week of gestation

    d. The 20th to 23rd week of gestation

12. Which of the following are valid units for the S-value used in MIRD?

    a. mR-mCi/h-cm

    b. R-cm^2/mCi-h

    c. mGy/MBq-s

    d. μCi-h

13. Radionuclides that do not cross the placenta

    a. do not irradiate the fetus and are harmless.

    b. can still irradiate the fetus with X-rays and gamma rays.

14. For Tc-99m, what is the S-value when the spleen is both the source organ and the target organ?

    a. 8.6 E–07 mGy/MBq-s

    b. 9.2 E–07 rad/μCi-h

    c. 9.2 E–07 mGy/MBq-s

    d. 3.3 E–04 rad/μCi-h

15. The half-life of F-18 is 110 minutes. What is the decay constant, λ, for this radionuclide?

    a. 0.0063 per second

    b. 0.0091 per minute

    c. 0.54 per hour

    d. 0.0063 per minute

16. The absorbed dose in the fetal thyroid from I-131 administered to the mother ranges from 230 mGy/MBq at a gestational age of 3 months to a maximum of _____ mGy/MBq at 5 months gestational age.

    a. 530

    b. 320

    c. 580

    d. 100

CHAPTER 14

ENVIRONMENTAL RADIATION

KEYWORDS

Natural background, man-made radiation, background sources

TOPICS

- State the magnitude and source of natural background radiation
- State the fraction of environmental radiation in the United States that is due to medical exposure
- List the health effects of background radiation
- Compare risk versus benefit in various occupations and activities

INTRODUCTION

Everyone is constantly exposed to radiation from the environment. Environmental radiation comes from the sky, the earth, and the air we breathe and can be categorized as natural or artificial. In 2009, the National Council on Radiation Protection (NCRP) published NCRP Report 160, which is a summary of the radiation exposure to the United States population in 2006. Background radiation can be divided into two sources: man-made and natural background. The average total effective dose to a person living in the United States in 2006 was 6.2 mSv, of which medical exposure was 3.0 mSv. Table 14.1 shows the estimated effective doses to an individual in

Radiation Biology of Medical Imaging, First Edition. Charles A. Kelsey, Philip H. Heintz,
Daniel J. Sandoval, Gregory D. Chambers, Natalie L. Adolphi, and Kimberly S. Paffett.
© 2014 John Wiley & Sons, Inc. Published 2014 by John Wiley & Sons, Inc.

TABLE 14.1 Estimated Effective Doses per Individual in the U.S. Population (from NCRP 160)

	mSv	%
Internal, inhalation (radon and thoron)	2.3	36.5
External, space	0.3	5.3
Internal, ingestion	0.3	4.6
External, terrestrial	0.2	3.4
Natural background dose	3.1	
CT	1.5	23.5
Nuclear medicine	0.8	12.3
Interventional fluoroscopy	0.4	6.9
Conventional radiography and fluoroscopy	0.3	5.3
Medical dose	3.0	
Other		
Consumer products	0.1	2.2
Industrial, security, medical, educational, and research	<0.1	<0.1
Occupational—average	<0.1	0.1
Total effective dose	6.2	100

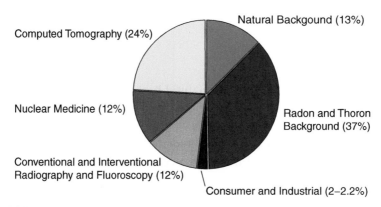

Figure 14.1 Graphical illustration of the estimated dose to the U.S. population in 2006.

the United States as published in NCRP Report 160. Figure 14.1 shows the relative magnitude of various environmental radiation sources.

NATURAL BACKGROUND RADIATION SOURCES

Figure 14.2 illustrates the major sources of natural background radiation. They are internal, cosmic, and from rocks and dirt from the earth. The amount of these sources can vary considerably. Locations at higher altitude or in regions with high radioactive minerals have higher background radiation levels.

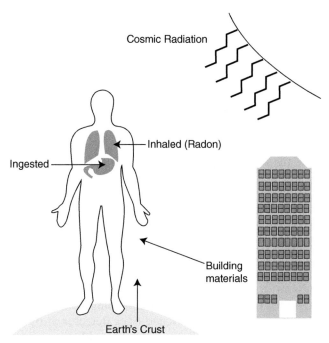

Figure 14.2 The figure shows many of the man-made sources or radiation that the public is exposed to daily.

TABLE 14.2 Effective Doses from Background Radiation	
Source	Effective Dose (mSv)
Space (cosmic)	0.33
Terrestrial	0.21
Potassium K-40	0.15
Ingested thorium and uranium series	0.13
C-14, Rb-87	0.01
Inhalation radon 222-Rn	2.12
Inhalation thoron 220-Rn	0.16
Total	3.11

Table 14.2 lists the magnitude of the prominent sources of natural background radiation. The effective dose (E) from all of these sources is about 3.11 mSv/year. Seventy-three percent comes from internal inhalation mostly from radon. Eleven percent comes from external sources including outer space, followed by 9% from internal ingestion, and 7% by external terrestrial.

INHALATION SOURCES

Radon is produced through the decay of uranium and thorium that are found naturally in the earth's crust. One of the products of this decay is ^{222}Rn, which is an inert noble gas that is capable of moving from the ground into the air we breathe. Another product is ^{220}Rn, which is called thoron. On average, ^{222}Rn contributes 2.12 mSv/year and ^{220}Rn contributes 0.16 mSv/year.

^{222}Rn also known as radon is produced by the decay of 226 radium. Radium has a half-life of 1622 years. Radon decays to 218 polonium by alpha decay with a half-life of 3.8 days. Radon is a gas that decays to a solid, so when it is inhaled, the decay products stay in the body. Most of the dose to the body comes from alpha particles in the trachea, bronchus, and lungs.

Radon is a gas, as such diffuses from its point of origin. The amount of radon activity depends on the local concentrations and the soil porosity. Radon concentrations in open air are low because there is rapid mixing. However, in buildings, it moves by diffusion. Radon itself poses little biological danger. However, its daughter products are alpha emitters, are solids, and contribute to the internal dose in the tracheobronchus and lungs. Radon gas exposure can be higher in buildings because it is heavier than air and is often trapped in basements.

Radon gas is the largest component of natural background radiation. The Environmental Protection Agency (EPA) estimates that radon is the primary cause of lung cancer deaths in nonsmokers. BEIR IV (1998) report estimates that radon inhalation is thought to contribute 10% of the fatal lung cancer in the United States.

Radon gas is easily measured by an etched track detector or by using a small jar filled with activated charcoal. Outdoor levels are low with an average level of 7 Bq/m^3 and typical indoor levels with an average of 45 Bq/m^3. Indoor concentrations vary by location and building material. Areas near uranium mining usually have higher concentrations of radon gas. The EPA action limit for the radon gas in a home is 4 pCi/L, which is equal to 148 Bq/m^3. Ninety-five percent of the homes in the United States are under this action level.

Figure 14.3 shows the distribution of radon concentration in living areas in the United States. The coastal areas have the lowest concentrations with less than 37 Bq/m^3 while the central part of the United States has the highest with greater than 148 Bq/m^3.

INTERNAL SOURCES

Foods rich in potassium contain a small fraction of ^{40}K, which is made in the upper atmosphere and has a half-life of 1.3 billion years. ^{40}K has a natural abundance of 0.0117%, about 4400 nuclei of ^{40}K decay per second in the human body. Table 14.2 shows that ^{40}K contributes 0.15 mSv to the annual effective dose. The dose contributions from radon-220, lead-210, and polonium-210 are less than that of ^{40}K. Radium in the body is found mostly in the bone, as it is close to calcium in its atomic structure. It enters the body by ingestion of food.

As a side issue, food irradiated for preservation does not become radioactive from the irradiation process. Therefore, there is no residual radiation that would contribute dose to the population.

COSMIC RADIATION

Cosmic radiation comes from the sun and outer space. Cosmic radiation contributes approximately 0.33 mSv/year. Most of it comes from directly ionizing radiation—90%

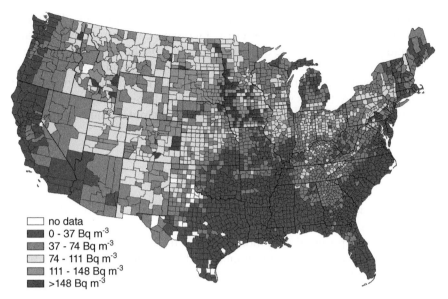

Figure 14.3   The radon concentration in areas in the United States as shown in NCRP 160. The darker areas indicate higher radon concentrations.

protons and 9% alpha particles. While most cosmic radiation is either deflected by the earth's magnetic field or absorbed by the atmosphere, a small amount reaches the earth's surface to which we are exposed. The atmospheric attenuation of cosmic radiation is equivalent to about 10 m of water. Cosmic radiation is not uniform on earth. It is highest at the north and south poles and minimum at the equator.

The exposure to this type of radiation is higher for people living above sea level. For example, people living in Albuquerque or Denver will have an increased cosmic ray dose of 0.29 mSv/year above those people living at sea level. People living above 2500-m (~8000 ft) elevation will have an additional 0.70 mSv/year higher than people living at sea level.

Cosmogenic radioisotopes contribute some to the daily background exposure. These isotopes are produced by cosmic radiation interacting with the upper atmosphere. Of all the isotopes bombarding us, only tritium (^{3}H), beryllium (^{7}Be), carbon (^{14}C), and sodium (^{22}Na) contribute significantly. ^{14}C is the major contributor at 0.01 mSv/year. Recall that ^{14}C has a half-life of 5730 years and is used for "carbon" dating of living organisms. While an organism is alive, it exchanges ^{14}C with regular carbon in the organism and reaches equilibrium. When it dies, this exchange stops, and the carbon to ^{14}C ratio is no longer in equilibrium. The ratio of nonradioactive carbon to carbon can be used to date the material.

PRIMORDIAL AND TERRESTRIAL

The primordial earth was very radioactive. However, the shorter-lived isotopes have since decayed away. Primordial and terrestrial radiation are present in rocks and soils and occur when naturally radioactive isotopes of uranium, thorium, and potassium decay within the earth's crust. Geologic concentrations of uranium, thorium, and potassium geologic deposits typically have higher background radiation levels. In some areas, the largest contributor to background radiation in the soil is from ^{40}K. Other high background locations in the world include Brazil, India, Iran, and areas in China. Activities such as mining enhance these background levels, such as uranium mining in New Mexico and Colorado or potash mining in northern Florida.

MAN-MADE RADIATION

There are two types of "man-made" radiation: technology modified and technology produced by man.

An example of exposure due to modification is the exposure from radon. Radon is a natural isotope, but the exposure is enhanced by building practices that trap the radon gas. Examples of exposure due to man-made production of radioactive sources include X-ray devices and nuclear fission in reactors and nuclear weapons.

Fallout radiation is one of the forms of technology-produced radiation. It is a result of past atmospheric nuclear bomb tests. During the 1950s and 1960s, many test explosions released radioactive products into the atmosphere, and these materials have been transported around the world and eventually fall back to the earth. Since 1945, there have been approximately 502 atmospheric and 1876 underground atomic tests conducted around the world. This amounts to 504 megatons (MT) of TNT. Although classified, there are about 13,000 MT of nuclear weapons still in existence. Each weapon contains about 4 kg of plutonium. The testing so far exposes the world population to about 900 mSv over a lifetime, which is equivalent to three additional years of background irradiation during their lifetime. Of this effective committed dose, ^{14}C accounts for about 70%, ^{137}Cs accounts for 14%, and ^{90}Sr (a bone-seeker) accounts for 3.2%, even though the last atmospheric nuclear weapons test was in 1962. This dose over a typical lifetime is almost inconsequential.

Nuclear power production also contributes to global exposure. The exposure comes from uranium mining, milling, fuel fabrication, reactor operation, waste storage, and waste disposal. This accounts for about 0.0001 mSv/year per person. Because people living close to nuclear power plants are concerned about their exposure, the U.S. Nuclear Regulatory Commission (NRC) has limited the total release from a power plant to be less than 0.050 mSv/year at the boundary of the facility. The nuclear power industry has an excellent safety record, and the total dose contribution from nuclear power to the population has been very small.

There have been several nuclear power plant accidents. The largest was Chernobyl, which contributed significant exposure to the people of the Soviet Union, and Europe. Most recently, the Fukushima nuclear power plants in Japan damaged by a large earthquake and tsunami released radioactive material from their plants. Most of the contamination came from iodine-131 along with cesium-134 and cesium-137. In the United States, the largest nuclear accident was at Three Mile Island Power Plant. The magnitude of the collective exposure to the population of western Soviet Union and northern Europe from Chernobyl was 30,000 times greater than the exposure to the people living within 80 km of the Three Mile Island accident.

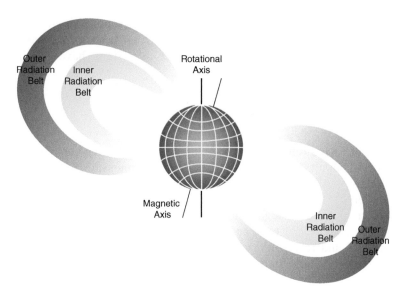

Figure 14.4   Radiation from the atmosphere and the Van Allen belts.

Conventional power plants contribute more radiation to the environment than nuclear power plants. One of the biggest sources of this type of radiation is from the fly ash residue from coal-fired power plants. This is an inhaled source of radiation that contains ^{40}K and other primordial radioactive elements. Most of the radiation exposure is concentrated near the power plant. It is estimated that the annual exposure from the coal-fired plants is 0.015 mSv/year to persons living nearby.

People traveling by air are exposed to additional radiation. Airline crews and frequent flyers accumulate significant annual doses. Flight crews can receive between 1.8 and 3.6 mSv/year, while frequent flyers receive 0.9 mSv/year. Those people flying the supersonic aircraft can receive up to 10 times this dose, since they travel at a higher altitude.

The earth is encircled by two radiation belts called the Van Allen belts. There are two belts: one at about 100–10,000 km and one at 20,000–600,000 km. Protons and electrons in these belts can produce dose rates of tens of Sv/day. Astronauts and satellite operators are concerned about these high-radiation fields. The radiation levels are not uniform in these belts, and flight paths are often modified to minimize the radiation exposure from these belts. The lowest belt occurs in the south Atlantic anomaly. The belts are pictorially shown in Fig. 14.4. The Hubble Space Telescope, among other satellites, often has its sensors turned off when passing through regions of intense radiation. Manned space missions beyond low earth orbit leave the protection of the geomagnetic field and transit the Van Allen belts. A satellite minimally shielded in an elliptic orbit (200 by 20,000 miles) passing through the radiation belts will receive about 25 Sv/year. Almost all radiation will be received while passing the inner belt.

The population also receives small amounts of exposure from consumer products such as smoke detectors, wristwatches, and television sets. Many smoke detectors contain americium-241, which is an alpha emitter. Wristwatches that glow in the dark contain tritium, which is a low-energy beta emitter. Dose from one of these watches is negligible. Older cathode ray television sets emitted X-rays from the screen and the high-voltage circuit. However, stringent EPA rules have limited this exposure, and the new flat screen LCD televisions have eliminated it completely.

OCCUPATIONAL EXPOSURE

There are about 3.8 million people in the United States wearing personnel monitoring badges and about 1.2 million people receiving measurable exposures. The average effective dose for those receiving exposure is 1.13 mSv/year. The majority of these workers come from the medical field with an average exposure of 0.75 mSv/year. Airline crews have the highest average exposure of 3.07 mSv/year followed by workers in the commercial nuclear power field with 1.87 mSv/year. Other fields often monitored and receiving exposures are in education, research, the government, U.S. Department of Energy (DOE), and the U.S. military.

SMOKERS

In the United States, it is estimated that about 17% of the population are smokers, and the average user smokes 20 cigarettes/day (one pack). From the many researchers, it is estimated that the annual exposure to these smokers would range from 0.1 to 0.7 mSv/year with an average of 0.36 mSv/year.

MEDICAL RADIATION EXPOSURE

Medical radiation exposure is the largest man-made contributor to environmental exposure. It accounted for 3.0 mSv/year in the United States in 2006. Table 14.3 shows the breakdown of the types of procedures and their contribution to the total exposure. Notice that computed tomography (CT) accounts for almost half of the total medical exposure, while it accounts for less than 30% of the total procedures. Radiation therapy procedures are not included in this dose because the population is very small and the doses vary considerably.

TABLE 14.3   Percentage of Total Medical Exposure to General Public (from NCRP 160)

Medical Procedure	Percent Total Exposure
Computed tomography	49
Nuclear medicine	26
Interventional fluoroscopy	14
Conventional radiography and fluoroscopy	11

BENEFITS OF RADIATION

The benefits of radiation fall into two categories: a benefit to the individual and a benefit to society. To individuals working with radiation, either in production or application of radiation, one benefit is their paycheck, and in many professions that use radioactive sources, an additional benefit is the knowledge they are helping others. A patient having an X-ray or nuclear medicine examination has the benefit of the diagnosis, regardless of the answer. Nondestructive testing of industrial equipment using sources of radiation are proven and safe quality control mechanism used in the manufacture of items such as aircraft engines, and high-pressure vessels, this brings individual satisfaction. Individuals who have had radiation therapy to treat their cancer can testify to the relief in learning their cancer has been eradicated. Many new drugs in use today have been developed using radioactive tracers during their testing and evaluation.

Society benefits from the use of radiation to improve health care, to find defects in manufactured parts, and to generate electricity. Electricity generated by nuclear power does not emit CO_2 into the atmosphere and now produces more than 20% of the electricity used in the United States. The use of radiation in quality assurance testing reduces the effect of catastrophic failures of defective welds and joints. We no longer read of boiler and pipeline explosions, which were common in the late 1800s. Smoke detectors used in almost every home use a small radioactive source to detect fire. Tracer radioactive materials are also used in agriculture, industry, and different forms of research. Radiation is used to sterilize medical equipment and to improve the characteristics of plastics.

In many cases, the decision regarding the risks and benefits from radiation is an individual decision.

RISK OF TYPICAL RADIATION EXPOSURES

Each diagnostic X-ray procedure carries a small risk. This is a stochastic risk. There is no threshold for this risk. For example, the risk of 10 μSv is a 1 in 8 million risk of dying of cancer if the effects of large dose effects are extrapolated linearly to zero dose. A typical chest X-ray examination gives an effective dose of about 200 μSv. A person would get this amount of radiation from

- 3 days living in Atlanta
- 2 days living in Denver or Salt Lake City
- 7 hours on some beaches in Brazil or India
- 1 year of watching TV
- 1 year of sleeping next to another individual.

The loss of life expectancy from a 10 μSv dose is about 1.2 minutes.

Other comparisons of loss of life expectancy are shown in Table 14.4, which come from the article by B. Cohen entitled "LLE—Loss of Life Expectancy."

TABLE 14.4 Estimates of Effective Dose and Risks from Diagnostic Examinations

Examination	Effective Dose	Life Shortening[a]
Head AP and LAT	51 μSv (5.1 mrem)	11 minutes
Chest AP and LAT	82 μSv (8.2 mrem)	18 minutes
Abdomen AP	490 μSv (49 mrem)	1.8 hours
Lumbar spine AP and LAT	700 μSv (70 mrem)	2.5 hours
Pelvis AP	500 μSv (50 mrem)	1.8 hours
IVP	175 μSv (18 mrem)	40 minutes
Barium enema		
6 spot films and 1 min fluoro	3700 μSv (370 mrem)	14.3 hours
Mammographic exam	480 μSv (48 mrem)	1.75 hours
Fluoroscopy	720 μSv/min (72 mrem/min)	2.5 h/min of fluoro
CT scans		
Head	2.3 mSv (230 mrem)	8.3 hours
Chest	14.3 mSv (1400 mrem)	2.1 days
Body	15.4 mSv (1500 mrem)	2.3 days
Other risks		
15% overweight		777 days
Nonsmoker living with a smoker		50 days
Eating 2-lb broiled meat per week		1 day

Natural background radiation in Albuquerque is about 3000 μSv, 3 mSv, or 300 mrem per year.
[a] Ten millisieverts results in a life shortening of 1.5 days.
AP, anterior posterior; LAT, lateral; IVP, intravenous pyelogram.

SUMMARY

The total effective dose from all background radiation in the United States as of 2006 is 6.24 mSv/year. The medical contribution to the total is 3.0 mSv/year. The nonmedical background radiation level is 3.24 mSv/year. This level has remained constant for many years. The largest single component of the natural background is from radon and thoron at 2.28 mSv/year. That leaves less than 1 mSv/year from all the other sources of background radiation. The traditional sources of background radiation vary considerably depending on geographic location. Many studies have been completed to determine if there is a relation between background radiation levels and the incidence of cancer or other radiation-related effects. *No study has shown any correlation between geographic location and cancer incidence.*

The medical component is now being added to the background radiation levels. This component varies by country and technology level. In the United States, it is 3.0 mSv/year and rising. Medical exposure is not a low-level exposure to a large population, but rather a collection of acute high-level exposures to a small population. This will not have the same biological effect as low continuous natural background. The age distribution is also skewed toward the older population as compared with the general public. Three millisieverts per year has been calculated using the person-Sv approach and therefore could be seen as deceiving.

Summary points are as follows:

- Natural background is considered not hazardous because humans have been living with background radiation levels for millions of years.
- The total effective dose from all background exposure is 6.24 mSv/year.
- The contribution to the total effective dose from medical exposure is 3.0 mSv/year, with the largest single contributor being CT.
- The total annual exposure does not include the contribution from smoking or occupational exposure.
- There are no known ill effects traceable to people living in high background areas of the world.

BIBLIOGRAPHY

Cohen BL. Catalog of risks extended and updated. Health Phys. 1991 September; 61(3):317–35.

EPA. Calculate your radiation dose. Washington, DC: U.S. Environmental Protection Agency; 2011 [updated July 8, 2011; cited March 29, 2013]. Available from: http://www.epa.gov/rpdweb00/understand/calculate.html.

Mettler FA, Upton AC. Medical effects of ionizing radiation. 3rd ed. Philadelphia: Saunders/Elsevier; 2008.

National Council on Radiation Protection and Measurements. National Council on Radiation Protection and Measurements. Scientific Committee 6-2 on Radiation Exposure of the U.S. Population. Ionizing radiation exposure of the population of the United States: Recommendations of the National Council on Radiation Protection and Measurements. Bethesda, MD: National Council on Radiation Protection and Measurements; 2009.

United Nations. Scientific Committee on the Effects of Atomic Radiation. Effects of ionizing radiation: United Nations Scientific Committee on the Effects of Atomic Radiation: UNSCEAR 2006. New York: United Nations; 2008.

QUESTIONS

Chapter 14   Questions

1. According to the BEIR IV report, radon is responsible for ___ of all fatal lung cancers.
   a. 10%
   b. 30%
   c. 50%
   d. 90%

2. The average effective dose from background to a person living in the United States in 2006 was _____ mSv per year.

   a. 6.2

   b. 3.0

   c. 2.2

   d. 1.0

   e. 0.62

3. The largest contributor to medical exposure is

   a. chest X-ray.

   b. CT scan.

   c. nuclear medicine study.

   d. fluoroscopy.

4. What is the largest contributor to natural background radiation that is not man-made?

   a. Radon gas

   b. Cosmetic radiation

   c. Thoron gas

   d. Radium-226

5. The EPA estimates that radon is the number _____ cause of lung cancers in nonsmokers.

   a. one

   b. two

   c. five

   d. ten

6. An individual receives the largest exposure from

   a. working as a transatlantic flight attendant.

   b. one day in the sun.

   c. working as an X-ray technologist.

   d. working in a nuclear power plant.

7. Which area in the United States gets the largest background radiation from radon gas?

   a. Los Angeles

   b. Seattle

   c. Albuquerque

   d. Upper Midwest

8. The average background radiation in the United States is _____ mSv per year.
   a. 0.5
   b. 1.0
   c. 3.0
   d. 4.0
   e. 5.0

9. The average medical dose to the public in the United States is _____ mSv per year.
   a. 0.5
   b. 1.0
   c. 3.0
   d. 4.0
   e. 5.0

10. The radiation exposure received during a transcontinental flight is approximately _____ mSv.
   a. 0.5
   b. 1.0
   c. 3.0
   d. 4.0
   e. 5.0

11. The risk of an adverse biological response from mammography is
   a. unknown.
   b. large.
   c. small.
   d. moderate.

12. People living at what elevation have a higher incidence of fatal cancers?
   a. 1000 ft
   b. 5000 ft
   c. 15,000 ft
   d. There is no measured increase with altitude.

13. A head CT exam has produced the same biological effect as
   a. 1 year of background radiation at sea level.
   b. a mammographic exam.
   c. chest X-ray exam.
   d. one body CT exam.

14. Nuclear medicine procedures account for about what percentage of all medical exposures to the public?
   a. 10%
   b. 25%
   c. 40%
   d. 50%

15. How many people in the United States get a measurable occupational exposure?
   a. 120,000
   b. 600,000
   c. 1,200,000
   d. 6,000,000

16. The average citizen in the United States receives how much radiation per year from nuclear power plants?
   a. 0.0001 mSv
   b. 0.001 mSv
   c. 0.01 mSv
   d. 0.1 mSv

CHAPTER 15

REGULATIONS AND RISK

KEYWORDS

ICRP, BEIR, NCRP, UNSCEAR, NRC, linear no-threshold, dose–response, Life Span Study, relative risk, absolute risk, regulations, nominal risk, sunk cost bias

TOPICS

- Risk for radiation-induced stochastic effects
- Sources of data for long-term risk of exposure to ionizing radiation
- Linear and nonlinear models of risk
- Risks associated with activities in radiology compared with risks associated with other activities
- Organizations that evaluate radiobiological data and make recommendations regarding radiation protection
- Regulatory agencies and regulations

INTRODUCTION

The purpose of radiation protection regulations is to ensure the safe use of ionizing radiation. This involves balancing the benefits of radiation applications with the risks. Regulations are established by national or state governments and have the force of

Radiation Biology of Medical Imaging, First Edition. Charles A. Kelsey, Philip H. Heintz,
Daniel J. Sandoval, Gregory D. Chambers, Natalie L. Adolphi, and Kimberly S. Paffett.
© 2014 John Wiley & Sons, Inc. Published 2014 by John Wiley & Sons, Inc.

law with civil and or criminal penalties for violations. Regulations historically require long and complex procedures prior to becoming law. Recommendations are promulgated by extra-government organizations interested in radiation safety. They do not have the force of law but usually are the basis for government regulations. This chapter covers both regulations and recommendations regarding safe radiation use.

The benefits of radiation in medicine come from improved diagnostic information. The risk comes primarily from an increased risk of cancer. Regulators must weigh the benefits and risks of using ionizing radiation for workers, patients, and the public. Current regulations do not place limits on the amount of radiation delivered to a patient. This is because the benefit and risk to an individual are evaluated by the physician ordering the procedure. Regulations usually divide exposures to humans into exposures to the general public and exposures to those working with radiation. Radiation exposure limits to radiation workers are higher than the limits for the general public because they presumably are receiving an additional benefit (their job) in return for the slightly higher risk associated with the higher allowed radiation exposure.

EXPRESSIONS OF RISK

Risk is often expressed as the probability or likelihood that an event will occur. In this section, we will discuss the probability of long-term, stochastic, detrimental biological effects occurring in a person's lifetime. These stochastic effects include genetic damage and carcinogenesis.

Committee reports such as Biological Effects of Ionizing Radiations (BEIR) VII and International Commission on Radiological Protection (ICRP) 103 state risk from radiation exposure as either absolute risk or relative risk. Absolute risk is expressed as the number of occurrences of a disease in a population. Relative risk is often expressed as a fraction or percentage. The relative risk is defined as the ratio of the rate of disease in an exposed population divided by the rate of disease in an unexposed population:

The ERR is excess relative risk and is equal to the relative risk minus one.

The EAR is the excess absolute risk and is equal to the rate of disease in exposed population minus the rate of disease in unexposed population.

Example of a numerical application of absolute risk and relative risk:

Consider a population with a natural absolute risk for incidence of a disease of 20,000 cases in every 100,000 individuals. After this population is exposed to ionizing radiation, there are 20,300 disease cases observed.

$$\text{The ERR is } (20,300/20,000) - 1 = 1.015 - 1 = 0.015 = 1.5\%.$$

The EAR is $(20,300/100,000) - (20,000/100,000) = 300/100,000$ or 300 in 100,000.

ORGANIZATIONS

There are four national and international organizations that evaluate epidemiological and radiobiological data and make recommendations regarding exposure to ionizing radiations. The recommendations are usually adopted by regulatory agencies and incorporated into national regulations. These organizations include the following:

The BEIR (Biological Effects of Ionizing Radiations) Committee. The committee was formed by the National Research Council of the National Academy of Sciences. The goal of the council is to advise the U.S. government on the effects of ionizing radiation on human health. A recent report from the BEIR Committee is BEIR VII Phase II (2006). One objective of the BEIR VII report was "to develop the best possible risk estimate for exposure to low-dose, low linear energy transfer (LET) radiation in human subjects."

International Commission on Radiological Protection (ICRP). This is a multinational, independent organization of experts in radiologic protection. The recommendations and guidelines produced by the commission are incorporated into the regulations and policies of many nations. A noteworthy publication in the field of radiation protection is ICRP 60 (ICRP 1990). A later report, ICRP 103 (ICRP 2007) has now been issued and supersedes ICRP 60. In the later report, data from the years since the issue of ICRP 60 was evaluated. The result was that the basic recommendations of ICRP 60 were unchanged except that the estimated risk of hereditary effects was lowered in ICRP 103.

United Nations Scientific Committee of the Effects of Atomic Radiations (UNSCEAR). The committee is responsible for advising the General Assembly of the United Nations regarding ionizing radiation. The reports of the committee are widely used for evaluation of risk and formulation of policy.

National Council of Radiological Protection and Measurements (NCRP). This organization was founded by the U.S. Congress. Its mission is to advise the U.S. government in matters pertaining to ionizing radiations. Its mandate specifies that it should cooperate with the ICRP and other agencies in the field of radiation protection.

These organizations have established recommendations based on data from human exposures to radiation, animal studies, and other laboratory data.

SOURCES OF DATA

A primary source of data used in committee reports such as BEIR VII and ICRP 103 is from the Life Span Study (LSS) in which the incidence of disease in the survivors of the nuclear weapon attacks on Hiroshima and Nagasaki has been tracked. The LSS data have been used to estimate quantitative risks of exposure to ionizing radiation.

The LSS data are unique for several reasons. The exposed population is large and includes approximately 100,000 individuals. People of all ages and both sexes were exposed to ionizing radiation during the attacks. The range of radiation exposures was large and included many who received relatively low doses (5–100 mSv) of radiation. The low doses are in the same range that can be expected from some diagnostic medical procedures. The LSS is also unique in that incidence and mortality data for cancer and other diseases have been tracked for nearly 70 years.

DOSE–RESPONSE MODELS

Dose–response models are used to estimate the quantitative risk associated with an exposure to ionizing radiation. Obtaining a suitable model for risk associated with low doses has been controversial. For many survivors of the attacks on Nagasaki and Hiroshima, the exposure to radiation resulted in a high dose delivered at a high-dose rate. Occupational exposures and most radiological exposures involve low doses and low-dose rates. Yet the high dose, high-dose rate data from the LSS are still the primary source of data used for the estimation of risk factors due to low doses and low-dose rates.

To relate the high dose, high-dose rate data to low dose, low-dose rates, the dose and dose-rate effectiveness factor (DDREF) is used. Both the ICRP and BEIR Committee use a DDREF value of approximately 2. This used to account for the fact that the body repairs some radiation damage if the radiation exposure is spread over a longer time period. The assumption is that exposure to high doses and high-dose rates, such as found in nuclear weapon attacks, is approximately twice as likely to produce stochastic detrimental effects as low dose, low-dose rate exposures. In Fig. 15.1, the difference in the slope between the linear no-threshold (LNT) (high-dose rate) line and the LNT (low-dose rate) line in the figure is the DDREF.

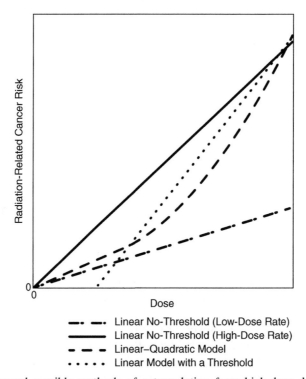

Figure 15.1   Several possible methods of extrapolation from high-dose data to low-dose data. The linear no-threshold (low-dose rate) line is equivalent to the linear no-threshold (high-dose rate) line divided by the DDREF. Adapted from BEIR VII Phase II (2005). Modified from Brenner et al. (2003).

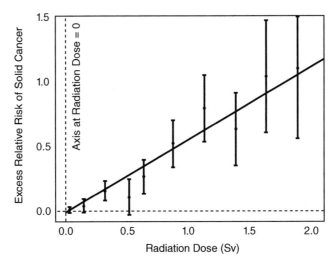

Figure 15.2 Excess relative risks of solid cancer for survivors of nuclear weapon bombings of Japan. The error bars represent approximate 95% confidence intervals. Adapted from BEIR VII Phase II (2005).

There are several dose-rate models that may be used to extrapolate from the high-dose data to the low-dose range where most occupational and radiological exposures are found. In the linear–quadratic model, the dose–response is nearly linear at low doses and then the slope increases at increasing doses. Some diseases, notably leukemia, are best modeled with this type of curve fit.

The linear models include the linear with-threshold and LNT models. In both linear models, the risk is assumed to increase linearly for all doses. In the linear with-threshold model, there is a nonzero, threshold level at which the ERR and EAR drops to zero. The ERR and EAR remain at zero for all doses less than the threshold. Evidence suggests that if a threshold truly exists, it is at low doses.

The model that is currently used by the BEIR Committee and the ICRP to model the risks for solid cancers is the LNT model. In this model, there is no threshold and the line crosses the origin. In the LNT model, it is assumed that *any* exposure to ionizing radiation carries a risk proportional to the dose. The LNT model is easy to use and is also the most conservative at relatively low doses (less than 500 mSv). In the latest reports, the ICRP and BEIR Committee still maintain that they do not have enough reason to depart from the LNT model. It should be noted that the ICRP and BEIR VII Committee state that the LNT dose–response model should only be used for radiation protection purposes. The model should not be used for epidemiological purposes or for estimation of risk to an individual.

There is some evidence that the LNT model does not provide good estimates of the dose–response in the low-dose range. Notice in Fig. 15.2 and Fig. 15.3 that the error bars in the low-dose range actually extend below 0.0 ERR. This could possibly indicate that low doses actually have zero risk or even less than zero risk. In other words, low doses of radiation could have a beneficial impact on health. The hypothesis that low doses of radiation actually reduce the risk of disease is known as hormesis. There is some evidence that exposure to low doses of radiation impart some degree of radioresistance to the organism being irradiated. The existence of

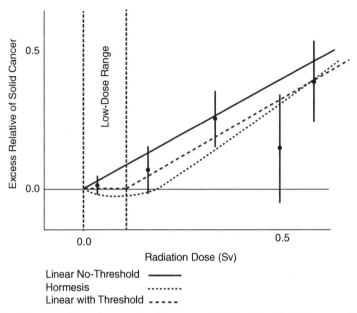

Figure 15.3 Close-up of low-dose region for excess relative risks of solid cancer for survivors of nuclear weapon bombings of Japan. The error bars represent approximate 95% confidence intervals. Adapted from BEIR VII Phase II (2005).

hormesis in humans is inconclusive and has generally not been incorporated into radiation protection policy.

A simple method of assessing risk of a radiological procedure is to use the collective effective dose and the nominal risk coefficients. The collective effective dose is the sum of all of the effective doses for individuals who underwent a specific procedure. The nominal risk coefficients are based on models of ERR or EAR data. The nominal risk coefficients are themselves only a generic, single value for the risk of fatal cancer and are not specific for factors such as age and sex. This type of estimate only provides a crude estimate of the risk of a procedure but can be useful for comparing procedures. The current ICRP 103 (ICRP 2007) nominal risk coefficients are shown below for low-LET radiations, that is, X-rays, gamma rays, and electrons:

- For the general public and low-dose rates and low doses, the estimate for lifetime fatal cancer risk is 5.5% per Sv and for heritable (genetic) effects is 0.2% per Sv.
- For the working population and low-dose rates and low doses, the estimate for lifetime fatal cancer risk is 4.1% per Sv and for heritable effects is 0.1% per Sv.

The nominal risk value for the general public is higher than the nominal risk for the working population because the general public includes children while the working population does not. Because of their relatively large population of undifferentiated cells and longer expected lifetime, children have a higher risk for stochastic detrimental effects than adults for a given amount of exposure. The ICRP estimates that the lifetime cancer risk can be two to three times greater for young children and infants than for adults.

The nominal risks presented in ICRP 103 in conjunction with the average collective effective dose of a procedure can be used to estimate the risk associated with a radiological procedure. This risk is for a population undergoing the procedure and should only be used for comparison of procedures for radiation protection purposes. The ICRP emphasizes that the effective dose to an individual should not be used to calculate the risk of detrimental effects for an individual or for epidemiological purposes. However, a comparison of risks from radiological exposures to the risks associated with other activities may be useful when explaining to patients the relative risk of a procedure. In Table 15.1, the collective average effective doses are from a study by Mettler et al. Data regarding risk due to nonradiological causes is from the National Safety Council, Injury Facts 2011 edition. Here, the average effective dose is multiplied by the nominal risk coefficient, 4.1% per Sv.

As shown in Table 15.1, the risks associated with some common activities such as driving a motor vehicle are much greater than the risks from the 2-mSv exposure due to a head computed tomography (CT) scan. Although this may be a useful comparison, it should be noted that the values in Table 15.1 are for a population of exposed individuals. The estimation of risk for an individual is a complicated process that involves age, sex, and other factors.

Another way to illustrate risk is to express the average effective dose from a procedure in terms of equivalent background exposure. Every place on earth has some natural background radiation. This background varies from location to location depending on environmental variables such as elevation and geologic composition. In the United States, the average annual effective dose due to naturally occurring background is 3.1 mSv. Thus, an average head CT is equivalent to

TABLE 15.1   Risk from Several Medical Procedures Compared with Other Risks

	Average Effective Dose (mSv)	Excess Lifetime Risk of Cancer Death
Procedure		
PA and lateral chest X-rays	0.1	1 in 240,000
Mammography	0.4	1 in 61,000
Head CT scan	2	1 in 12,000
Pelvic CT scan	6	1 in 4,000
Abdomen CT scan	8	1 in 3,000
Lung perfusion (5 mCi Tc-99m MAA)	2	1 in 12,000
Lung ventilation (20 mCi Xe-133)	0.5	1 in 48,000
F-18 FDG WB PET scan (20 mCi)	14.1	1 in 1,700
Estimated lifetime risks of death		
Lightning strike		1 in 84,000
Drowning		1 in 1,100
Motor vehicle accident		1 in 90
Cancer		1 in 7

PA, posterior–anterior; PET, positron emission tomography.

(2 mSv)·(1 year/3.1 mSv) or 0.65 years of exposure to naturally occurring background radiation.

SUNK COST BIAS

A consequence of using a linear dose–response model is that the incremental risk due to an incremental dose is the same at all points along the line. The risk estimates derived from the LNT model are independent probabilities. In other words, the risk of stochastic effects associated with a procedure does not depend on a patient's previous radiation exposures. Once an imaging procedure has been performed, there is no action that can be done to mitigate the risk from the procedure.

When faced with independent probabilities, there is a common misconception that the previous outcomes somehow affect the probability of the current measurement. For instance, let us say a fair coin is flipped 10 times and every flip results in tails being up. A person may think that the 11th flip should result in heads because heads "is due." In reality, the probability of heads landing up on the 11th attempt is still 50%. The probability of heads landing up is not influenced by the previous history of flips. This cognitive pitfall is referred to as sunk cost bias or "gambler's fallacy."

Sunk cost bias can be a potential pitfall in the weighing of risk versus benefit of an imaging procedure. For example, two nearly identical patients present with identical symptoms. One patient has had many CT scans in the past year. The other has had none. For both patients, the risk from the next CT scan is the same. Thus, the risk in the risk versus benefit analysis is the same for both patients. Keep in mind that this is for stochastic detrimental effects. The damage from deterministic effects *does* depend on a patient's previous history. In some high-dose procedures, damage to the skin or some organ may exist but may be latent or otherwise not visible. Subsequent procedures may increase the cumulative dose to the organ above the threshold dose. At this point, the damage may visibly manifest is some manner.

RADIATION PROTECTION RECOMMENDATIONS AND REGULATIONS

The ICRP has a system of radiation protection that has been used as a basis for radiation protection programs in many countries. In the latest version of this system, exposures are divided into three categories: planned exposure situations, emergency exposure situations, and existing exposure situations. Planned exposure situations are those in which the use of radiation is deliberate. Emergency exposure situations are those in which actions are necessary to reduce or prevent unwanted consequences. Existing exposure situations include exposure to naturally occurring background radiation and situations such as exposure after an emergency event.

The ICRP system of radiation protection is based on three principles. These are the principles of justification, optimization, and limitation. The principle of justification states that any decision regarding an exposure situation should result in more benefit than harm. The principle of optimization states that in any planned reduction of exposure, economic and societal impacts need to be addressed. This essentially is the same as the principle of ALARA mandated by the U.S. Nuclear Regulatory

Commission (NRC). ALARA is an acronym that stands for as low as reasonably achievable. ALARA is the principle of reducing exposures when it is reasonable and practical to do so. The principles of justification and optimization should be applied to all three exposure situations as described by the ICRP. The principle of limitation requires that doses do not exceed dose limits. Dose limits are only applied to planned exposure situations and are not applied to patient exposures.

The occupational dose limits and dose limits for exposure of the public are lower than levels likely to produce detrimental effects. The levels are set to protect workers, and the public yet allow for the beneficial use of ionizing radiation. While there are limits for workers and the public, it should be mentioned that there is no limit to the amount of radiation a physician may prescribe for a patient.

Historically, the ICRP began using a risk-based approach for setting recommended dose limits in the 1970s. The recommendations were set such that the incremental risk of death to a radiation worker was no greater than the risk of traumatic injury to workers in "safe" industries. Based on the risk of death to workers in safe industries and data from the survivors of the atomic bombings of Japan, the ICRP arrived at a recommended maximum annual dose limit of 50 mSv/year. Since that time, the ICRP has refined its recommendations. Its current recommendation is that radiation exposure be limited to 100 mSv in any 5-year period with a maximum of 50 mSv in any 1 year. The NCRP has set its recommended limit on whole body dose to an average lifetime dose of 150 mSv/year with a maximum of 50 mSv in any 1 year.

The NRC has adopted into regulations many of the recommendations of the ICRP and NCRP. The major radiation protection guidelines in the United States are found in the Code of Federal Regulations. The following are the annual dose limits for occupational workers in the United States. For the entire body, the annual dose limit is 50 mSv total effective dose equivalent (TEDE). The TEDE is the sum of internal and external exposures and is essentially the same as the effective dose. For organs other than the eye, the limit is 500 mSv. For the lens of the eye, the limit is 150 mSv. The annual limit to the skin of the whole body or extremity is 500 mSv. Once a pregnant occupational worker declares her pregnancy, the dose to the embryo or fetus must be monitored. The dose equivalent to an embryo or fetus must not exceed 5 mSv for the entire pregnancy. The TEDE for members of the public may not exceed 1 mSv/year except in special circumstances. The regulatory limit for exposure to the public is lower than the average exposures from natural background radiation encountered in the United States. Overall, these annual dose limits are the same or very similar to the annual dose limits recommended by the ICRP and NCRP.

The U.S. federal agencies that regulate activities commonly associated with the medical use of ionizing radiation include the NRC, Department of Transportation (DOT), and the Food and Drug Administration (FDA). Other federal agencies such as the Environmental Protection Agency (EPA) may also impact the operation of a medical facility.

The NRC is responsible for the regulation of the purchase, receipt, use, and disposal of radioactive materials produced by nuclear reactors and particle accelerators. This includes all radionuclides used in nuclear medicine. Agreement states accept responsibility for the regulation of all radioactive materials. Most states in the United States are now agreement states. In an agreement state, the state regulations must be at least as strict as those set forth by the NRC. The FDA regulates and monitors the manufacture, distribution, safety, and effectiveness of pharmaceuticals and radiopharmaceuticals. The FDA enforces the Mammography Quality Standards Act (MQSA) regulations and regulations pertaining to other X-ray-producing devices used in radiography, CT, and fluoroscopy. The DOT controls the packaging and interstate movement of hazardous materials, including radioactive materials.

It should be mentioned that some organizations in the United States such as the American College of Radiology (ACR) and The Joint Commission publish recommendations regarding exposure to radiation. While these organizations do not have the power to make law, they have considerable economic power. Health care organizations that do not meet the accreditation standards set forth by these organizations may experience a negative financial impact.

CONCLUSIONS

The risk due to exposure to ionizing radiation is assumed to be proportional to the absorbed dose. Several international and national organizations have extensively examined radiologic data and made dose–risk estimations. The dose–risk relationship in the low-dose region is controversial because much of the data are from high-dose situations. Some question the validity of extrapolating these data to the low-dose regime with the LNT model. Regardless, this is the method most often used to create risk estimates for radiation exposure. It is also the basis for the regulatory limits that are included into federal and state regulations. Regulations are designed to ensure that the public and radiation workers are not exposed to harmful levels of radiation while still allowing beneficial uses of radiation.

BIBLIOGRAPHY

Brenner DJ, Doll R, Goodhead DT, Hall EJ, Land CE, Little JB, Lubin JH, Preston DL, Preston RJ, Puskin JS, Ron E, Sachs RK, Samet JM, Setlow RB and Zaider M. Cancer risks attributable to low doses of ionizing radiation: Assessing what we really know. P Natl Acad Sci USA. 2003 Nov;100(24):13761–6.

Durand DJ, Dixon RL, Morin RL. Utilization strategies for cumulative dose estimates: A review and rational assessment. J Am Coll Radiol. 2012 July;9(7):480–5.

Eisenberg JD, Harvey HB, Moore DA, Gazelle GS, Pandharipande PV. Falling prey to the sunk cost bias: A potential harm of patient radiation dose histories. Radiology. 2012 June;263(3):626–8.

International Commission on Radiological Protection (ICRP). The 1990 recommendations of the International Commission on Radiological Protection. ICRP Publication 60. Pergamon Press; 1990.

International Commission on Radiological Protection (ICRP). The 2007 Recommendations of the International Commission on Radiological Protection. ICRP Publication 103. New York: Pergamon Press; 2007.

Mettler FA, Jr., Huda W, Yoshizumi TT, Mahesh M. Effective doses in radiology and diagnostic nuclear medicine: A catalog. Radiology. 2008 July;248(1):254–63.

National Research Council (U.S.). Committee to assess health risks from exposure to low level of ionizing radiation. Health risks from exposure to low levels of ionizing radiation: BEIR VII Phase 2. Washington, DC: National Academies Press; 2006.

National Safety Council. Research and Statistics Dept. Injury Facts. Itasca, IL: The Council; 2011, p. v.

QUESTIONS

Chapter 15   Questions

1. The concept that exposure to low levels of ionizing radiation may be good for an organism is known as
   a. homeostasis.
   b. the bystander effect.
   c. heterodynamic peristalsis.
   d. hormesis.

2. For the working population, what is the nominal risk coefficient for heritable effects from low doses and low-dose rates of low-LET radiation?
   a. 0.1% per Sv
   b. 5% per Sv
   c. 16 % per Sv
   d. 25% per Sv

3. Members of a population undergo a medical procedure. The rate of incidence of a particular cancer in the exposed population is 500 in 100,000. The rate of incidence of the same type of cancer in an unexposed population is 300 in 100,000. What is the excess relative risk (ERR) for the medical procedure?
   a. 200 in 100,000
   b. 0.005
   c. 1.67
   d. 0.67

4. What federal agency is responsible for enforcement of federal regulations regarding mammography (MQSA)?
   a. DOT
   b. FDA
   c. EPA
   d. NRC

5. Which of the following procedures produces the greatest excess risk of inducing a fatal cancer? Assume that the LNT dose–response model is valid.
   a. Positron emission tomography (PET) scan with 20 mCi of F-18 FDG
   b. Abdomen CT scan
   c. Head CT scan
   d. Chest X-ray (posterior–anterior [PA] and lateral)

6. Why are the ICRP nominal risk coefficients higher for the general population than for the working population?
   a. The general population has more smokers and overweight people. This contributes to a higher mortality rate.
   b. The general population includes children who have a higher risk for radiation-induced detrimental effects.
   c. The working population is better educated about the risks of radiation and is better able to avoid radiation exposure.

7. The ICRP system of radiation protection is based on which three principles?
   a. Justification, maximization, and deregulation
   b. Minimization, shielding, more shielding
   c. Justification, optimization, and limitation
   d. Time, distance, and shielding

8. Which risk model is used by the ICRP, BEIR, and the NCRP when making recommendations on dose limits to the public and occupational workers?
   a. Linear–quadratic
   b. Linear with-threshold
   c. Linear no-threshold
   d. Quadratic no-threshold

9. Members of a population undergo a medical procedure. The rate of incidence of a particular cancer in the exposed population is 500 in 100,000. The rate of incidence of the same type of cancer in an unexposed population is 300 in 100,000. What is the excess absolute risk (EAR) for the medical procedure?
   a. 200 in 100,000
   b. 0.005
   c. 1.67
   d. 0.67

10. What population is being studied for the Life Span Study (LSS)?
    a. Children in the United States that have been exposed to radiation in medical procedures
    b. Many of the survivors of the nuclear weapon attacks in Nagasaki and Hiroshima
    c. People who were exposed to radiation in medical procedures prior to current regulations (before 1960)
    d. Radiation workers injured in radiation accidents; this includes the workers exposed during the Chernobyl accident.

11. The DDREF is

   a. a factor that is used to take into account the dose and dose rate for producing stochastic detrimental effects. It is approximately two.

   b. the slope of the survival curve in the high-dose rate region.

   c. the agency responsible for setting occupational dose limits in the United States.

   d. a dose–response model that has a linear portion and a quadratic term. The result is a nonlinear model.

12. In the United States, what is the occupational annual dose limit, TEDE, for radiation workers in Système International (SI) units?

   a. 50 mGy

   b. 50 mSv

   c. 500 mrem

   d. 5 Sv

13. What is the ICRP nominal risk coefficient for the general population and low-dose rates and low dose for lifetime fatal cancer risk?

   a. 4.1% per Sv

   b. 7.5% per Sv

   c. 0.2% per Sv

   d. 5.5% per Sv

14. The LNT dose–response model is characterized as

   a. being linear, exposures below a threshold level have no associated risk.

   b. being nonlinear, exposures below a threshold level have no associated risk.

   c. being linear, even very low exposures to radiation carry some associated risk.

   d. being nonlinear, even very low exposures to radiation carry some associated risk.

15. In general, as an individual's exposure to ionizing radiation increases, his or her risk of developing a stochastic detrimental effect such as cancer

   a. increases.

   b. remains unchanged.

   c. decreases.

16. In the United States, what is the annual dose limit for patients?

   a. 50 mGy

   b. 50 mSv

   c. 500 mrem

   d. There is no regulatory limit on the annual dose a patient may receive.

CHAPTER 16

BIOLOGICAL EFFECTS OF ULTRASOUND

KEYWORDS

Diagnostic radiology, biology of diagnostic radiology, ultrasound imaging, biological effects of ultrasound, ultrasound equipment

TOPICS

- Basics of ultrasound in medical imaging
- Equipment and techniques to acquire ultrasound images
- Biological effects of ultrasound
- Thermal properties of ultrasound
- Acoustic properties of ultrasound
- Cavitation

INTRODUCTION

Ultrasound produces biological effects by two tissue interactions: heating and cavitation. Heating is caused by the mechanical friction of the tissue moving during passing of the ultrasonic wave. Cavitation is the production and collapse of small bubbles in the inter- and intracellular tissue fluid. Before discussing these mechanisms and their potential biological effects, it is useful to briefly discuss the properties of medical ultrasound and how it is clinically applied.

Radiation Biology of Medical Imaging, First Edition. Charles A. Kelsey, Philip H. Heintz,
Daniel J. Sandoval, Gregory D. Chambers, Natalie L. Adolphi, and Kimberly S. Paffett.
© 2014 John Wiley & Sons, Inc. Published 2014 by John Wiley & Sons, Inc.

ULTRASOUND PROPERTIES AND PROCEDURES

The primary reason for the popularity of ultrasound is because it does not use ionizing radiation, which makes it especially appealing in obstetrical imaging. Procedures such as estimation of fetal age and determination of fetal position and placental localization can be accomplished with no ionizing radiation exposure to the fetus. Ultrasound is also used in cardiac imaging for determination of ejection fraction, detection of pericardial effusion, detection of wall motion abnormalities, and detection of vascular stenoses. In radiology, ultrasound is used for the diagnosis of many vascular and abdominal diseases, including bladder tumors, renal abnormalities, vascular abnormalities, and line placements.

Higher-power ultrasound can also be used to kill biological tissue. High-intensity focused ultrasound (HIFU) procedures are used to treat cancer patients. By focusing high-power ultrasound onto a target area, the temperature is raised enough to kill the target tissue. More moderate ultrasound power levels are used in diathermy and hyperthermia to produce local heating of tissue. It is used in physical therapy and sports medicine to deliver moderate heat directly to damaged tissues to increase and improve healing of tears, strains, and bruises.

PROPERTIES OF ULTRASOUND WAVES

Unlike X-rays and gamma radiation, ultrasound is a pressure wave, not an electromagnetic wave. It produces no direct ionization. Ultrasound is a series of pulsed sound waves. Sound is mechanical energy that travels as pressure waves through a medium. That is, the pressure increase and decrease during each ultrasound wave cycle. This pressure wave exerts mechanical forces causing molecules to move back and forth from their original stationary position. Ultrasound waves used in medical imaging have frequencies from 1 to 20 MHz. Low-frequency sound waves penetrate deeper into tissue than high-frequency sound waves. The pressure in a 5-MHz ultrasound wave increases to maximum and decreases to a minimum 5 million times each second. This is above audible sound that has frequencies of 2–20,000 Hz.

As shown in Fig. 16.1, the sound frequency is shown by the oscillating wave. As the magnitude of the wave decreases, the energy is absorbed by the medium. The energy loss heats the medium. The magnitude of the velocity the wave travels at in the medium depends on the acoustic properties of the medium, which include its density, elasticity, and compressibility. Water is a good transmitter of sound, whereas air is a poor transmitter at ultrasound frequencies and bone is a very good sound transmitter. This is important because ultrasound frequencies can travel reasonable distances in tissue and water, but do not penetrate lung or air cavities. The sound frequency is transmitted in packets, as shown in Fig. 16.2. The frequency of the packets is called the pulse repetition frequency (PRF).

When the sound wave interacts with an interface between two different materials, some of the sound wave is transmitted though the interface, and the remainder is reflected back. The amount of reflection depends on the difference in the acoustic properties of the two tissues. The larger the difference between the two tissues, the

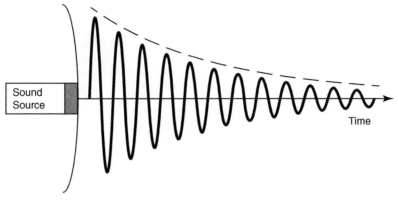

Figure 16.1   A sound wave as it interacts with a medium. Notice the magnitude decreases with depth.

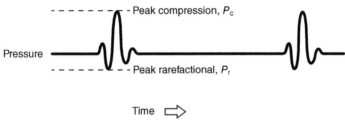

Figure 16.2   A typical pulsed ultrasound beam with time. This is the waveform used in clinical real-time imaging. Short pulses of fixed frequency and duration are used to generate a dynamic image. The ultrasound pulse deposits energy as it traverses the patient.

more sound wave is reflected. This reflected wave is used to form the ultrasound image. Signals from deep within the body take longer to return to the transducer.

There are two frequencies associated with an ultrasound wave. The first is the ultrasound frequency, and the second describes how many ultrasound pulses are sent out each second. The second frequency is called the pulse repetition frequency (PRF), which describes the number of pulses per second sent into the patient. Changing the ultrasound frequency often requires changing the transducer head, which is applied to the patient's skin. Changing the PRF is accomplished by changing a setting on the control panel. If the depth of a user-defined region of interest is changed, modern scanners will often automatically adjust the PRF to compensate for the change in pulse travel time. Increasing the depth of the region of interest decreases the PRF because a greater time must be allowed for the deeper echoes to return. The PRF is usually in the range between 100 and 12,000 Hz. An increase in the PRF results in an increase in the ultrasonic power sent into the patient.

Ultrasound images are presented in two modes: B- or 2D mode and M-mode. A 2D scan presents in a two-dimensional image of the anatomy. It is a still frame mode

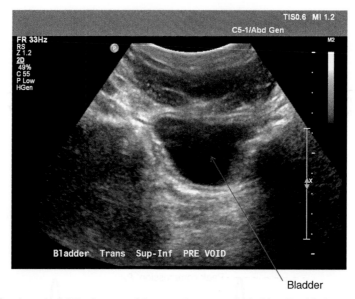

Bladder

Figure 16.3 A typical 2D ultrasound image of a normal bladder. In this image, the object lines represent an interface point in the tissue media. The dark area in the middle is the bladder filled with urine. It has almost no echoes because it is a homogeneous liquid. The labeling on the image shows the MI and TI, which are discussed in the text.

just showing the anatomy. The M-mode is a B scan with motion. The M-mode was the first ultrasound modality to record display moving echoes from the heart, and thus the motion could be interpreted in terms of myocardial and valvular function. A typical ultrasound M mode image is shown in Fig. 16.3.

Doppler ultrasound scanning is used to measure a moving structure or flowing blood in the body. These images are formed by analyzing the Doppler shift in the reflected signals. The images appear similar to conventional normal 2D images but show moving structures as a color overlay on the anatomical grayscale image. Figure 16.4 shows a typical Doppler ultrasound image of the abdomen.

The wave form at the bottom of Fig. 16.4 shows the pulsation in the blood flow. Pulsed Doppler requires higher power levels than regular M-mode scans because only part of the reflected signal is used to obtain the Doppler information.

Ultrasound beam power is the amount of acoustic energy per time. Beam intensity is the beam power per unit area and is specified in mW/cm^2. To describe the ultrasound beam, there are four quantities of intensity. These are described in Table 16.1 and vary with time and distance (space). The four are necessary because the beam varies with time (the pulse) and space as the beam is not necessarily fixed in space and the beam varies in size with depth.

Spatial peak–pulse average (I(SPPA)) has the highest value because it reports peaks in magnitude and space. Spatial average–time average (I(SATA)) has the lowest magnitude because it reports averages in both magnitude and space. The Food and Drug Administration (FDA) regulations use spatial peak–time average (I(SPTA)) because heating occurs only during the "pulse on" time as shown in

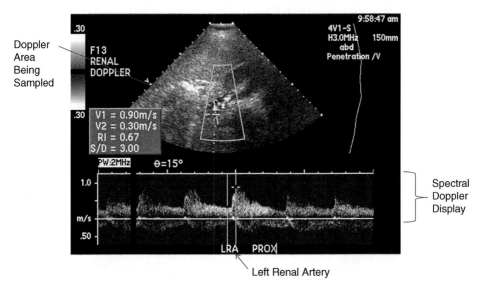

Doppler
Area
Being
Sampled

Spectral
Doppler
Display

Left Renal Artery

Figure 16.4   Pulsed Doppler image of the abdomen showing the anatomical structures and color images of flowing blood in the renal artery.

TABLE 16.1 Definition of Intensity Terms	
I(SATA)	Spatial average–time average
I(SPTA)	Spatial peak–time average
I(SATP)	Spatial average–time peak
I(SPPA)	Spatial peak–pulse average

TABLE 16.2   Typical Output Values for Ultrasound Scanners

Operation Mode	Acoustic Power (MPa)	I(SPTA) (mW/cm²)	I(SPPA) (mW/cm²)	Power (mW)
B-mode	1.68	18.7	174	18
M-mode	1.68	73	174	3.9
Color pulsed Doppler	2.59	234	325	80.5

Adapted from Zagzebski (1996), table 9-1.

Fig. 16.3. Table 16.2 shows the typical properties of ultrasound scanners used in the clinical environment.

ULTRASOUND IMAGING EQUIPMENT

Figure 16.5 is a picture of a modern universal clinical ultrasound unit. It is usually portable so it can be taken directly into a patient's room. It has a keyboard for logging patient and image information. The display shows the ultrasound image in

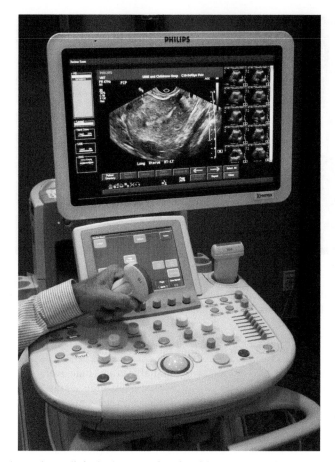

Figure 16.5 A modern clinical ultrasound unit with a zoomed image showing a typical transducer.

real time. Several different ultrasound transducers or probes can be used with the unit depending on the body area being imaged.

The ultrasound signal is sent and received by the transducer. The transducer is constructed of a piezoelectric crystal that oscillates at a specific frequency when a voltage is applied. This generates the ultrasound signal. The transducer is pulsed on and off at the PRF. During the off cycle, the transducer receives the reflected sound signal. The reflected sound is converted into an electrical signal that is processed and then displayed as an image on the screen.

The frequency, power, and pulse sequence are all variable and chosen by the operator. The display shows all of the parameters set by the operator. The location and orientation of the transducer is controlled by operator, so it is really freehand imaging. It is important that the operator describes the image to the physician, so the image contains a lot of descriptive information such as RT OB Liv, or right oblique liver. Good communication between the ultrasound technologist and the physician is needed.

The ultrasound unit also displays two important safely parameters. These are the thermal index (TI) and mechanical index (MI). These values are shown in Fig. 16.3.

The TI is the ratio of the acoustical power produced by the transducer to the power required to raise the temperature in the tissue by 1°C. The unit calculates the TI value based on an internal algorithm taking into account the acoustic power, ultrasound frequency, beam area, tissue attenuation, and tissue absorption. A TI of one means the ultrasound beam would raise tissue at the specified location by 1°C.

The MI is a quantity describing the likelihood of the beam to producing cavitation in the patient. An MI of 1 means a 100% likelihood of cavitation.

The MI is given by

$$MI = PNP/\sqrt{(f_c)},$$

where PNP is the peak negative pressure of the ultrasound wave in megapascal (MPa) and f_c is the center frequency of the ultrasound wave.

BIOLOGICAL EFFECTS OF ULTRASOUND WAVES

The ultrasound wave is a pressure wave that is transmitted through tissue by mechanically vibrating the molecules in the tissue. Given enough intensity and long enough exposure, ultrasound is capable of producing measurable effects in tissue. As mentioned earlier, at diagnostic levels, there have been no measurable biological effects reported in the literature.

There are two mechanisms that produce biological effects in tissue: heating and cavitation.

As the sound beam propagates through tissue, it is attenuated. Most of the attenuation is caused by absorption, which deposits energy as it traverses tissue. At low power levels, most of the heat is dissipated. At higher power rates (exceeding 1000 mW/cm^2), the heat is not dissipated, producing local heating. This can be used for therapeutic applications, which will be described later. Color Doppler ultrasound uses the highest power level of all diagnostic procedures. If a biological problem could happen, this procedure is one to watch. The operator much watch the TI described earlier.

Ultrasound beams of high intensity can produce cavitation. Cavitation is the formation of microbubbles produced by the interaction of the ultrasound field and the molecules in the tissue. These bubbles are formed by the sound field oscillations and grow as the intensity of the beam increases with time. At low power levels, a stable cavitation level is reached. If the intensity is high enough, high temperatures can be generated inside causing the bubbles to burst, producing unknown damage to the tissue. This is known as transient cavitation. The MI is a measure of the energy level needed to produce cavitation.

The biological effects are directly related to the sound intensity and power. There are two frequencies of concern in diagnostic ultrasound. The first is the actual sound frequency, which varies from 2 to 20 MHz, and the second is the pulsed repetition frequency or refresh rate. The PRF varies from 100 to 12,000 Hz. Color pulsed

Doppler uses the highest power level of all diagnostic studies and the highest PRF. Therefore, it has the highest possibility of producing biological damage.

The eye is more sensitive to sound because it has poor blood circulation compared with the rest of the body. The following regulations reflect this sensitivity. The fetal dose should be limited because of the sound interaction with the eyes of the fetus. Therefore, the maximum power limits during fetal exams should be that of the eye.

ULTRASOUND REGULATIONS

The current FDA regulations for diagnostic ultrasound units were established in 1976 and revised in 1992. There are only two limits, and they are listed as follows:

Limits of the whole body (nonophthalmic)

$$I(SPTA) \leq 720 \, mW/cm^2$$

$$MI \leq 1.9$$

$$TI \leq 6.0$$

Limits for the eye (ophthalmic)

$$I(SPTA) \leq 50 \, mW/cm^2$$

$$MI \leq 0.23$$

$$TI \leq 1.0$$

The FDA limits the SPTA to 720 mW/cm^2 because the cooling capacity of tissue is relatively high and most of the time in an ultrasound cycle is spent in the listening mode. Heating occurs only during the "pulse on" time. The limits for the eyes are much less than the whole body mode. That is because the depth is shallow, the PRF can be higher, and there is less blood flow in the eye to remove the heat.

The TI limit can be compared with a 7-W night light, which is 7000 mW. If a transducer is 1 cm^2, then the whole body limit is about 10% of the power from a night light. The power limit to the eye is less than 1% of the night light.

OTHER TYPES OF MEDICAL ULTRASOUND PROCEDURES

As we have discussed, ultrasound waves can heat tissues and produce cavitation. By using higher-powered ultrasound pulses, ultrasound can be used to treat patients. The three main techniques used are HIFU, diathermy, and hyperthermia used to treat cancer patients.

HIFU is just what the name says. A high-intensity ultrasound beam is focused to a location often deep in the body. With the right amount of energy, the tissue is heated in order to destroy diseased or damaged tissue through ablation. In the clinical setting, HIFU is typically performed in conjunction with an imaging procedure to enable treatment planning and target placement before applying ablative energy levels of ultrasound energy. In HIFU therapy, ultrasound beams are focused on diseased tissue. Due to the high energy deposition at the focus, the temperature within the tissue can raise to levels from 65 to 85°C, destroying the diseased tissue by coagulation necrosis. The desired volume is treated by scanning the beam to cover the volume desired. This technique has been used to treat cancer of the prostate, bone, breast, liver, pancreas, rectum, and kidney. The most effective to date is the treatment of prostate cancer. The treatment of prostate cancer is done as an outpatient procedure using a transrectal probe for guidance and takes less than 3 hours. HIFU is also used to treat arrhythmia and atrial fibrillation for patients with cardiac disease.

Diathermy means "heating through." This is usually done by electromechanical stimulation; ultrasound has been used for local heating of tissue in physical therapy. This heating increases the blood flow and speeds up the metabolism. The heat makes the fibrous tissues in tendons and scars more easily stretched thereby relieving stiff joints and promoting relaxation of muscles.

Hyperthermia is used to treat cancer. Much like diathermy, hyperthermia is used to heat cancerous tissues. The local temperatures during hyperthermia can be as high as 45°C. This temperature must be held for a reasonable time in order to damage and kill cancer cells. Hyperthermia is almost always used with other forms of cancer therapy, such as radiation oncology and chemotherapy. Clinical trials are being conducted to evaluate the effectiveness of hyperthermia.

SUMMARY OF RADIATION EFFECTS OF ULTRASOUND

- Diagnostic procedures when done properly do not pose a significant biological risk.
- The lens of the eye is one of the most sensitive tissues to ultrasound waves.
- Thermal heating is one of the biological effects produced by ultrasound.
- Cavitation is another biological effect produced by ultrasound.
- Ultrasound can be used to heat tissue, thereby used to treat cancer and other tissue disorders.

SAFETY STATEMENT

The American Institute of Ultrasound in Medicine (AIUM) states that "There are no confirmed biological effects on patients or operators caused by exposure from present diagnostic ultrasound instruments. Although the possibility exists that such biological effects may be identified in the future, current data indicate that the benefits to patients of the prudent use of diagnostic ultrasound outweigh the risks, if any, that may be present."

Keeping this in mind, the chapter describes how an ultrasound unit is used and how the interaction of the ultrasound beam can affect tissue.

BIBLIOGRAPHY

Hedrick WR, Hykes DL, Starchman DE. Ultrasound physics and instrumentation. 4th ed. St. Louis, MO: Elsevier Mosby; 2005.

National Council on Radiation Protection and Measurements. Biological effects of ultrasound: Mechanisms and clinical implications. Bethesda, MD: The Council; 1983.

Salvesen KA. Ultrasound in pregnancy and non-right handedness: Meta-analysis of randomized trials. Ultrasound Obstet Gynecol. 2011 September;38(3):267–71.

Zagzebski JA. Essentials of ultrasound physics. St. Louis, MO: Mosby; 1996.

QUESTIONS

Chapter 16   Questions

1. The intensity parameter used to measure cavitation is
  a. SATA.
  b. SATP.
  c. SPTA.
  d. SPTP.

2. The intensity parameter used in the FDA intensity limit is
  a. SAPA.
  b. SATP.
  c. SPTA.
  d. SPTP.

3. The intensity parameter used to monitor pulsed Doppler imaging is
  a. SAPA.
  b. SATP.
  c. SPTA.
  d. SPTP.

4. In the intensity measure SPTP, the S stands for
  a. single.
  b. spatial.
  c. special.
  d. sepal.

5. In the intensity measure SPTP, the P stands for
  a. primary.
  b. photon.
  c. probe.
  d. peak.

6. In the intensity measure SPTP, the T stands for
   a. temporal.
   b. tumor.
   c. treble.
   d. truncated.

7. The MI value displayed on the U.S. Monitor refers to the ____ value.
   a. median index
   b. modal index
   c. mechanical index
   d. mechanical inversion

8. The MI value is related to the
   a. highest positive pressure in the ultrasound wave.
   b. pulse repetition frequency.
   c. central frequency of the ultrasound wave.
   d. tissue mechanical viscosity.

9. FDA regulations require the MI to be _____ 1.9.
   a. less than
   b. greater than
   c. equal to

10. In the clinic, a lower MI indicates a _____ biological effect.
    a. higher
    b. lower
    c. indeterminate
    d. There is not enough information to determine.

11. The MI indicates which biological affect?
    a. Heating
    b. Cavitation
    c. Boiling
    d. Ionization

12. Switching to a lower PRF should produce _____ MI value.
    a. a lower
    b. a higher
    c. an unchanged

13. Acoustical power is given in
    a. pascals.
    b. nW/cm^2.
    c. joules.
    d. milliwatts.

14. Which of the following quantities is the largest?

    a. I(SATA)

    b. I(SPPA)

    c. I(SATP)

    d. I(SPTA)

15. The ultrasound imaging mode that produces the highest power in tissue is

    a. pulsed Doppler.

    b. M-mode.

    c. B-mode.

    d. transverse scanning.

16. The AIUM statement on biological effects states that for focused ultrasound beams, there are no known effects on mammalian tissue at I(SPTA) at values lower than

    a. 10 mW/cm^2.

    b. 100 mW/cm^2.

    c. 1000 mW/cm^2.

    d. 10,000 mW/cm^2.

BIOLOGICAL EFFECTS OF MAGNETIC RESONANCE IMAGING

KEYWORDS

Magnetic resonance, biological effects, superconducting magnet, static magnetic field, magnetic field gradient, projectile effect, RF fields, RF coil, RF ablation, gradient coil, peripheral nerve stimulation, implanted medical device

TOPICS

- Basic components of a magnetic resonance (MR) scanner and the types of magnetic fields each component produces
- Potential biological effects of static magnetic fields and field gradients during interactions with magnetic objects
- Interaction of radiofrequency (RF) magnetic fields with normal tissue and electrically conducting materials
- Biological effects of time-varying magnetic field gradients
- Potential impacts of magnetic resonance imaging (MRI) on subjects with implanted medical devices

INTRODUCTION

Regarding biological effects, the first thing to note about magnetic resonance imaging (MRI) is the lack of ionizing radiation. During a normal magnetic

Radiation Biology of Medical Imaging, First Edition. Charles A. Kelsey, Philip H. Heintz, Daniel J. Sandoval, Gregory D. Chambers, Natalie L. Adolphi, and Kimberly S. Paffett.
© 2014 John Wiley & Sons, Inc. Published 2014 by John Wiley & Sons, Inc.

resonance (MR) scan, the patient's body absorbs energy; however, the absorbed energy is in the radiofrequency (RF) portion of the electromagnetic spectrum. As explained in Chapter 3, RF electromagnetic energy, when absorbed by body tissues, causes heating but not ionization. In addition to mild heating, there are other biological effects that may result during MRI. Some of these are routinely encountered (such as audible noise); others occur very infrequently (such as RF burns). Although extremely rare, improper MR procedures have resulted in serious injury or death. In general, MRI is safe and imparts absolutely no ionizing radiation dose.

In order to appreciate the range of potential biological effects of MRI, it is necessary to first become familiar with the basic components of an MR scanner, and the purpose and type of magnetic field produced by each component.

BASIC PRINCIPLES OF MRI

The ability to noninvasively image the body by MRI is based on the manipulation and detection of the magnetic properties of hydrogen nuclei. Hydrogen is the most abundant element in the body, and the hydrogen nucleus has a magnetic moment, with magnetic behavior similar to that of the electron or a compass needle. The electron is a "spin ½" particle, meaning that it is observed in one of two states, referred to as "up" and "down." Similarly, the spin of the hydrogen nucleus (i.e., proton) assumes either an "up" or "down" orientation with respect to an externally applied magnetic field. Note that electron spins are what create magnetism in magnetic materials, such as iron. The hydrogen magnetic moment, however, is about 2000 times weaker than that of the electron, and therefore hydrogenous materials (e.g., plastic, water, and tissue) do not stick to magnets. Fortunately, the very weak magnetism of hydrogen nuclei is adequate to enable MRI.

MRI involves first aligning the hydrogen spins using a strong external magnetic field, and then perturbing the spin direction in a way that produces a voltage in a detection coil. The polarizing field is typically provided by a large donut-shaped superconducting magnet that produces a strong, constant magnetic field in the center of the donut. Figure 17.1a is a photograph of a typical clinical MR scanner, and Fig. 17.1b shows a cutaway indicating the location of the various hardware components discussed in this chapter.

The perturbation of the hydrogen spins and subsequent voltage detection are performed by the much smaller RF coil, which basically acts as a two-way radio antenna that transmits and receives RF signals. (In modern MRI systems, the transmit and receive functions may be performed by separate circuit elements, or there may be multiple parallel receive circuit elements, but the ensemble of RF circuits is still referred to as "the coil.") The RF coil is wrapped around (or placed against) the part of the body that is being imaged.

Additionally, during the MRI acquisition, another set of coils (the "imaging gradient coils" or "gradients") surrounding the patient are pulsed on and off in a way that encodes information about spatial position in the voltage signals detected from the hydrogen spins. The encoded spatial information in the voltage signals is decoded using computer algorithms (e.g., fast Fourier transform) to create a two-dimensional or three-dimensional image. Because the MR signals generated from hydrogen in different tissue types differ in magnitude and duration, the differing signal

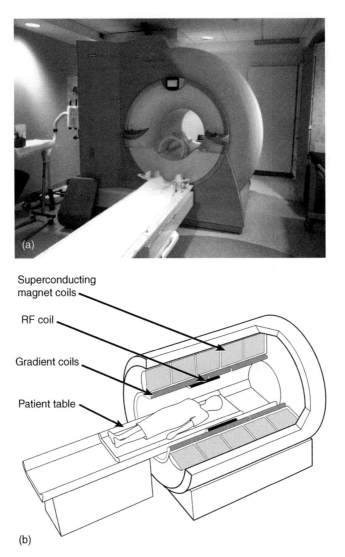

Figure 17.1 (a) Photograph of a clinical MR scanner. (b) Cutaway diagram showing the essential components of an MR scanner, including the main magnet, RF coil, and gradient coils.

intensities from different tissues (e.g., muscle and fat) enable anatomic structures to be distinguished.

To summarize, MRI utilizes three main hardware components—(1) the main magnet (to align the spins), (2) the RF coil (to perturb the spins and detect voltage signals), and (3) the gradient coil set (to encode spatial information into the voltage signals). Each hardware component generates magnetic fields with different characteristics that result in different biological effects, as discussed in the following section.

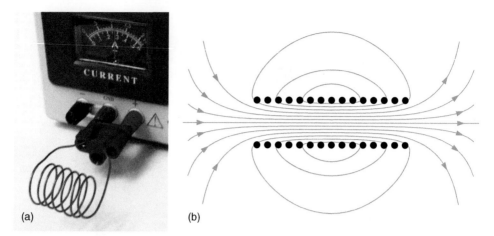

Figure 17.2 (a) A current-carrying wire, wrapped to form a solenoid, produces a magnetic field. (b) The gray lines represent the magnetic field of a solenoid, while the black dots represent the current-carrying wires (in cross section).

BIOLOGICAL EFFECTS OF MRI

Main Magnet: Static Magnetic Field and Field Gradient Effects

The main magnet creates a magnetic field that is extremely strong, >1 tesla (T), spatially uniform across the patient's body, and constant over time. The most common field strengths for clinical whole body magnets are 1.5 and 3 T. Whole body magnets with field strengths of 7 T or greater are used in research, but are not yet clinically approved. For comparison, the Earth's magnetic field is about 0.00005 T = 0.5 gauss (G) (1 T = 10,000 G).

Whole body MRI magnets are generally superconducting solenoids. A solenoid is a coiled current-carrying wire (see Fig. 17.2a); the field inside of a cylindrical solenoid is uniform and parallel to the axis of the coil, as depicted by the gray magnetic field lines in Fig. 17.2b. A superconducting solenoid is immersed in liquid helium (at a temperature of –269°C) to maintain the superconducting state. Super-conductivity (the flow of electrical current without resistance) is what maintains the magnetic field indefinitely without a constant input of electrical energy. In other words, the magnet is not "plugged in" during normal operation. Once the solenoid is magnetized, the magnetic field is maintained at a constant value over time, ideally for the entire life of the scanner (hence the term "static" field). As in computed tomography (CT), the patient is imaged in the center of the donut, but the length of the cylinder is much greater in an MR scanner than in a CT scanner. Thus, a common biological effect of MR is claustrophobia, which is occasionally serious enough to contraindicate MRI for some patients.

Brief exposures to static magnetic fields are not known to have any significant biological effects on mammals. This makes sense because mammals do not naturally have ferromagnetic materials in their bodies that would interact with static fields. Normal tissue does not interact with static fields, and therefore, tissue is essentially transparent to static fields (i.e., there is no attenuation). Ferromagnetic materials (so called because they typically contain iron) interact strongly with magnetic fields due to cooperative effects of the electron spins in the material. However, not all iron-containing substances are ferromagnetic. For example, the iron-containing hemoglobin in your blood exhibits very weak magnetism (it does not participate in cooperative magnetic effects) and is not significantly affected by MRI magnetic fields. *Generally, the strong static magnetic field created by the main magnet only causes significant biological effects by interacting with* foreign *ferromagnetic objects inside or near the patient.*

Torque   Just as the Earth's magnetic field will orient a compass needle, the strong static field in an MR scanner will exert a torque (twisting force) on elongated magnetic objects to orient the long axis of the object parallel to the magnetic field. Because the torque is proportional to the strength of the magnetic field, the torque generated by an MR magnet is tens of thousands of times stronger than the torque caused by the Earth's field. For example, if a child has swallowed a straight pin, the child should not undergo MRI, because the pin would rapidly rotate to align with the main magnetic field. For this reason, people with a known history of injury involving penetrating metallic objects may be screened using X-ray imaging prior to undergoing MRI.

Translational Force   The translational magnetic force (the force that causes a magnetic object to move toward a magnet) is proportional to the spatial *gradient* of the magnetic field. A spatial gradient is a change in the magnetic field strength as a function of position. Note that a perfectly spatially uniform magnetic field does not cause any translational force, even if the field is extremely strong. However, the field of an MRI magnet is only spatially uniform in the center of the bore. In Fig. 17.2b, the magnetic field lines from a solenoid are shown. The gray lines represent the magnetic field, and the black dots represent the turns of wire forming the solenoid (in cross section). The magnetic field is strong (denoted by the density of the lines) and uniform (denoted by parallel lines) inside the solenoid, but the field becomes rapidly weaker (lines are less dense) and nonuniform (lines are not parallel) as one moves outside of the solenoid. In general, the field strength of any magnet, including MRI magnets, decreases as one moves further away from the magnet. Magnetic forces (e.g., the pull of a refrigerator magnet) are caused by the spatial variation of the magnetic field near the magnet.

Projectile Effect   A rare but significant biological effect of the main magnetic field occurs when someone accidentally brings a ferromagnetic object (e.g., a pair of scissors or an oxygen bottle) into the MRI suite. The object can become a dangerous projectile due to the strong attraction of the object to the "mouth" of the magnet bore, the location where the field strength is changing rapidly with distance (i.e., where the gradient is the strongest). Note the position of the gas cylinder in Fig. 17.3, which shows the result of bringing a non-MR-safe object into an MRI suite. If the ferromagnetic object is either sharp or massive, this phenomenon can result in serious injury, or even death, to patients or others in the MR suite. Note that the

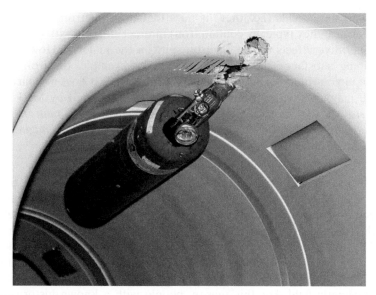

Figure 17.3   A non-MR-safe oxygen bottle, stuck in the bore of an MR scanner at the position where the field gradient is the strongest. Careful screening of everything entering the MR scanner room is necessary to prevent serious accidents.

serious biological effect is caused by the impact with the projectile and is not a direct effect of the magnetic field on the subject.

How do projectile accidents happen? Keep in mind that the magnetic field decreases as a function of distance (d) with a $1/d^3$ dependence, and the spatial gradient decreases with a $1/d^4$ dependence. This very strong dependence of the gradient strength on distance means that the magnetic force on an object can be nearly imperceptible at one point in the room (perhaps a meter or so from the main magnet), but the force becomes extremely strong if the object is moved just a few centimeters closer. Thus, the danger with objects becoming projectiles is related to how suddenly the force changes from insignificant to dangerous. If a person is walking toward the magnet carrying a magnetic object, the time between first feeling the force and the object clanging uncontrollably into the mouth of the magnet is typically less than the person's reaction time—by the time a problem is perceived, the force is too great to overcome.

Diligence in screening patients (and accompanying persons, medical personnel, custodial and maintenance workers, and security and emergency personnel) for ferrous objects prior to entering the MR suite is the single most important safety precaution in the MR environment. If an MRI subject requires emergency medical treatment, the recommended course of action is to remove the patient from the MR scanner room prior to commencing treatment, because emergency treatment typically involves personnel and equipment that have not been screened for MR safety. It is faster and safer to move the patient to an area of low magnetic field than it is to either shut down the magnet (emergency shutdown requires minutes) or to attempt to screen all of the personnel and crash cart equipment.

Clearly, a patient with metal *inside* his or her body (e.g., shrapnel or a medical implant) should not enter the MR suite unless the implanted material or device is verified to be MR safe, in writing. Note that many common metals (aluminum, brass, copper, lead, titanium) are nonmagnetic, while iron and steel generally are ferromagnetic (i.e., *strongly* magnetic). Most stainless steels are ferromagnetic, although there are some grades of stainless steel that are only weakly magnetic. Most modern medical implants are designed to be non-ferromagnetic with MRI in mind; however, it is important to note that the normal functioning of magnetically or electrically active medical implants (such as pacemakers, defibrillators, or insulin pumps) may be adversely affected by the static magnetic field in an MR scanner, even if the device is not strongly attracted to the magnet. Therefore, persons with such implants should not enter the MR suite unless the device is verified to be MR safe.

Due to medical implant safety concerns and to prevent accidents involving ferrous foreign objects, access to the area around an MR scanner must be restricted to prevent exposure of unscreened persons to magnetic fields greater than 5 G (approximately 10 times the Earth's field).

The RF Coil: Oscillating Magnetic Field Effects

The second important MRI component, the RF coil, is used to transmit energy into the patient (to manipulate the hydrogen spins) and also to receive signals from the hydrogen nuclei that are ultimately processed to form the image. The RF coil is basically a radio antenna that can be made in various sizes and geometries ("birdcage," "pancake," etc.) depending on the part of the body to be imaged. (See examples of different RF coil geometries in Fig. 17.4.)

The term "radiofrequency" is used because the RF coils are designed to produce a magnetic field that oscillates at the same frequency as the oscillation of the hydrogen spins. Thus, the interaction of the RF magnetic field and the spins is a resonant effect, hence the term "magnetic resonance." The oscillation frequency is 63 MHz

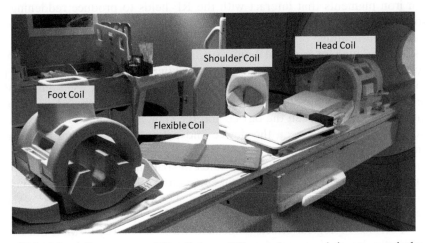

Figure 17.4 Magnetic resonance RF coils have different shapes and sizes to match the part of the body to be imaged.

in a 1.5-T scanner or 126 MHz in a 3-T scanner. (Compare this with the FM band of your radio, which is 88–108 MHz.) The amplitude of the RF magnetic field is generally tens of gauss, orders of magnitude weaker than the main magnetic field. *According to basic electromagnetic theory*, oscillating *magnetic fields produce electric fields, and the induced electric fields interact with tissue*. (Note that normal tissue contains ions, such as Na^+, that interact with electric fields.) During normal MRI acquisition, the RF power deposited in normal tissue causes very mild heating. During MRI, the rate of energy deposition in the patient (the specific absorption rate, or SAR) is limited by the Food and Drug Administration (FDA) to 4 W/kg averaged over the whole body over 15 minutes, for subjects with normal thermo-regulatory function. The FDA limit is 3 W/kg to the head and 8 W/kg over any 1 cm^3 of tissue (e.g., in the extremities) over a 5-minute period. MR scanner software is designed to keep the energy absorption within the FDA limits, based on the patient's body weight, which is entered into the scanner by the MRI technologist, and the type of MR acquisition sequence being used. Limits on SAR place limitations on how quickly the image acquisition can be performed by limiting the RF transmitter duty cycle.

As explained earlier, normal RF heating during MRI is not a biological hazard; however, if the patient has a metallic (i.e., electrically conducting) implant or a metallic device in contact with the body, the interaction of the RF field with the metallic object can lead to excess energy deposition at the site of the metallic object. As described earlier, oscillating magnetic fields create electric fields that can induce currents in conducting objects. Loops of wire or sheets of conducting material can support circulating currents, while elongated conductors may act like antennas, so these types of conductive structures are particularly problematic. When a current (I) flows in a conductor with resistance (R), the rate of heat pro-duction is given by I^2R. This heat production can result in localized burns, so MR safety screening must include the identification (and removal when possible) of electrically conducting objects (e.g., jewelry or drug patches) from the patient. Electrical conductors also tend to be good thermal conductors, which compounds the burn risk. Occasionally, permanent cosmetics (tattoos, permanent eyeliner, etc.) contain iron pigments that interact with the RF fields to produce reddening and irritation at the site of the cosmetic alteration. Ice packs can be used to reduce the risk of overheating.

Besides screening for personal items, extreme care must be used in the placement of necessary medical devices, such as electrocardiography (EKG) leads. Many pre-cautions can be taken to avoid burns from medical equipment used during MRI. These include keeping the device and electrical leads outside of the RF coil, placing insulating materials between the device and the skin, applying cold compresses to the points of contact between the device and patient, and avoiding unnecessary looping of any wires.

Due to the normal salt levels in body fluids, the patient's body is a weak electrical conductor. Therefore, care should be taken to ensure that the patient's arms and legs not be allowed to form loops (e.g., knees should be separated, ankles should not be crossed, hands should not be touching other body parts). However, in general, the most serious biological effects associated with RF energy in MRI are usually caused by the interaction of a *foreign* electrically conducting object with the RF field, not a direct effect of the RF field on the body.

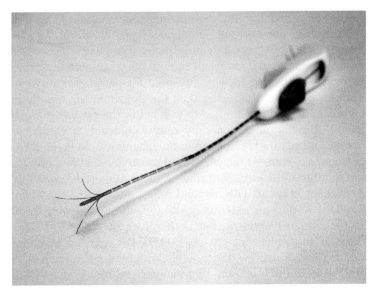

Figure 17.5   RF ablation catheter. When exposed to an externally applied RF electromagnetic field, significant heat is generated by the sharp ends of the catheter wires (where the induced electric field is greatest). The result is ablation of the diseased tissue in contact with the ends of the catheter.

RF Ablation   Although burns from RF fields interacting with metallic structures are undesirable in the MR setting, the heat generated by the interaction of elongated electrical conductors and RF energy (at frequencies in the ~300 kHz–1 MHz range) is used therapeutically. RF ablation utilizes RF energy focused by an electrically conductive catheter (see Fig. 17.5) to thermally destroy diseased tissue, such as tumors, damaged nerves, varicose veins, or abnormal cardiac tissue. This procedure is especially useful in situations where traditional surgery would lead to excessive bleeding (e.g., in nonresectable liver tumors) or other types of damage. Note that by employing RF frequencies above 100 kHz, peripheral nerve stimulation (another potential biological effect of oscillating magnetic fields) is avoided.

Imaging Field Gradients: Time-Varying Magnetic Field Effects

Finally, the third important component of the MR scanner is the imaging gradient coil set. The spatial field gradients produced by these coils (of order 10 mT/m) enable spatial localization of the MR signals from the hydrogen nuclei. The imaging gradients are much weaker in magnitude than the static field gradient at the mouth of the main magnet. However, in terms of biological effects, the important property of the imaging gradients is that they are switched on and off very rapidly (in milliseconds or tens of milliseconds) during the MRI acquisition sequence. The switching frequency of the gradients (of order 100–1000 Hz) results in two main effects in humans exposed to MRI—peripheral nerve stimulation and loud audible noise.

The time variation of the amplitude of the magnetic gradient fields induces electric fields, and therefore tiny currents, in conducting paths within the MR-scanner-sensitive volume, including the conducting paths formed by the patient's nerve fibers. The induced neural currents result in mild nerve stimulation, which may be perceived as tingling or mild pain. The threshold for peripheral nerve stimulation is at least an order of magnitude lower than the threshold for stimulating *cardiac* muscle, and gradient switching is limited to well below the cardiac stimulation level. Peripheral nerve stimulation is generally only significant at frequencies below 100 kHz. The much more rapid oscillation of the magnetic field in the RF coil occurs at too high a frequency (tens of megahertz) to cause nerve stimulation.

Unpleasant audible noise occurs during gradient amplitude switching, because the imaging gradient coils actually expand and contract slightly when they are switched on and off, so they are essentially vibrating at the switching frequency. The frequency of the expansion/contraction is therefore of order 100–1000 Hz, well within the range of human hearing (20–20,000 Hz). The resulting mechanical vibration results in sounds perceived variously as clicking, buzzing, or banging, depending on the imaging sequence that is used. Fast imaging techniques that rely heavily on large-amplitude, short-duration gradient pulses (e.g., echo planar imaging) tend to be the loudest. Ear protection may be provided to the patient and staff or accompanying persons in the MR scanner room during such sequences.

Peripheral nerve stimulation and audible noise are perceived as being more unpleasant for some patients than others; however, under normal circumstances, neither of these biological effects of gradient switching is life threatening or results in any lasting harm to patients.

Implanted Medical Devices

Implanted medical devices are a special concern when considering MRI, because the devices may be subject to one or more of the magnetic field effects described above. The implant may be affected by the static field or static field gradient, the RF field, and/or the time-varying imaging gradients—depending on the construction of the implant and whether it has active electrical or magnetic components. The result of exposure to MRI magnetic fields may be damage to the device, injury to the patient, or both. For example, if the implanted device contains ferromagnetic materials (such as the magnets used to position cochlear implants), the device may become misadjusted, it may dislodge, or it may even injure the patient if the force on the device is great enough. If the device is sensitive to electromagnetic interference (EMI), the RF fields may cause the device to function improperly (such as a defibrillator misfiring) or the device may stop working altogether, which may have serious consequences for the patient. If the device contains electrically conducting materials (such as a metal plate, wire, or foil), interaction with the RF field may lead to excessive energy deposition resulting in damage to the device and/or burns. Therefore, patients with medical devices that cannot be removed should not undergo MRI unless it can be verified (in writing) that the medical device or implant has been tested as MR safe. Furthermore, the testing must have occurred under the same conditions (same magnetic field strength, same maximum RF amplitude, gradient amplitude and switching times, etc.) that will be used in the subsequent MR examination.

Other Considerations

Pregnancy   Pregnant subjects are generally advised to delay MRI if doing so will not compromise the subject's health. That said, there is no documented evidence of harmful effects of MR to the fetus, so avoidance of MR is simply a precaution. In some cases, performing MR may be advised in lieu of performing an imaging procedure that involves ionizing radiation exposure, as there are clearly documented effects of ionizing radiation on the developing fetus.

Contrast Agents   As in CT, some MRI procedures involve the use of intravenously injected contrast agents. In general, MR contrast agents (i.e., gadolinium chelates) are better tolerated and give rise to fewer side effects and allergic reactions compared with the iodinated contrast agents used in X-ray imaging. However, there is an infrequent but severe complication of gadolinium contrast that occurs in patients with compromised renal function. The condition is known as nephrogenic systemic fibrosis (NSF) and can be avoided by verifying renal sufficiency prior to receiving MR contrast.

Cryogens   In the event of an emergency shutdown or malfunction of a superconducting MR magnet, the magnet may become resistive and dissipate all of its stored energy as heat, causing the cryogenic liquid helium (and liquid nitrogen in some magnets) to boil and be released as gas. Because there are tens to hundreds of liters of liquid cryogens, and gas occupies roughly 1000 times the volume of liquid, the main biohazard in this case is asphyxiation, in the event that too much of the room air is displaced by helium and/or nitrogen gas. Modern MR facilities are designed with appropriate airflow and ventilation to virtually eliminate this risk.

CONCLUSIONS

There are a number of unique biological effects associated with MRI, but there is no ionizing radiation associated with this imaging modality. The various types of magnetic fields used in MRI (static, RF, and time-varying gradients) are not directly harmful to subjects when normal safety procedures are followed. However, interactions of electrically conducting or magnetic objects with the magnetic fields produced during MRI can result in potentially harmful effects, notably burns or impacts with fast-moving projectiles. To avoid injury or device malfunction, persons with implanted medical devices must remain in areas where the magnetic field strength is below 5 G, unless the device is verified to be MR safe.

SUMMARY

- An MR scanner consists of three main magnetic field-producing components: the main magnet, the RF coil, and the gradient coil set.
- The main magnet produces a strong, static magnetic field that aligns the hydrogen nuclear magnetic moments in the subject.

- The static field does not cause significant bioeffects, but the interaction of magnetic objects or implants with the static field can result in significant rotational and translational forces.

- The RF coil produces a weaker magnetic field that oscillates with a frequency of tens of megahertz (RF range) for the purpose of manipulating the nuclear spins and detecting signals.

- Exposure of normal tissue to the RF magnetic fields results in mild heating, but the interaction of the RF field with electrically conducting objects, internal or immediately external to the patient, may lead to burns. Conducting loops formed by the body itself should be avoided, as induced loop currents may lead to excessive heating during exposure to RF.

- RF ablation is a therapeutic technique that utilizes external RF fields and a conducting probe inserted into a particular location in the body to thermally destroy diseased tissue at the site of the probe.

- The imaging gradient coil set produces spatial magnetic field gradients that are rapidly switched on and off. The imaging gradients are used to encode spatial information in the signal detected by the RF coil to enable an image to be formed.

- The switching frequency of the imaging gradients (of order 100–1000 Hz) produces audible noise, which may be uncomfortable for the subject. The switching of the imaging gradients can also cause peripheral nerve stimulation, perceived by the subject as tingling or mild pain.

- Implanted medical devices can interact with all of the different types of magnetic fields produced during MRI. The interaction may result in injury to the patient and/or malfunctioning of the device. Implanted devices must be verified in writing to be MR safe prior to MRI.

BIBLIOGRAPHY

FDA US. MRI (magnetic resonance imaging). 2010 [updated August 25, 2010; cited October 25, 2013]. Available from: http://www.fda.gov/MedicalDevices/DeviceRegulationand Guidance/GuidanceDocuments/ucm073817.htm.

Kanal E, Barkovich AJ, Bell C, Borgstede JP, Bradley WG, Froelich JW, et al. ACR guidance document for safe MR practices: 2007. Am J Roentgenol. 2007 June;188(6):1447–74.

Schaefer DJ, Bourland JD, Nyenhuis JA. Review of patient safety in time-varying gradient fields. J Magn Reson Imaging. 2000 July;12(1):20–9.

Shellock FG, Crues JV. MR procedures: Biologic effects, safety, and patient care. Radiology. 2004 September;232(3):635–52.

Voigt T, Homann H, Katscher U, Doessel O. Patient-individual local SAR determination: In vivo measurements and numerical validation. Magn Reson Med. 2012 October; 68(4):1117–26.

Weinberg IN, Stepanov PY, Fricke ST, Probst R, Urdaneta M, Warnow D, et al. Increasing the oscillation frequency of strong magnetic fields above 101 kHz significantly raises peripheral nerve excitation thresholds. Med Phys. 2012 May;39(5):2578–83.

Woods TO. Standards for medical devices in MRI: Present and future. J Magn Reson Imaging. 2007 November;26(5):1186–9.

QUESTIONS

Chapter 17   Questions

1. The biological effects of magnetic resonance imaging (MRI) are caused by
   a. ionizing radiation.
   b. static magnetic fields only.
   c. time-varying magnetic fields only.
   d. static and time-varying magnetic fields.

2. The physical basis of clinical magnetic resonance is the generation of signals by manipulations of
   a. hydrogen nuclear magnetic moments.
   b. electron spins.
   c. hydrogen nuclear reactions, which create detectable photons.
   d. electron–hydrogen interactions.

3. Strong static magnetic fields
   a. cause significant biological effects in mammals.
   b. cause significant biological effects when the field strength is greater than 1 T.
   c. cause significant biological effects primarily when the magnetic field interacts with foreign ferromagnetic objects.
   d. do not cause any biological effects.

4. The three main magnetic-field-producing components of an MR scanner are
   a. the main magnet, the secondary magnet, and the power supply.
   b. the main magnet, the power supply, and the magnetic processor.
   c. the main magnet, the RF coil, and the gradient coil set.
   d. the RF magnet, the gradient magnet, and the imaging magnet.

5. Under normal conditions, the RF energy deposited in the patient during MRI causes
   a. ionization.
   b. nerve stimulation.
   c. audible noise.
   d. mild heating.

6. Ferromagnetic objects interact strongly with static magnetic fields. *None* of the following materials is ferromagnetic:
   a. Plastic, glass, aluminum, brass
   b. Plastic, glass, aluminum, stainless steel
   c. Plastic, glass, stainless steel, iron
   d. Glass, lead, titanium, steel

7. Magnetic field gradients with switching times of tens of milliseconds result in which biological effect(s)?
   a. Audible noise
   b. Nerve stimulation
   c. Burns
   d. a and b

8. Under what conditions should a patient with an implanted medical device enter the MR scanner room?
   a. If the device does not contain any ferromagnetic components
   b. If the patient provides written verification that the device is MR-safe
   c. A patient with an implanted device can never enter the MR scanner room
   d. If the device is not electrically or magnetically active

9. RF ablation is used
   a. to destroy diseased tissue.
   b. to generate the signal detected during MRI.
   c. to improve MR contrast.
   d. to decrease the RF exposure to the patient during MRI.

10. The strength of the main magnetic field in clinical MRI is typically
    a. <1 T.
    b. 1–3 T.
    c. 3–10 T.
    d. >10 T.

11. In MRI, the RF coil is used
    a. to manipulate the nuclear magnetic moments and detect a signal.
    b. to localize the signals by encoding spatial information into the MR signal.
    c. to polarize the nuclear magnetic moments.
    d. to reduce biological effects.

12. The oscillating magnetic field created by the RF coils
    a. oscillates at too low of a frequency to cause any biological effects.
    b. causes peripheral nerve stimulation.
    c. causes the projectile effect.
    d. causes current to flow in electrically conducting objects, which may result in burns.

13. The maximum magnetic field strength allowed in areas accessible by members of the general public is
    a. 5 T (50,000 G).
    b. 0.5 T (5000 G).
    c. 5 mT (50 G).
    d. 0.5 mT (5 G).

14. A pregnant subject
   a. should never be discouraged from having an MRI exam, because MRI does not use ionizing radiation and is completely safe.
   b. should decide whether to have an MRI exam in consultation with her doctor, based on risk/benefit considerations, such as the urgency of her medical condition.
   c. may be advised to undergo MRI, in lieu of an X-ray or CT exam.
   d. Both b and c.

15. Implanted medical devices are known to interact with
   a. static magnetic fields and field gradients.
   b. RF magnetic fields.
   c. imaging magnetic field gradients.
   d. All of the above.

16. Time-varying magnetic fields cause biological effects because they induce
   a. static magnetic fields that interact with ferromagnetic objects.
   b. field gradients that rotate elongated magnetic objects.
   c. electric fields that cause current to flow in electrically conducting objects, such as the body itself or implanted devices.
   d. ionization that causes gamma rays to be emitted.

ANSWERS TO ODD-NUMBERED QUESTIONS

CHAPTER 1   ANSWERS

1. c
3. c
5. a
7. c
9. d
11. b
13. b
15. d

CHAPTER 2   ANSWERS

1. c
3. a
5. b
7. c
9. d
11. c
13. d
15. c

CHAPTER 3   ANSWERS

1. c
3. b
5. d
7. a
9. a
11. d
13. b
15. c

CHAPTER 4   ANSWERS

1. b
3. c
5. a
7. c
9. a
11. d
13. b
15. d

Radiation Biology of Medical Imaging, First Edition. Charles A. Kelsey, Philip H. Heintz, Daniel J. Sandoval, Gregory D. Chambers, Natalie L. Adolphi, and Kimberly S. Paffett.
© 2014 John Wiley & Sons, Inc. Published 2014 by John Wiley & Sons, Inc.

CHAPTER 5   ANSWERS

1. a
3. c
5. c
7. d
9. b
11. b
13. c
15. b

CHAPTER 6   ANSWERS

1. d
3. b
5. d
7. d
9. d
11. b
13. b
15. a

CHAPTER 7   ANSWERS

1. a
3. b
5. b
7. a
9. b
11. a
13. d
15. b

CHAPTER 8   ANSWERS

1. c
3. b
5. b
7. b
9. a
11. c
13. a
15. a

CHAPTER 9   ANSWERS

1. b
3. b
5. b
7. a
9. d
11. b
13. b
15. c

CHAPTER 10   ANSWERS

1. a
3. d
5. d
7. c
9. b
11. c
13. b
15. a

CHAPTER 11   ANSWERS

1. c
3. a
5. b
7. d
9. c
11. b
13. b
15. a

CHAPTER 12   ANSWERS

1. b
3. b
5. c
7. c
9. c
11. d
13. a
15. c

CHAPTER 13   ANSWERS

1. d
3. a
5. a
7. d
9. a
11. c
13. b
15. d

CHAPTER 14   ANSWERS

1. a
3. b
5. a
7. d
9. c
11. c
13. a
15. c

CHAPTER 15   ANSWERS

1. d
3. d
5. a
7. c
9. a
11. a
13. d
15. a

CHAPTER 16   ANSWERS

1. d
3. c
5. d
7. c
9. a
11. b
13. d
15. a

CHAPTER 17   ANSWERS

1. d
3. c
5. d
7. d
9. a
11. a
13. d
15. d

INDEX

Radiation Biology of Medical Imaging, First Edition. Charles A. Kelsey, Philip H. Heintz,
Daniel J. Sandoval, Gregory D. Chambers, Natalie L. Adolphi, and Kimberly S. Paffett.
© 2014 John Wiley & Sons, Inc. Published 2014 by John Wiley & Sons, Inc.

Printed and bound by CPI Group (UK) Ltd, Croydon, CR0 4YY

16/04/2025

14658537-0001